Let's Stop
"Killing"
Our Children

Let's Stop "Killing" Our Children

HEALTHY LIFESTYLE AND DISEASE PREVENTION START IN THE WOMB AND IN THE CRIB

A Simplified Survival Guide for Parents and Society to Save Our Children

PHILIP S. CHUA, MD, FACS, FPCS

Copyright © 2011 by Philip S. Chua, MD, FACS, FPCS.

Library of Congress Control Number: 2011908669

ISBN: Hardcover   978-1-4628-7754-6
            Softcover   978-1-4628-7753-9
            Ebook   978-1-4628-7755-3

This book was printed in the United States of America.

scalpelpen@gmail.com

To order additional copies of this book, contact:
Xlibris Corporation
1-888-795-4274
www.Xlibris.com
Orders@Xlibris.com
95816

Table of Contents

Preface

I chose to title this book *Let's Stop "Killing" Our Children* to highlight, using this metaphor, the fundamental value of starting healthy lifestyle and prevention of diseases from the crib, or even before conception of the child. Maintaining good health and warding off diseases must start from even before infancy. In this regard, parents have the essential role of serving as good examples for their children by living healthy lifestyles themselves. Through personal discipline, parents can save these young lives from avoidable morbidity and premature death as they grow older.

This book is an anthology of health-related articles and commentaries about our environment and other social issues I've had published on various websites and in newspapers in the United States and abroad. These are aimed to educate, challenge, and inspire the public on health issues and offer preemptive strategies in dealing with diseases in general. Medical data in this collection have been updated to achieve this publication's intended goal of serving as a household health reference.

Some postmortem studies on accident victims age five and younger revealed that their young arteries already had some evidence of arteriosclerosis (hardening of the arteries), a condition expected only among adults, especially those who are 40 and older. While the thin layer of arteriosclerotic plaques lining the intima (inner wall) of their coronary arteries were minimal and not enough to cause any blockage, it was, nonetheless, convincing proof that adult coronary heart disease, which often leads to heart attack, starts in the preschool age.

How do we explain this scary and surprising discovery?

As a cardiac surgeon, I fully understand that diseases, like coronary artery blockage, heart attack, stroke, and even diabetes and cancer, do not develop overnight. While genetic predisposition is a factor in the causation of diseases, epidemiology teaches us that, in general, a healthy lifestyle significantly outweighs hereditary factors. The children of parents who had heart attacks, stroke, diabetes, or cancer due to their unhealthy lifestyles are not necessarily doomed to suffer the same fate.

Children, starting from infancy, who are properly trained and guided about health and personal discipline by their parents or guardians grow up to be more health-conscious. In general, they are more healthy compared with those who are not conscientiously supervised. Unguided children merely continue their unhealthy habits into adulthood.

I strongly feel that it is the inherent responsibility of parents to lead, teach, inspire, and discipline their children about healthy habits and behavior from birth to the time they leave home and fly solo. Dereliction of duty by default, or pampering children in the name of love, on the part of the parents, eventually predisposes these individuals to diseases otherwise preventable and cut short their lives, denying them their natural maximal potential for well-being and longevity.

With the title *Let's Stop "Killing" Our Children* I am putting the onus squarely on parents whose innocent, helpless children are under their wisdom, guidance, and protection, all of which will determine their children's future health and life.

A cardiologist friend of mine, who reads my health column, jokingly said, "I don't read the *New England Journal of Medicine* anymore. I just read Philip's column to get medical updates."

As complimentary as that tease was, I am the first to admit that the contents of this modest book can never equal the talent, skills, and experience of your physician and that they are certainly far from being a substitute for medical literature. The thrust of this health reference guide is prevention through education. I wrote each column in layman's terms and with a bit of editorial slant to highlight the pertinent issues and achieve the individual column's objective.

Medical literature is replete with data which show that each year, millions upon millions of preventable deaths involve, not only those in their '60s and '70s, but people in their mid-'40s and '50s, in the prime of their life. With abandon, many of us seem to have programmed our life to cruise on an automatic self-destruct, slow-suicide mode. This passive "surrender" pervasive in our society today is what my health education crusade is trying to change.

Since this is a compilation of my previously published weekly medical columns over time, there are repetition of facts, data, issues, statements, commentaries in a few articles in this book. I did not delete them to keep each column intact. For the redundancy, I beg for your kind indulgence.

If this book is able to inspire one soul or save even one life, the countless hours, all the research and hard work I have put into this public health campaign for healthier lifestyle and into this book would have all been worth it.

Philip S. Chua, MD, FACS, FPCS
June 21, 2011

Foreword

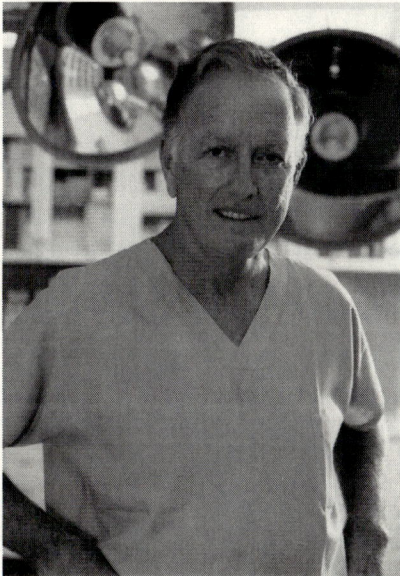

In his book *Let's Stop "Killing" Our Children*, Philip S. Chua, MD, FACS, FPCS, cardiac surgeon emeritus in Munster, Indiana, focuses on disease prevention starting from the crib and highlights the fundamental obligation parents have in teaching children how to live a healthy lifestyle by setting good examples.

My acquaintance with Dr. Chua began in 1972 when he pursued a fellowship in cardiovascular surgery at the Texas Heart Institute (THI) in Houston. There, he gained experience with the surgical treatment of cardiac and vascular diseases in both children and adults. At THI, he was recognized for his professional and technical skills. After leaving Houston, he developed a successful clinical practice in Northwest Indiana, where he continued to demonstrate the same skills and organizational ability.

Dr. Chua has an innate compassionate side, which has prevailed throughout his professional life. As a result, he has frequently returned to his home country, the Philippines, to do cardiac surgery and repay what he considers his debt to his native country for the basic medical education he received there. In the United States and abroad, he has worked diligently to write, compile, and publish articles about health and societal issues, which he considers his personal public health educational campaign for healthier lifestyle and the prevention of diseases.

The title *Let's Stop "Killing" Our Children* may be a bit startling, but it serves Dr. Chua's purpose in attracting attention to the roles of society and parents in guiding children toward a healthier lifestyle to prevent premature morbidity and mortality. I applaud Dr. Chua for his outstanding attitude and dedication. His book should stimulate a focus on healthy lifestyle and disease prevention here and abroad.

Denton A. Cooley, MD, FACS
Founder, Surgeon-in-Chief, and President Emeritus
Texas Heart Institute
Houston, Texas 77225-0345

Dedication

I heartily dedicate this book to my wife, Farida I. Chua, a pediatrician, who taught me not only about children but also how wonderful life can be and how to savor it; to our five loving children, who are also physicians, Sheillah Gentile, Felipe I. Chua, Portia Chua Gonzales, Rachel Chua (Brown), and Emily Greenlee, who are our pride and joy and who have never ceased to inspire us; to our four amazing sons-in-law, Anthony N. Gentile, Luisito C. Gonzales, Jim Milton Brown III, and Jeremy D. W. Greenlee, who, together with our children, have shared their respective medical expertise and served as my specialist consultants in writing and editing some of the articles in this book; and to our ten fabulous grandchildren, Evan Anthony Gentile, Sydney Elizabeth Brown, Samantha Chua, Aidan Everett Gonzales, Jacob Woodfill Greenlee, Jimmy Milton Brown IV, Brendan Alexander Gonzales, Alaina Anne Greenlee, Anna Elise Greenlee, and Colin Alexander Greenlee, our inspiring vision of tomorrow who make growing old truly a privilege for us and an enriching journey to the future.

Finally, I extend this dedication to all my other relatives and friends, for their love and loyalty, and to all of my patients, who placed their lives in my hands with inspiring confidence and appreciation—an ultimate honor that humbles me, and for which I am most grateful.

Dedication

To my mother,
Maxima Sia Chua,
of Raleigh, North Carolina,
who taught me love, patience,
and compassion, and
who, at her age of 92,
still amazes and inspires me.

*

In loving memory of
my father,
Jose Salas Chua,
a victim of heart attack at 46,
my rock and my compass
to this day.

*

To all my brothers and sisters
and their families, whose
love and respect
I value dearly.

Acknowledgment

The main sources of data and statistics in this book include *The New England Journal of Medicine, Clinical Evidence, The Journal of Pediatrics, British Medical Journal, Journal of Thoracic Cardiovascular Surgery, American Journal of Cardiology, American Journal of Emergency Medicine, Circulation, Texas Heart Institute Journal, Pediatrics, Annals of Thoracic Surgery, Journal of the American Medical Association, Journal of the American College of Cardiology, CA—A Cancer Journal for Clinicians, Annals of Surgery, Annals of Internal Medicine, Clinical Geriatrics, Mayo Clinic Health Letter, WebMD, The Cancer Journal, News-Medical, The Johns Hopkins News-Letter, Breakthrough Digest Medical News, Medical News Today, Merck Manual, Obstetrics and Gynecology, Medline Plus, Today in Medicine, Health News, Prevention, Physicians' Desk Reference, the Center for Disease Control and Prevention, National Institute of Health, US Department of Health and Human Services, US Food and Drug Administration*, and various other medical and surgical subspecialty journals. I acknowledge all these references with gratitude, appreciation, and reverence, including those I may have inadvertently missed.

Disclaimer

The main objective of this book is to educate, challenge, and inspire people, especially parents, whose way of life inevitably impacts the health of their children. This would promote living a healthy lifestyle to prevent illnesses and disabilities and achieve a happier and more productive life for themselves and for their offspring.

The discussion of the details of the various illnesses presented in this book, including, but not limited to, the diagnosis, treatment, and prognosis, are general medical information and not intended to be applicable to, or appropriate for, anyone. The data, statistics, and personal comments presented here are not a substitute for, or inferred to be superior to, the professional opinion and recommendation of your physician. Your own physician knows your overall condition well and is your best ally when it comes to your health.

Perspective

Let's Stop "Killing" Our Children

Let's Stop "Killing" Our Children is a challenge I pose to society in general and to parents and guardians in particular. This is not an indictment, but an invitation to a more scientific perspective and dialogue on parents' and society's role and obligation in disease prevention for the ultimate benefit of mankind.

When we build anything priceless, we make doubly sure that the structural integrity of the foundation is as solid and as lasting as it could be.

When we prepare to bring forth a child into this present world of potential infirmities and disabilities, we want to avoid possible congenital defects, or damage to its DNA no matter how minor or subtle, due to our thoughtlessness, carelessness, indifference, or patent unhealthy behaviors detrimental to the fetus.

The prospective parents, especially the mother, should live a healthy lifestyle conducive to child-bearing long before and during pregnancy, even beyond delivery.

We want the best environment and ideal conditions as possible for our future child in order to protect its DNA and maximize the ability of this new life to ward off infection and diseases as they are born, climb out of the crib, and grow to adulthood, middle age, and beyond.

Autopsy findings on children, as young as four and five, who were victims of accidents, already had evidences of arteriosclerosis (hardening of their arteries), a condition we expect to see only in adults. There must be something we, parents, are doing wrong.

This leads to my proposal that we need to institute a pre-emptive and proactive health strategy that starts from "Ground Zero," even before conception starts, because, after all, the race does not start in the middle of the track. The postmortem findings above are self-evident.

During the first lap, when the baby is born, it must be nurtured with a healthy diet, the best one being mother's milk, from one who lives a healthy lifestyle and with a team mate who is likewise health-aware and protective of the infant.

We often wonder why most formula-fed babies, or those taking formula supplement, appear to be heavier, more rotund, even before their first birthday, compared to those totally breast-fed, quantity being equal.

The reason for infant obesity is the character and quality of milk they are fed. Since six decades ago, the consumer's need for milk in the country increased so much that producers had to resort to shortcuts in milk production by reducing the grazing area per cow, to accommodate more, and also by feeding them wheat, corn, and soy, with hormones to fatten them, plus antibiotics and other additives. These feeds are totally deficient in omega-3 and contain high level of omega-6, which causes an unhealthy imbalance in of the ratio of omega-3 and omega-6 in the human body. Normally it should be 1:1, but in this case, it is 1:15 or as high as 1:40. Omega-6 causes our body to store fats and induce inflammation, which promotes high cholesterol level, hardening of the arteries, and blockages in them, reducing blood supply to vital organs, such as the brain and the heart muscles. Formula-overfeeding makes matters even worse.

This unhealthy imbalance leads to obesity, and later in life, to hypercholesterolemia and an increased risk for the development of diabetes, cardiovascular diseases, Alzheimer's, and a variety of cancers.

Canada and many countries in Europe are more stringent in their laws against using hormones, and antibiotics and other additives in animal feeds. They also favor milk and meat from pasture-raised or grass-fed, not corn-fed, cows, for the health reasons we stated above. The United States is still lagging behind in this regard.

So, we have to remember that whatever junk foods the sources of milk, either the mother or the cows, eat, the baby drinking the milk from either, also gets the same junk in its system.

Grass-fed cows yield quality milk and meat with healthy balance, a 1:1 ratio of omega-3 and omega-6. The same goes true with the eggs and meat from chickens that eat healthy feeds, without hormones and other additives. Chickens fed with corn, which is a most common practice today, produce eggs with lower levels of essential fatty acids as they did more than half a century ago. A New England Journal of Medicine article reported that eggs from corn-fed chickens have twenty times more omega-6 than omega-3, a most unhealthy ratio.

Before babies climb out of the crib, their obesity cannot be blamed on the hamburger and French Fries stands. But thereafter, when we, parents, unwisely introduce them to these "vendors of saturated fats," "the heart attack food stores," as some people correctly label them, the dilemma begins. A bad habit is born! And many of us parents, out of our love to please our children, too often succumb to their "demand" for a fix of unhealthy saturated fats.

Unfortunately, the damage to their tender bodies are not immediately obvious. They show up thirty or forty or fifty years later, when obesity sneaks in, arthritis begins to hurt, blood pressure starts to climb, blood cholesterol and blood sugar levels shoot up, and coronary arteries and arteries to the brain start to clog up, causing heart attack or stroke, or Alzheimer's.

When children develop a taste for red meat and other fatty foods, which are not really essential food items and which we can actually live without, they lose interest in, and even "hate," anti-oxidant-loaded and immune system- boosting vegetables, nuts, whole grains, fruits. At this point, they are well on their way to obesity, arthritis, diabetes, high blood pressure, heart attack, stroke, and even cancer, as they grow to middle age.

The same adverse effects come from children's lack of parent-inspired discipline and interest in physical exercises and their addiction to the couch, television, as they binge on unhealthy carbs (chips, soft drinks, ice cream, sweets, etc.) and processed foods. Just like what many of us parents, their model and idol, do.

The worse scenarios are, of course, when they take up the nasty habit of smoking, undisciplined drinking, or using illegal drugs.

Tons of medical evidence show that a low-fat, low-carbohydrate diet of fish, generous amount of vegetables, hi-fiber whole grain, nuts, and fruits, plus daily exercise, good hydration, adequate sleep and relaxation, medical consultation when needed, are actually the "secret" fountain of youth we have all been searching for. It is not illusive; it is right here under our noses. We are simply ignoring it.

The parental pre-emptive approach early on to prevent the risk for diseases through loving but firm discipline and persuasive inspiration through good examples set by the parents themselves, could lead children to a safer path and a healthier fate in their adulthood.

While it is never too late to start a healthy lifestyle even by those of us with high blood pressure, obesity, diabetes or heart disease, it is self-evident that to pre-empt all these infirmities would have been a wiser beginning. That would have made everything less complicated and safer at this stage in our life. That initial step is what I described as ground zero, at the DNA level, decades before what our current and widely practiced strategy is doing.

I strongly believe that healthy lifestyle and disease prevention for every child should start before conception, in the womb, and in the crib. This puts the onus squarely on society and our government, on parents and guardians of young children, who are totally "at the mercy" of national health policies and these adults, whose good or bad habits and behaviors will be inevitably emulated by the children. It is in the five formative years of the children up to age 12 when instilling proper discipline and behavioral modification are most effective.

Almost all diseases known to man today are self-induced or self-inflicted, and are, therefore, obviously preventable. Unfortunately, many of us seemed to have unwittingly programmed our mindset and behavior to a self-destruct and slow-suicide mode. This negative surrender and fatalistic attitude are what this book aims to change.

In the past half a century, society has failed to significantly prevent ailments and conditions afflicting man. The pandemic of obesity, arthritis, diabetes, cardiovascular diseases, and cancer are evidences that our conventional preventive strategy is miserably ineffective and inadequate. Could this be because we are starting in the middle of the race, when our enemies are already well ahead of us?

To be honest with ourselves as parents, we must the ask this other logical question, Who is responsible for this health dilemma?

Anyone not positively contributing to the well-being of a child under his/her care, for whatever reason, including love, is literally cutting short the life span of that youngster. In addition, poor lifestyle choices on our part as parents are bad examples which negatively affect our children.

Unless we wisely recognize, accept, and remedy our fundamental flaws in parenting, our adult children, like those of the past generations before them, will continue to suffer the ravages of preventable diseases and premature death.

In view of this, it behooves society as a whole, including governments, and parents to seriously re-evaluate our current conventional strategy in dealing with disease prevention, if we are to contain, if not eradicate, the most common major diseases afflicting man around the world today.

A well-structured pre-emptive and proactive strategy can go a long way in our quest for health, well-being, happiness, and longevity.

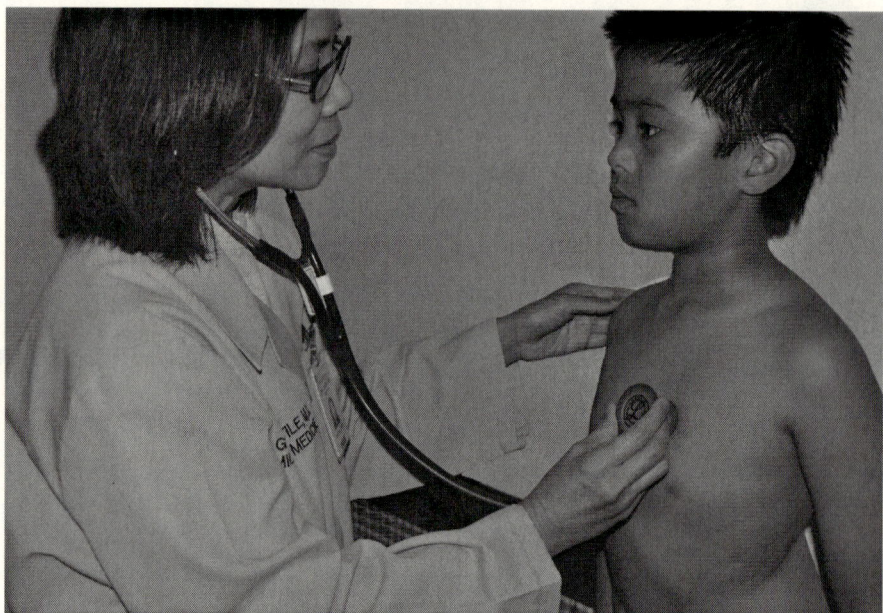

A regular well-child medical check-up, including uptodate immunizations, starting from infancy, is essential in preventing diseases and maintaining children's health.

Healthy lifestyle Starts in the Womb, "Dieting" Begins in the crib

The future health of a child as an adult begins way before conception. The lifestyle of the parents, especially the mother, determines the genetic integrity and development of the fetus. A healthy pregnant woman whose habits and behavior are protective of the growing life in her womb, and who undergoes regular prenatal check-ups, maximizes the infant's health and well-being.

Contrary to scientific facts, a chubby kid is somehow considered as a healthy child by some. Numerous TV commercials today use plump children in their food and vitamin ads. This sends a wrong message and is a disservice to the public, especially to our youngsters. Nothing is farther from the truth.

Overweight children, as shown by countless studies, are more likely to develop a cluster of health problems and their complications, compared to their peers with normal weight. The greater the weight excess, the higher a child's body mass index (BMI) - a measure of weight in relation to height - the greater the risk of acquiring the so-called metabolic syndrome early in life. Obesity, in children and in adult, is a pandemic and a significant health danger.

The Risk Factors and Some Alarming Stats

The risk factors that characterize metabolic syndrome are elevated triglycerides (blood fats), blood sugar, and blood pressure; low HDL (high-density lipoproteins, the good cholesterol); ad abdominal obesity. These precede the development of type 2 diabetes and cardiovascular diseases.

Two out of every 3 Americans are overweight, and about half of them have gone on, or on their way, to being obese. About 15% of children between ages 6 and 19 (that's one out of 6) are overweight, and another 15% are on their way there. Two decades ago, there were only 5% overweight kids in the USA. Among those 20 and older, 30% are overweight today compared to 15.1% twenty years ago. From 1996 to 2001, there were 2 million obese teenagers and young adults. Interestingly, about 1 out of 4 dogs and cats are tipping up the scale too. Statistics in Asian countries are catching up with those of the Western world.

Diabesity (diabetes and obesity) is upon us globally, but this common entity is preventable to a significant extent. About 39% of children who are moderately obese and almost 50% of those severely obese develop the metabolic syndrome. Obviously, we are not over feeding only ourselves to death but also our children and our pets.

The increase in the incidence of diabetes has also catapulted: from 2.8% in 1980 to 4.2% in year 2000. This and cardiovascular illnesses parallel the rate of the increasing waistline of America. Fifty percent of all obese adults have high blood pressure.

Educating Children's Taste Buds

All of us learned to love foods we were exposed to as children. Our preferences today were acquired when we were young. Dieting, which means choosing the proper food items and controlling the total calorie intake, should actually start in the crib.

Breast milk, when adequate, is the ideal food for the baby for at least year. If formula is needed, as a supplement, or as a primary source of nutrition, it must be milk formula from grass-fed cows, free of hormones, antibiotics and other additives.

The solid food started at age 4 months should consist of vegetables and fruits, and at 6 months, fish could be gradually introduced and serve as the primary source of protein. Red meat is not an essential food item at any age. Baby foods available today can be healthier. Yogurt, according to Frank Greer, a pediatrician and former chairman of the American Academy of Pediatrics, may be started at 6 months old, unless the infant has milk allergy or intolerance.

As early as a year old, toddlers should be exposed to meals consisting mainly of vegetables, fish, and fruits. If they are not fed red meat and other high cholesterol and high carbohydrate food items, they will not develop a taste and a craving for them. This invariably means the meals we prepare for ourselves should be exactly the healthy food items we want our children to learn to love. Our choices, habits, and behavior are examples they will inevitably emulate. If they are exposed to a healthy lifestyle, which includes regular physical exercises besides eating the right quality and quantity of food daily, they subconsciously tend to adopt the same wholesome way of living.

Individuals who do not like fish and vegetables, and prefer red meats and carbohydrates, were obviously exposed predominantly to the latter as they climbed out of the crib. Statistics show that children of parents who smoke, drink, or do not exercise are more prone to develop the same habits. Discipline, behavior, and preferences acquired during the first five years of life are ingrained in the child and carried over into adulthood.

In essence, what our children grow up to be is, to a significant extent, are our doing. Whatever children turn out to be is a reflection of their upbringing. That responsibility rests squarely on our shoulders, and not on society or on the environment. Sociology and psychology have shown that, as a rule, youngsters who have been taught and guided wisely developed personality, character, and integrity that served them well in making their choices or decisions throughout their lives.

Overfeeding, at any stage in the child's development, or even among us adults, is not healthy. Maintenance of the proper caloric requirement is fundamental.

The fact that pre-schoolers have been found to have hardening of the arteries at such tender ages only suggests we have been feeding our children too much cholesterol, fats, and carbohydrates, and too little vegetables, fish, and fruits starting from the crib. The kids' fascination with hamburger-and-fries stores, inspired by adults' less than wholesome example, is a significant part of the health dilemma.

A child who is overweight is obviously eating the wrong food and taking in more calories than he/she burns. To allow this to continue without proper and prompt intervention is to doom the child to a future marred by a string of health problems along the way. As a consequence of this seemingly trivial matter, the child could be so impacted by the exposure to unhealthy lifestyle and become a victim of otherwise preventable diseases and death in the prime of their life.

Not Only for Aesthetic

The extra pounds adversely affect the body shape but, more importantly, they are a most unhealthy baggage that takes its toll in terms of the development of otherwise preventable illnesses, like high blood pressure, diabetes, heart disease, stroke, infertility, osteoarthritis, gall bladder disease, and many forms of cancer. Obesity is not a primary cosmetic issue, but an essential health issue.

Timing of the Strategy

As we have stated in the previous article, dieting starts when the baby is born, not when he/she is a teenager. The brain is more receptive to teaching at that early stage, when tastes, preferences and habits are just beginning to develop. But it is never too late to start living healthier, no matter how old a person is. Adopting a healthy lifestyle is always prudent and wise at any stage in life.

Overfeeding, at any stage in the child's development, or even among us adults, is not healthy. The solid food started at age 4 months should consist of vegetables and fruits, and at 6 months, fish could be introduced and serve as the primary source of protein. Red meat is not an essential food item at any age. Yogurt, according to Frank Greer, a pediatrician and former chairman of the American Academy of Pediatrics, may be started at 6 months old, unless the infant has milk allergy or intolerance.

The Sensible Diet

I advocate a plain, simple, inexpensive, and sensible formula. We do not really need to spend on packaged diet meals. With a little imagination and creativity, one can prepare healthy meals with the desired caloric content similar to those on the frozen shelves of grocery stores. And your version will even be freshly cooked.

The basic principle to maintain a normal weight among those who already have the desired weight requires intake of calories to closely approximate the output of energy thru physical exercise. Quantity and quality are essential factors in weight control.

Quality: Eat foods that have been proven scientifically to be healthy. This includes fish, vegetables, nuts, whole grains, fruits: a low-fat/ low-cholesterol/high-fiber diet - minimizing red meats and eggs and dairy products. For adults, skim milk is preferred; for growing children, 2% milk; for infants, breast milk; and if supplement is needed, formula milk from grass-fed cows, as prescribed by the pediatrician. Carbohydrates (the "sweets," potato, bread, rice, non-diet pop drinks, ice cream, cakes, candies, etc.) are loaded with sugar and a great culprit causing obesity.

Drinking soft drinks (cola or uncola, regular or diet, with or without caffeine) could lead to metabolic syndrome. Low-carb diet is in. People will do well with low-carb diet for weight reduction. However, to substitute high-fat and high-cholesterol (red meats, eggs, etc.) for carbohydrates is blatantly unhealthy, tremendously increasing the risk of cardiovascular diseases and cancer.

The best diet is still one consisting of fish and high-fiber items like vegetables, nuts, whole grains, and fruits. The new Food Plate released by the USDA June 2, 2011 basically confirmed what I, among others, have been preaching and prescribing for decades. First Michelle Obama, who endorsed and presented the new Food Plate. will go down in history for this great contribution in nutrition and health.

For adults in mild active life, with normal weight, 1,500-1,800 calories a day should suffice to maintain normal weight. For children with normal weight, 2,000 calories a day should be tops and adjusted accordingly if the child is starting to be overweight for his height and age. Children who are overweight should be checked by a physician, who could prescribe a diet plan. The habit of pushing ourselves away from the dining table less than full, as I have stated somewhere in this book, will serve all of us well. A little less, in this case, is healthier than full or a bit too full.

We must remember that the quality, the type of food items, is as important to health as the quantity.

Saying "no" is love

We must learn to say "no" to our children where appropriate, for their own good, even if it hurts us inside. Instead of trying to be popular with our kids, let's protect them, even from themselves. Their appreciation will come later, when they have children of their own.

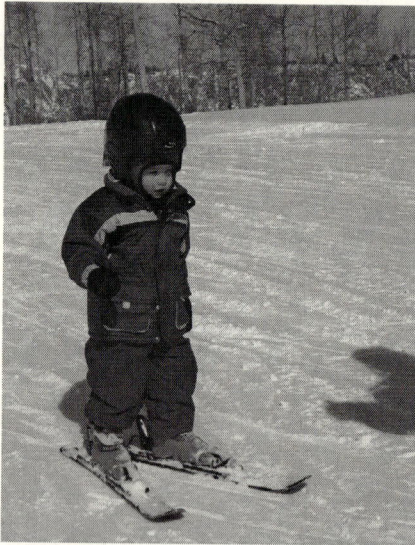

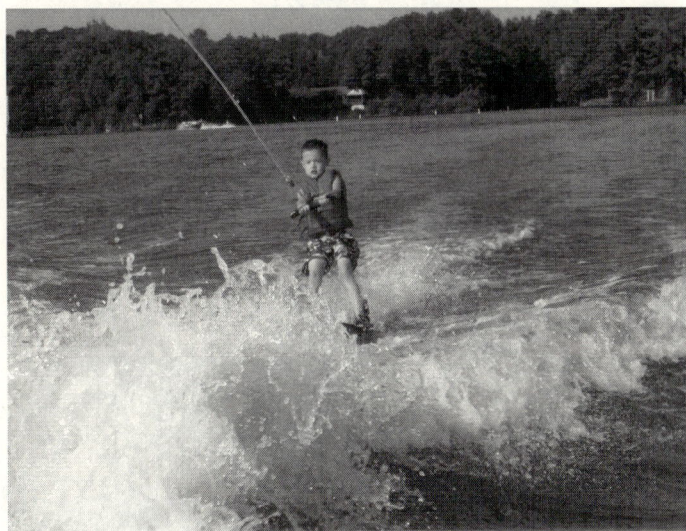
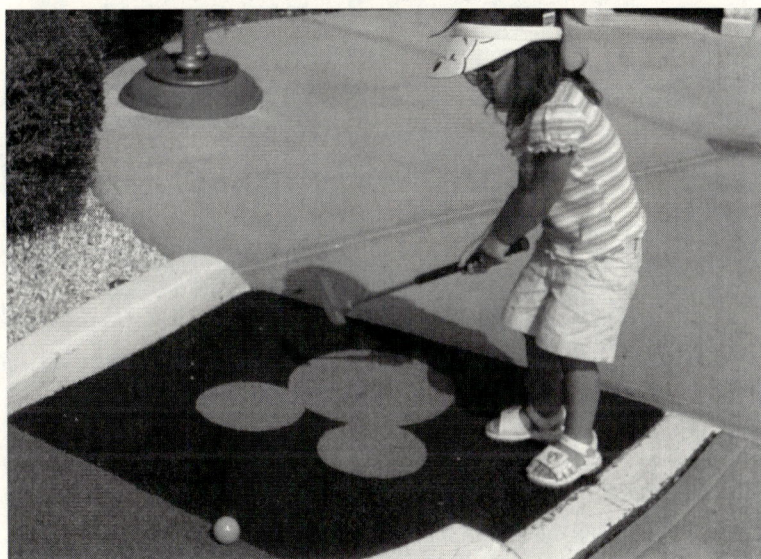

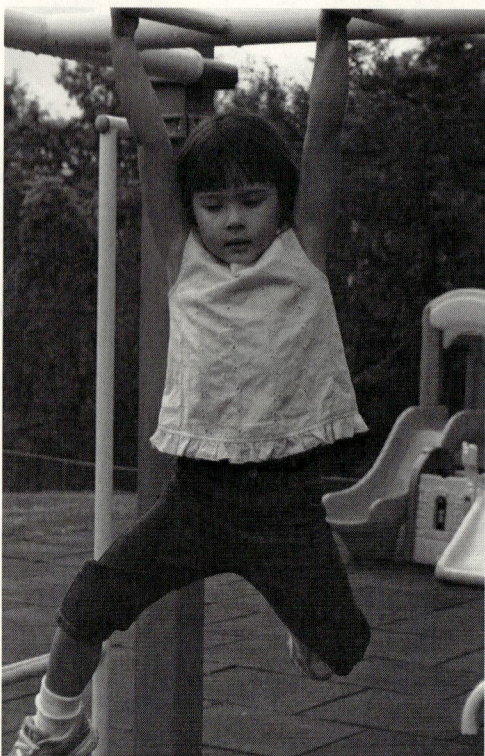
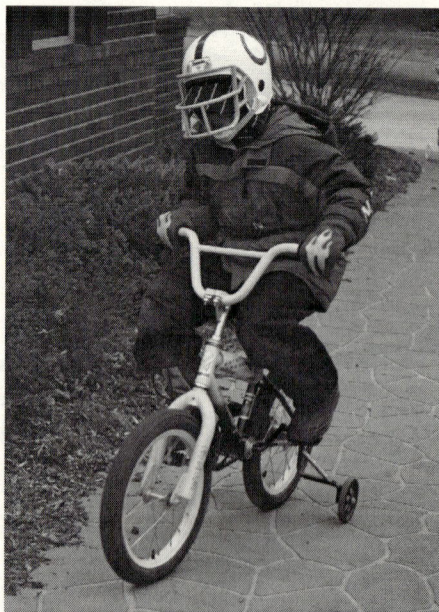
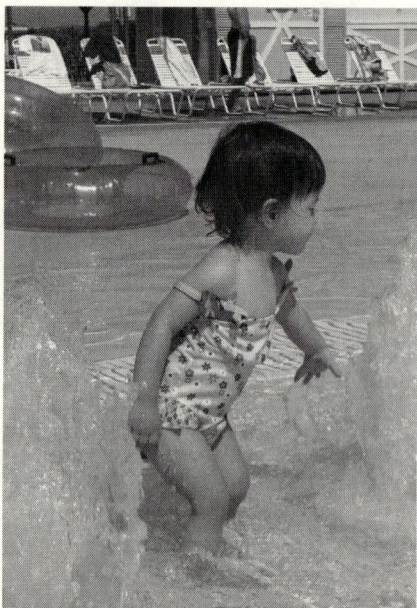

Sports for children will instill in them discipline and wholesome competitiveness, at the same time teaching them the value of physical activities.

Studies have shown that children, no matter how young, who indulge in sport(s), besides regular exercises, are overall healthier. They perform better in school, are more competitive, more positive and sociable, are less prone to do drugs, and have lower risks of depression. They are also more likely to watch their diet and do regular physical exercises when they grow up.

First Lady Michelle Obama Introduces "My Plate"

On Thursday, June 2, 2011, US First Lady Michelle Obama introduced *My Plate*, the new basic food guide to replace the outdated Food Pyramid of 1992.

The picture on the next page from The New York Times shows Mrs. Obama, Agriculture Secretary Tom Vilsack and Surgeon General Regina M. Benjamin, as they unveiled *My Plate* in Washington, DC.

"The new design called *My Plate* was conceived as a crucial part of Mrs. Obama's campaign against obesity, designed to remind consumers about the basics of a healthful diet," writes William Neuman of The New York Times

My Plate is simpler, easier to understand, and a more practical guide, whose main emphasis is on vegetables, whole grain, nuts, fruits, and less on carbohydrates and meat, unlike the Food Pyramid, whose wide base consisted of 6-11 servings of bread, cereals, rice and pasta groups, a heavy dose of carbohydrates.

Since proper diet is a most crucial regimen in a healthy lifestyle, Mrs. Obama's health crusade will go a long way in inspiring us to eat healthier, in controlling the epidemic of obesity, and in preventing diseases and premature deaths in the United States, if not in the whole world.

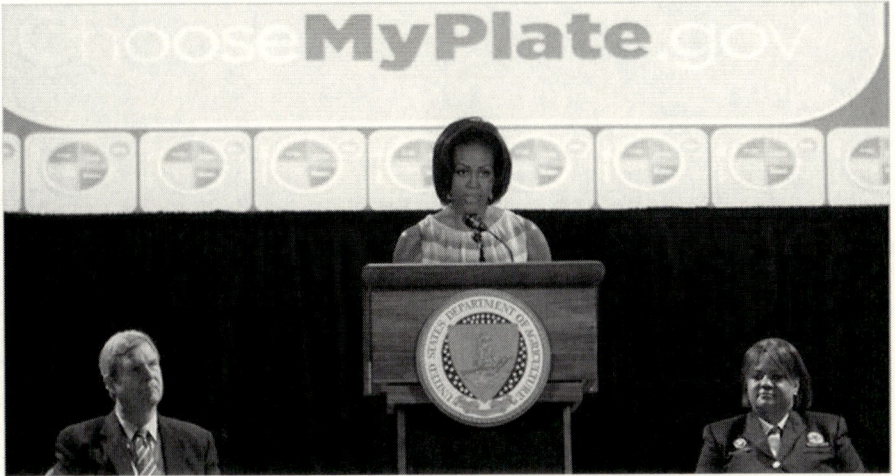

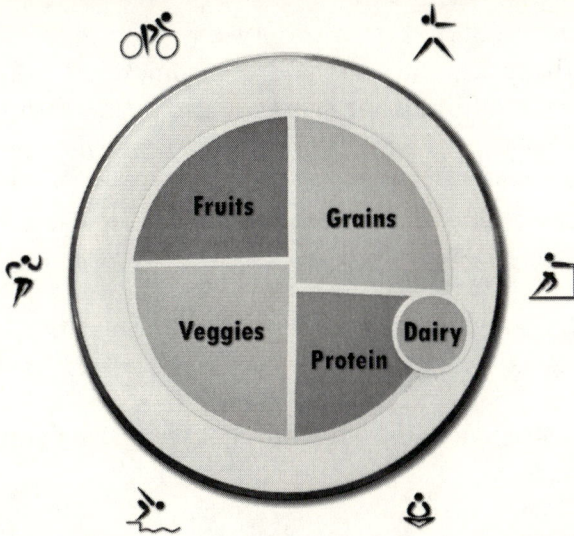

The new Food Plate, released June 2, 2011 by the US Department of Agriculture, replaces the original Food Pyramid of 1992. On this Plate, roughly 50% consists of vegetables and fruits, and the remaining 50%, grains (rice, bread, pasta, oat meal) and protein (fish, chicken, beef, pork).The vegetables and grains are about 30% each, and the fruits and proteins about 20% each. The average healthy total calorie intake ranges between 1800 to 2000 a day, lower for those trying to lose weight. Diet for diabetics is tailored to the individual's needs. Eating a lot of vegetables and minimizing pork and beef and other high cholestrol foods is prudent, and daily physical exercise is vital in our pursuit of good health.

Attitude Impacts Health and Life

Show me a man with a bad attitude, and I will show you one abandoned by his friends and scorned by strangers.

Here are some quotes of wisdom I have come across, which are inspiring for those who, like many of us, sometimes find themselves falling toward the pit of discouragement and despair. With the proper attitude, these sage proverbs lift our spirits by allowing us to view and accept the trials and tribulations in this world in their most positive and best light. Indeed, all of us need a psychological boost, an inspiration, every now and then. Here are some:

Anthony J. D'Angelo, in *The College Blue Book,* said "Wherever you go, no matter what the weather, always bring your own sunshine."

To quote Oscar Wilde, "If you don't get everything you want, think of the things you don't get that you don't want."

Voltaire expressed it beautifully when he stated, "Life is like a shipwreck, but we must not forget to sing in the lifeboats."

An ancient Persian saying puts a great perspective on our daily aches and pains in life: "I had the blues because I had no shoes, until upon the street, I met a man who had no feet."

And as some of us may curse some bad days we encounter and wish they never came, Cavett Robert offers these poignant words: "If you don't think every day is a good day, just try missing one."

Indeed, every day is a good day, although others are better and others not as good. But each day is a gift. Not waking up to another day is a deadly waste, but not appreciating another day is a tragedy. How each of us greets the day depends greatly on our attitude. Indeed, attitude impacts our health, our life, and our everyday happiness and success. A person with a chip on his shoulder, with a negative attitude or pessimistic view of life, will obviously be miserable most of the time. And the opposite is true, as Annette Goodheart brilliantly points out: "Just because you're miserable doesn't mean you can't enjoy life."

Happiness is basically an attitude. Gaining inner peace is an attitude. We have that God-given power to feel what we want to feel. We can even psyche ourselves. I do.

When I wake up each morning, I thank God for another wonderful day. I tell my mind ahead of time that it will be another good day. It may not be a perfect day, but a good, pleasurable, and productive one—a day I could enjoy being with my family, doing my computer work, writing my column, or simply praising someone, inspiring somebody, planting a tree, or enjoying the sunset and the beauty of the universe.

In a world plagued by war, economic crises, corruption, resource shortages, and natural disasters, a good attitude is one of our best weapons against helplessness, despair, and depression.

With all these complex problems confronting us, we often find ourselves in the gutter of hopelessness. Oscar Wilde suggests we look up at the heavens and "see the stars." Indeed, a positive attitude can help tremendously in conquering our fears, insecurities, and dilemmas. When we sometimes lose or fail, we should remind ourselves to get up and fight even harder. After all, "defeat is not bitter unless you swallow it," as Joe Clark states. To this, I will add my own: "No one can succeed in life without having the courage to fail," and "The greatest risk in life is not taking any risk at all."

Someone said, "You cannot adjust the direction of the wind, but you can adjust your sail." Very true, indeed. These are simple words of wisdom that could make our day, if not our life.

And all this leads me to quote a very popular soothing prayer that you may know, one that I say to myself almost every day: "God, grant me the serenity to accept the things I cannot change, courage to change the things I can, and the wisdom to know the difference."

My faith in God eliminates more than 75 percent of my worries day in and day out. I do not dwell on things I cannot change and allow fear and despair to paralyze my life. Worrying about things outside of my control is a waste of my time and emotion that takes a toll on my mental and physical health.

While we cannot cure the cancer of poverty, we, as individuals who are more blessed, can at least open our heart to help the homeless and the hungry and gain that sense of inner satisfaction and peace. As I have stated a few times in the past, let us not wait for surgery to open our heart. Let our good attitude and compassion for our fellow men reign.

As I live my life each day, I remind myself of an ancient proverb that says, "To everyone is given the key to heaven, the same key opens the gates to hell." It's indeed a matter of personal choice. And that choice inevitably depends on our attitude in life. Some people believe their fate is predestined and that they can't do anything about it. Others, inspired by a good attitude and a positive frame of mind, design, create, and charter their own destiny.

I strongly believe that leaving this world after this life is not a tragedy. Dying without significance, without making a difference, without leaving behind a good legacy, is.

Let's all develop a good attitude to help us enjoy life. It's a most potent prescription for health and happiness.

Let's Enjoy Life

In this topsy-turvy, muddled world of ours, where stress is the usual order of the day, we need a disciplined mind to keep and maintain our sanity.

For hundreds of years, philosophers, from Plato to Aristotle, Aquinas to Descartes, displayed their intellectual and moral struggle in search of the meaning of life, truth, discipline, and inner peace. Yoga, the art of living and transcendental meditation, practiced in the East for thousands of years, has been shown to have soothing, calming, and healthy effects on the mind and on the cardiovascular system.

Indeed, the marvelous human body produces endogenous, auto-regulated chemical substances triggered and controlled by the mind, which affect our entire system as exogenous drugs do. It is, therefore, paramount that we discipline our mind and body in order to take full advantage of this unique and beneficial built-in "pharmacy" in each of us.

One way to discipline our mind in dealing with daily stress in life is by behavioral modification with philosophical reinforcement. Expressing our gratitude to the Almighty when we wake up each morning—for the health and safety of our family and ourselves, for the home we live in, the food on our table, the job we have, and all the wonderful graces we have received over the years—provides us a more confident and stalwart outlook on life as we begin our day.

While our life is not perfect, we must realize and remind ourselves every day how lucky we are to be blessed with this bounty. These few seconds of bedside meditation each morning alone will instill positive thoughts in our minds at the very start of the day, enough to initiate the flow of opiate-like polypeptides, like enkephalins and endorphins, throughout our body, making us feel good and happy. And we do not even have to spend money for these "fixes" or go to the drugstore for them!

Life is only a dream and a fleeting one. Let's live it fully before we wake up one day and realize that we have missed it all. While we have time, we have to think and take care of ourselves, and not only of our loved ones. We should also pamper ourselves every now and then. We should do things we have always wanted to do that give us pure pleasure and joy. Take the trips we have always planned to take. Enjoy the wonders of nature. Make people laugh. Play with a child. Smell the flowers along the way. And as my wife often says, let's remember to "eat the dessert first," because life is uncertain and not eternal.

Many of us seem to see only the negative things in our life. Most often we forget to count our blessings. Like we train our physical being to be strong and healthy, so must we discipline our mind in coping with our daily stresses and in preserving a sense of joy and inner peace as we live each day.

Life is too short. Let us not endure it. Let's enjoy it.

Savor Life

Let us not hurry to our graves

by casting recklessly our fate

Not much time to abuse and waste

let all the empty gravesites wait

Savor life's overflowing cup

and every second we have left

'cause time pauses not for any man

Let joy consume us not by chance

for we shall live this life but once.

PSC 6-21-72

Parenthood

Every child is a blessing and having children, natural or adopted, is one of the greatest privileges a couple or a person can have. But just like any privilege in life, parenthood comes with serious obligations and responsibilities for both the mother and the father, or the adopting parent(s).

It does not require a man to be a genius or a superhero to impregnate a woman. Nor does pregnancy in a woman constitute being a mother. What makes a woman a mother is not the few minutes of romance or the short nine months of carrying the child, or even the actual delivery. It is the everlasting love, enduring sacrifice, and endless patience in caring for the child that defines motherhood. Childbearing is easy. Child rearing is something else. Any woman can get pregnant and deliver a child, but not everyone can be a mother.

Similarly, it takes more than just virility and prowess in bed for a man to be a father. Fatherhood requires the strength and courage to selflessly love another unconditionally.

Anything less in either parent makes the man nothing but a sperm donor and the woman only an incubator.

While most couples may be blessed with parenthood, some may strive harder to have a family. In today's world where unfortunate orphans and unwanted, or neglected, children abound, adoptive couples create forever families by considering adoption. After all, when all is said and done, we will all agree that procreation, conception, and delivery are only a miniscule part of true motherhood, and providing the sperm, only an iota of what fatherhood is all about.

Parenthood entails commitment to a lifetime contract between parents and child. It is entered into the very moment the man and the woman engaged in an act that could bring forth new life into the world. Conceivably, that same commitment has been faithfully kept and handed down from the very first family of humans on earth to our generation today. The reciprocal obligation, of course, is for the children to take care of their parents when the time comes.

That this covenant is a part of the laws of nature is evident even among animals, especially among mammals. It is a tragedy and a shame to realize that it is more pervasive among humans to neglect, hurt, and/or abandon their young than most animals. Similarly, it is a sad commentary, on the other end of the spectrum, that ingratitude and cruelty is all too common among some people of today, who wantonly desert their old and helpless parents in the sunset years of their lives when they need their children's love and care the most.

While parenthood is a grave responsibility filled with sleepless nights, sacrifice, and sometimes disappointment, it is nonetheless a joyous privilege. As long as we continue to honor this privilege, the world will remain a wonderful place to live in.

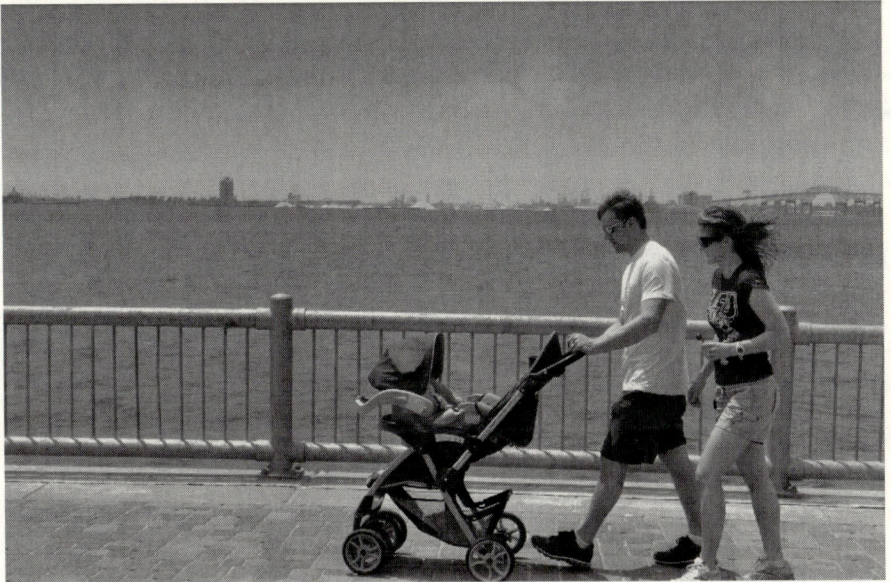

Stroller exercise is popular for health and family bonding.

A time to pause

We live in a complex, hurried, and stress-laden society. The carousel of life spins so fast we sometimes can't get off and get confused with our priorities and goals. In this world of instant this and instant that, of split-second e-mail, express grocery checkout counters, drive-up fast food, pharmacy, and banking, people give high fives instead of the old-fashioned handshake; and friendly conversation is reduced to "Hi!" and "Bye." Everyone seems to be in a hurry. People can't even say, "Just a second, please." They now say, "Just a sec," to save a split second of time. Everything is now, now, now. Instead of mailing handwritten letters, we now transmit e-mail messages with lightning speed, domestic and international. The whole world has shrunken smaller, and it seems even the hour has been reduced to less than 60 minutes, and the minute to less than 60 seconds.

We are all in a rat race. No time for visiting our parents, friends, and other loved ones. No time to be our brothers' keeper and save the poor. No time for exercises or R & R. No time for contemplation and soul-searching. No time to appreciate and smell the flowers along the way. No time to commune with nature. Simply no time, except for the wild and dizzying ride in the fast lane of today's society.

Several years ago, a husband and wife colleagues of mine gave me four books, among others, as Christmas gifts. One of these books was titled **Stopping**. Reading that book opened my mind and my eyes and provided me a wiser perspective in life, one that I never had the time to stop for and realize.

Looking back, from the time I stepped out of high school and the 18 years that followed (college, medical schooling, internship, residency training, and Fellowship), and the hectic medical practice thereafter,

I was always on the expressway of my life. Somehow, the speedy lane was the only path and direction I knew. I was caught in the vicious cycle of work, work, and work, unwittingly sacrificing the beauty of life itself. It now seems that part of my life had passed me by as I was whirling away, barely noticing it.

Not experiencing every minute of our life and savoring its beauty and wonders is really missing it all. And it would indeed be a great pity if, in the twilight years of our life, we woke up one morning and wondered, "Where have all the years gone? Did I enjoy life to the fullest, or did I miss it all?"

Pausing to live, love, and laugh is the way to get back to life and to have a life. Although in a zip-and-zoom mode, we sometimes have to put the brakes on, even if the inertia throws us overboard and wakes us up. Stopping the vertiginous circus, in order to live every moment in time, seems to be the saner and healthier way. For many of us it might be difficult to simply "slow down" gradually, because the habit we have developed over the years had conditioned our mind and body to "full speed ahead," and reducing the pace only leads to a poor compromise. What we have to do is to **just *stop*** as I have just learned from that book. At least to reorient our bearings in life and review our priorities, enjoy our family and friends, and this wonderful world as a whole.

Stopping the vicious cycle of work, work and work does not mean quitting altogether. All we simply have to do is to punctuate our routine at a prescheduled intervals with "non-work-related, fun-filled, pure-play" activities we have always wanted to do alone or with our loved ones "if we only had the time." Time management is not limited to our job, even in this mega trendy times. It also applies, and more appropriately so, to our life, mental health, and happiness. After all, we are here on earth to be fulfilled and to be happy. And happiness is not the destination in life. Happiness is the journey itself. Let's enjoy the travel to the fullest.

Are We Humans Really Civilized?

(Or are we for the birds?)

I was driving to work one early morning a few years ago in Munster, Indiana, when I noticed a flock of Canadian geese flying against a beautiful backdrop of a golden orange rising sun that was eagerly peeking over the clear horizon. The picturesque scene became even more poignant when I observed that the geese were flying in a perfect reversed V formation. One seemed to be the leader of the pack, at the very apex; and the rest, in an orderly fashion, followed in a reversed V formation. At one point, another goose flew ahead and assumed the "leadership" at the apex of the V. When the "leader" got tired, another flew to the apex, the former "leader" went behind the flank. They seemed to each take turns. Everything was smooth, easy, and quite orderly.

The reason came back to me as I recalled a book I once read. Birds, in general, have the instinct to know that the wind they fly against offers most aerodynamic resistance if they fly alone or on a straight frontal line. Flying in a reversed V-formation, with the apex cutting through the headwind, makes it a lot easier for the others behind to fly. The "leader" at the apex gets the most wind resistance, and less and lesser for those behind, who are covered by the birds in front of them. All of this appears to take place in an organized fashion, with no hesitation, no delays, no bickering, no pushing, no wrangling, as if each bird knew precisely its individual role and was graciously compliant.

How I wish we, humans, self-proclaimed the most civilized and most intelligent of all creatures on the planet Earth, would be as "civilized, compassionate, considerate, and orderly" as these birds. Imagine how wonderful it would be if we, brothers and sisters of the world, would stop fighting, hurting, destroying, and killing each other, and instead, understand, accept, help, and protect each other like these flying creatures of God.

Obviously, the transformation will not be easy, as the history of man has so far shown us. But human beings better start soon, before we unwittingly blow each other up, together with Mother Earth, into shameful particles of historical ash into the galaxy. The only legacy our species would leave behind then would be our *Homo sapiens* stupidity.

Destroying Our Planet

Our planet would be at an imminent grave risk of being destroyed, if global warming, more appropriately termed climate change, continued unabated. And like the multitudes of problems threatening the world, this major one is caused by its intelligent inhabitant, man himself, and his careless and irresponsible behavior, especially in the last two-hundred-some years. Human beings are not new to self-abuse, self-destruction, and to irreverence to his environment, in spite of their education, culture, and massive data in this age of exploding informational technology and mind-boggling advances in science and medicine.

Man's self-abuse and rape of his environment are almost certain to doom the world he lives in, unless he listens to Mother Nature and promptly starts to take a wise proactive strategy in dealing with his present ecologic dilemma. Man cannot afford to lose his only known sanctuary in the galaxy, because space exploration has not found a suitable substitute, a "spare" home for the earthlings yet. The change in the climate around the world and the frequent natural disasters occurring these days are signs and symptoms of a wounded planet.

Historically, the earth's climate has gone through various changes, from ice age to prolonged periods of heat waves. The factors involved include the alteration in the Earth's orbit, the degree of energy from the sun, and volcanic eruptions. The latter part of the 18th century ushered in the human factor: the industrial revolution which has contributed to more massive environmental pollution.

The human factor includes the carcinogenic fumes from cigarettes; carbon monoxide/dioxide from engine emissions; chemical contamination from the household agents, like soaps, bleaches, tile and toilet cleaners, etc.; factory air pollution and toxic waste products dumped into our rivers and lakes; deforestation and destruction of our greeneries; invasion of the original habitats of animals; disturbance in the natural order of things; and the environmental insults that urbanization brings with it in general. These changes in the landscape of nature have affected the health of our planet, causing global warming that is rising like a fever from an infection, and at an alarmingly faster rate than what it should be. All this is happening because of what we, its intelligent inhabitants, have done to the one and only "life-sustaining home" we know in the galaxy.

The burning of fossil fuels, such as coals and oil, and deforestation the past two centuries have led to the "greenhouse effect," where the toxic gases in the atmosphere has significantly increased to the point of trapping heat, like in a glass panel enclosure of a greenhouse, causing the earth's temperature to climb more rapidly than ever before in its history. The resultant man-induced depletion of the ozone layer (nature's protective "umbrella" shielding us from the harmful variety of sun rays) is likewise a great health hazard, a most plausible contributing factor in the alarmingly increasing rate of the various cancers killing people in the world today.

Although greenhouse gasses, at safe levels, are essential for life as we know it to keep our planet comfortably warm, abnormally high levels are far too dangerous for our planet. At the present, man's abuse of his environment has adversely affected many aspects of our life, including our means of subsistence, agriculture and aquaculture, to mention a couple.

Data from the National Oceanic and Atmospheric Administration and NASA "show that the earth's average surface temperature has increased by about 1.2 to 1.4 degrees Fahrenheit since 1900 . . . the warmest global average temperatures on record have all occurred within the past 15 years, with the warmest two years being 1998 and 2005." This indisputably means the human factor has contributed a lot to the causation of this dreadful and scary phenomenon.

Indeed, as guests on this planet we call home, we humans have not been ecology-conscious enough and environmentally friendly at all to Mother Earth. This has resulted in the gradual deterioration of our ecosystem.

What are the signs of a widespread and long-term trend toward global warming? The manifestations include unusually warmer weather and heat waves, glacier melting, Arctic and Antarctic warming, and ocean warming, rising sea level, and coastal flooding. Aren't the various volcanic eruptions, tsunamis, typhoons, and hurricanes, and evident weather changes enough hints for us?

If man does not do anything about this climate change soon, the resultant impact of this global warming, according to experts, will lead to the following "harbingers": diseases spreading more easily, spring arriving earlier, coral reef bleaching occurring, plant and animal range shifts and population changes taking place, downpours, heavy snowfalls, and giant tidal waves and flooding, droughts, and frequent fires.

While government initiatives by all nations around the globe are vital to the remedial solution to this potentially catastrophic dilemma that could make our world uninhabitable and wipe out civilization as we know it, our individual and concerted community behavioral modifications and proactive lifestyle changes could immensely help and positively impact on how much longer we can keep planet Earth a safe place to live in. The ball is in our court. Our fate is in our hands.

False Cancer Cures

A couple of years ago, an international vendor of herbal products denounced the United States Federal Trade Commission (FTC) for launching what it described as "a campaign of terror against companies selling natural cures for cancer."

This allegation was obviously worded to mislead and anger the consumers and pit them against the Federal Trade Commission. The FTC, like the US Food and Drug Administration (FDA), has the Congress-mandated obligation to protect the public from fraud and abuse. The FTC was simply doing its job of protecting the public by weeding out international and domestic manufacturers and traders who sell unproven products—herbs, pills, juices, potions, and lotions—they claim to be a cure for cancer.

Unfortunately, these "natural" or nonprescription products have not undergone the strict scientific tests and detailed scrutiny of the FDA. Every medical substance or drug used in the United States today has been exhaustibly tested in the laboratory and in clinical settings for its efficacy, safety, proper dosing, side effects, etc., before it gets the prestigious "security" stamp of approval by the FDA.

If these herbal products could really cure cancers as their vendors claim, then all cancers would have been eliminated from the surface of the earth and their manufacturers long awarded the Nobel Prize in Medicine. Unfortunately, nothing in their claims could be further from the truth today.

But the greater tragedy to the thousands of unsuspecting consumers is inflicted by manufacturers of herbal and "food supplement" by selling false hopes, victimizing cancer patients who are so desperate they would cling to anything, even to a knife, just to find a possible cure for the deadly malignancy that ails them. This act of greed is most cruel and unconscionable. Medical statistics have shown that all patients who resorted to these unproven alternative "cures for cancer" did not lose their fatal illnesses. All they lost were their lives and part of their savings. The anecdotal herbal treatment successes reported were nothing but cases of benign or nonmalignant conditions misdiagnosed (intentionally or otherwise) as cancers to begin with.

Today's great mind-boggling advances in medical diagnosis, therapeutics, and in science as a whole are indeed awesome. They provide promising opportunities for better health, more enjoyable life, and greater longevity. It behooves all of us to take full advantage of the wonders of modern medicine if we could and not succumb to charlatans' claims. In taking good care of our health and the only one life we possess, we have to be well-informed and wisely cautious and vigilant in protecting ourselves by adhering to what is scientific and proven, and to heed the sage advice, "Consumers beware."

"Please Help Me Die . . ."

This is one request every physician dreads to hear from a patient. No matter how hopelessly ill a person may be, even one dying from terminal cancer which has spread all over the body causing unabated pain and suffering, such a plea for mercy and final relief for the physician to prescribe higher dosage of intravenous pain killers and allow him/her to die with dignity nonetheless causes severe anguish and conflict on the part of the physician.

Trained to respect and save lives, not to kill, to adhere to the Oath of Hippocrates and its precept of "primum non nocere" (first, do no harm), and to alleviate pain and suffering, the physician in this situation faces a grave dilemma. As a scientist, he/she knows the hopeless nature of end-stage medical condition, that the quality of life at that point is dismal, and that the patient will only continue to languish in pain, with his loved ones suffering with him, day in and day out. Aware of these harsh realities and having compassion in his heart, the physician might be tempted to consider granting his patient's request. His final decision will certainly be dictated by his personal philosophy, moral conviction, medical standard of care, and the law of the land.

The most controversial issue of euthanasia, which has landed Dr. Jack Kevorkian (labeled Dr. Death) in jail for eight years and who died on June 3, 2011 at age 83, four years after his release, had been a subject of a recent survey among physicians in the United States.

Medscape Ethics Survey

"Doctors are sharply divided over the question of physician-assisted suicide," reports Wayne J. Guglielmo in the Medscape electronic

Exclusive Ethics Survey, covering August to September 2010, involving 10,000 US physicians of various specialties.

To the ethics question "Are there situations in which physician-assisted suicide should be allowed?" 45.8% responded affirmatively; 40.7% said, "No"; and 13.5% answered, "It depends."

Both ends of the spectrum of responses were quite direct, like stating, "Kill yourself, but don't involve me," and "I am a healer, not an executioner." The opposing group asked, "Did you ever watch a patient die a miserable death day by day?" and "We treat animals more kindly than people. This should be an absolute right of a terminally ill patient."

The report stated, "In between these two black and white extremes, physician respondents who are still uncertain about the issue expressed their continuing ambivalence in various shades of gray, a clear reflection of the competing ethical concerns they're struggling to balance."

One respondent stated: "As a physician, I do believe my job is only to keep a human being alive, but the quality of life is important as well." Another said: "I think there are times when it may be justifiable, but I don't think it should be legal." Another asked: "There is a thin line between 'comfort care' and 'physician-assisted suicide.' Who draws the line?"

Although debated for more than a century, the practice of euthanasia is still rare in the United States. Only 3 states legally permit physician-assisted suicide (referred to as Death With Dignity option): Montana permits it thru a trial court, and Washington and Oregon, through statutory law.

Fundamental Issue

This dilemma "not only raises fundamental questions about the nature of the profession itself but also about doctors' ethical obligations to their patients at the end of life," the report pointed out.

The survey revealed that "on one side, there are opponents of physician-assisted suicide who nevertheless draw a bright line between this practice and providing the palliative treatment necessary in order to alleviate a patient's pain, even if that treatment ends up suppressing respiration and hastening death . . . all agree that patient comfort is paramount."

The report further stated that in the United States today, "physicians who under treat pain sometimes place themselves in greater legal jeopardy than those who treat pain aggressively, even to the point of hastening a patient's death" among the terminally ill being given palliative care.

The law is clear-cut on the issue of "intent," even among those 3 states where physician-assisted suicide is concerned.

Distinction

"Palliative care and withdrawing life-sustaining support are legally and morally distinct from physician-assisted suicide," writer Guglielmo quoted Nancy Berlinger, PhD, deputy director and research scholar at the Hastings Center, an independent, nonprofit bioethics research institute in Garrison, New York. "While physician-assisted suicide is legal in only three states, palliative care is supported by a variety of measures in different states, where a legal and ethical consensus around its importance has formed," she emphasized.

According to the Pew poll, "Americans make a distinction between allowing a terminally ill patient to die and taking action to end someone's life." On the question of physician-assisted suicide, in fact, the 2006 poll found the public to be only slightly less divided on the question-46% in favor and 45% opposed—than the current Medscape survey shows physicians to be, Guglielmo writes. The 2010 Gallup Annual Values and Belief Survey confirms the public's ambivalence, noting a clear 46% to 46% split between those who find it "morally acceptable" and those who regard it as "morally wrong."

Proponents of physician-assisted suicide are questioning why abortion (which terminates the life of normal healthy fruit of conception) is allowed in several countries, while helping to end the life of a hopeless and suffering terminally ill person in great pains is illegal. They point out that in the name of love and compassion, it is universally accepted as humane to put animals, usually pets, to sleep when they are suffering and no longer have quality life; and yet the same society does not allow people to be similarly humane and compassionate and provide comfort to their loved ones under the same dire circumstances.

"Dying with dignity, in comfort and in peace, surrounded by loved ones is certainly a more charitable and more graceful alternative for the terminally ill constantly agonizing in severe pains, as the devastated family watch in tears," says a colleague.

Growing Old Is a Privilege

Quite often, people complain about growing old. They say they hate getting up there in age and living with the aches and pains of arthritis, diminished agility, and impaired vision, hearing, and memory.

The picture portrayed above is in general and invariably a description of what all of us, sooner or later, will face as we get nearer midlife and more so as we sail through the sunset of our life. As a cardiac surgeon, I feel that as long as one does not have a serious heart ailment or severely complicated illness like cancer, the changes our body and mind undergo as we grow older are as natural and "normal" as life itself. The cycle from birth to death is "predetermined," and none of us can escape it. In between those years, depending on our genes, and more so on our lifestyle, our health and longevity will vary accordingly.

In 1950-1955, global life expectancy at birth was estimated to be 46 years. This had risen to 65 in 2000-2005 and is supposed to reach 75 in 2045-2050. In well-developed countries, this rise in longevity is predicted to increase to 82 years by midcentury, while among less developed nations, where life expectancy is under 50 years today, the projection is 66 by 2045-2050.

In the United States, there are about 36 million who are 65 and older. By 2050, it will be about 87 million. One in 10,000 people live to be 100. In 2000, there were about an average of 75,000 centenarians, and this is expected to go up to 274,000 in 2025.

The life expectancy today of various races in the USA are as follows: Asian-American, 84.9; North Americans, 79; Middle America, 77.9; low-income whites in Appalachia, Mississippi Valley, 75; Black Middle Americans, 72.9; Western American Indians, 72.7; Southern low-income rural blacks, 71.2; and, high-risk urban blacks, 71.1 years. By state, Hawaii leads the nation with the longest life expectancy of 80 and Hawaiian women at 83.2. Minnesota follows at 78.8 and Utah at 78.7.

In Tomigusuku City, Japan, a report shows that in year 2000, women lived to 89.2 years and men, to about 82; and in Wara Village of Gifu Prefecture, men lived up to 80.6 years. Besides genetics as a factor, our diet, exercise, and lifestyle most significantly determine our quality of health and longevity.

With old age comes the signs and symptoms of normal wear and tear of any machine, and the human body is one machine that is no exception. As such, the immense tribulation that is inherent with growing old poses great limitations on the person physically, psychologically, and socially. How an individual copes with all these difficulties depends on the lifestyle he/she has lived and philosophical attitude in life. At 92, my mother still watches her diet and, about five years ago, replaced her decades old regimen of one-hour walking around the block with her daily home exercise, following the 2-mile aerobic exercise video *Walk by the Pound* by Leslie Samsone.

Alphonse Karr put it eloquently when he wrote, "Some people are always grumbling because roses have thorns; I am thankful that thorns have roses." Seeing only the donut hole and not the donut or a glass half full and not half empty, defines a person's point of view and outlook in life.

However challenging and oftentimes frustrating growing older might be, the blessing of a long and fairly healthy life is a privilege. While getting old is a problem, growing old is a blessing, in spite of all the aches and pains that come with the package. Life is tough and more especially so for the seniors. Growing old is, indeed, not for sissies or the faint of heart.

But let's be realistic and face it; we've got only one other option. That option is to stop aging. And the only way to achieve that alternative is to die young—not a palatable nor more attractive alternative, indeed. Since we cannot control and direct the winds in our voyage through this sometimes harsh ocean of life, we can at least, to quote a wise man, "adjust our sails" and find happiness and peace during our journey, wherever fate takes us.

Appreciate living life to the fullest with all our faculties and abilities to help ourselves. Enjoy laughing, sharing wisdom with our children and grandchildren. Strive to make a positive difference in our society. Savor smelling the flowers along the way and appreciating this magnificently wonderful world of ours (in spite of all man-induced imperfections and calamities). Experiencing the joys in life are, indeed, a sacred privilege. It is a blessing we should all look forward to with an upbeat frame of mind and one to be truly grateful. After all, not everyone is granted and blessed with this privilege.

So as we enjoy the youth of our life, let's lead a healthy lifestyle, show compassion for our less privileged fellow men, and set good examples for our children. As the years fly by, let us relish each day to the hilt, as if each day would be our last; and at the same time, let us pray for a life of good health, love, happiness, peace, and the privilege of growing old.

Diseases and Conditions

Acupuncture: A sticky issue

What is acupuncture?

Acupuncture is a Chinese method of encouraging the body to promote natural healing and improve bodily function by inserting super fine needles into precise acupuncture points in the body and/or applying heat or electrical stimulation at these specific points.

How old is this modality?

Acupuncture has been practiced for over 5,000 years. However, the first record of acupuncture was found in the 4,700 year-old *Huang Di Nei Jing (Yellow Emperor's Classic of Internal Medicine)*, which is considered the oldest medical textbook in the world. Acupuncture is said to have been theorized even earlier by Shen Nung, the father of Chinese medicine, who also documented his theories on the heart, circulation, and pulse over 400 years before Europeans had any concept about them.

What is the basis for acupuncture?

The popular classical Chinese explanation on how acupuncture works states that channels of energy run in regular patterns through our body and over its surface. This energy force is known as Qi (pronounced chee). The channels through which the energy flows are called Meridians, which are compared to rivers flowing to the body to irrigate and nourish the tissues. Blood flow and nerve impulses also follow Meridians. An obstruction to the movement of this energy leads to a backup in the flow (like a dam) to one part of the body and restricts it in others, eventually causing disease. The Meridians can be influenced by needling the acupuncture points to unblock the obstruction and reestablish the regular normal flow pattern.

What is the modern explanation for its action?

There are two major concepts in modern science which attempt to explain how acupuncture works: (1) Needling the acupuncture points stimulates the nervous system to release chemicals in the muscles, spinal cord, and brain. These natural chemicals will either alter the experience of pain or trigger the excretion of other hormones or chemicals in the body that will lead to internal auto-regulation; and (2) In Traditional Chinese Medicine (TCM), *yin* represents "-" (negative) and *yang* represents "+" (positive). The main principle is to keep the *yin* and the *yang* balance or bring the *yin and yang* back to the normal balance. *Yin-yang* balance is the healthy state of the body. When the positive and negative charges in the bio-electrons are not balanced, disease occurs. Acupuncture is claimed to be able to force the bio-electrons to resume their normal movement patterns and balance.

What are the other related acupuncture procedures?

Electro-acupuncture is administered through acupuncture needles, using very small electrical impulses, and generally for analgesia (pain control). The power used is only a few microamperes, but the frequency of the current varies from 5 to 2000 Hz. Other methods to stimulate acupuncture points are now being used, like laser and sonogram (sound waves). Another is moxibustion, a treatment using heat applied to acupuncture points. Cupping is another form, where suction from a jar made of metal, wood, or glass (where partial vacuum has been created) is used to stimulate acupuncture points. One of the most popular is acupressure, where no needles are used.

What are the effects of acupuncture?

No definite scientific proofs are available, but claims have been made that some of the good effects of acupuncture are raising the level of hormones, prostaglandins, white blood counts, gamma globulins, opsonins, and overall improvement in the body's immune system; stimulating the secretion of endomorphins (enkephalins) which alleviate aches and pains; affecting the neurotransmitters (serotonins and noradrenalins); closing the "motor gate" through which pains passes so pain is halted and is not felt.

Does acupuncture cure any disease?

While acupuncture has been known to relieve aches and pains from injuries or arthritis, there are no convincing medical studies to prove that organic diseases have been cured by acupuncture. Migraine headaches, anxiety and other psychological disorders, smoking or alcohol addiction, and low-back aches are some conditions where acupuncture appears to be effective in some cases. Cancer, obviously, cannot be cured by acupuncture; but the myth persists.

Can acupuncture substitute for general anesthesia?

There have been anecdotal reports that abdominal and chest surgeries have been done under acupuncture with the patients awake and talking. Again, there are no documented evidences that these are true. The proponents reported the first successful use of electroacupuncture in 1958 in China for tonsillectomy. Analgesia (pain control) seems to be the most popular action of acupuncture, where it is effective to a certain extent for certain people. I tried acupuncture for my tennis elbow about 30 years ago. Insertion of the hairlike acupuncture needles was practically painless except for mild stinging sensation. I did not obtain any relief. A friend of mine who had it done that same day said he did.

How can acupuncture hurt people?

When sick people become fanatical about acupuncture or about any other nonconventional form of medical treatment, resulting in the delay in diagnosis and treatment of their illness by a physician, the situation can lead to unnecessary increase in the risk, complications, and mortality. Some preventable deaths due to delayed diagnosis and treatment have been reported among patients who had rejected modern medicine in favor of acupuncture and alternative herbal drugs in the treatment of their ailments.

Cutting-edge medical technology is here. Let us allow the proven advances to help us prevent or treat diseases and maintain good health.

Does your child have ADHD?

What is ADHD?

Once called hyperkinesis or ADD (attention deficit disorder), ADHD (attention deficit hyperactivity disorder) is now the preferred name for a behavioral disorder that is noted in early childhood. Adults could have this same condition too.

When was this syndrome discovered?

Information from the US National Institute of Mental Health reveals ADHD was first described by Dr. Heinrich Hoffman in 1845, a physician who wrote books on medicine and psychiatry. He also wrote stories and poems for his 3-year-old when he could not find suitable materials for children. One of these books was titled *The Story of Fidgety Philip*, an accurate description of a little boy with ADHD. Fifty-seven years later, in 1902, Sir George F. Still presented to the Royal College of Physicians in England a series of lectures on this genetic dysfunction we now call ADHD.

How prevalent is this condition?

In the United States, between 3 and 5 percent of children or about 2 million have ADHD. In a classroom of 25 to 30 children, at least one will have this behavioral syndrome, which becomes obvious in the preschool and early years in school. ADHD often continues to adulthood, and if not treated, may cause insurmountable problems leading to failure to succeed or achieve the full potential of the individual. About 25% of close relatives in the families of ADHD children also have ADHD.

What causes ADHD?

Neurobiology and genetics play a major role. Environmental agents like alcohol and/or cigarettes use by the mother (during pregnancy) or by both parents as the baby grows up play a vital role. Lead exposure (as among those who live in old buildings), food additives, and sugars have also been implicated.

What are the types of ADHD?

Basically three types are recognized: hyperactive-impulsive (does not show significant inattention), inattentive (does not show significant hyperactive-impulsive behavior), and the combination (with all the principal characteristics). ADHD could also be accompanied by other disorders, such as learning disabilities, oppositional defiant disorder, conduct disorder, anxiety and depression, bipolar disorder (cyclic mood: intense highs and lows), and Tourette syndrome (nervous tics and repetitive mannerisms like eye blinks, facial twitches, and grimacing).

What are the signs of ADHD?

Children afflicted with ADHD are hyperactive, inattentive, impulsive, restless, unable to focus on a project or complete tasks, and may even be disruptive. They have learning disabilities as a result of ADHD. Many of these kids are very capable and intelligent and excel in some activities but having inordinately great problems with others. If untreated, these children become victims of the social and academic consequences of ADHD. Early diagnosis and therapy (before adolescence) greatly improve their chances of "recovery and cure."

What is hyperactivity?

Besides being inattentive, the children with ADHD are restless, anxious, and keep on moving, unable to sit still, and talk a lot continuously. They tap their feet, bouncing from one activity to the other, unable to control their talking while the class is going on, even if told to keep quiet. They possess a ball of inexhaustible energy. Their mind drifts, and they are unable to finish what they are doing; and if they do, there are a lot of mistakes. They get bored easily and cannot concentrate on what they are doing. But if they love television shows, they are able to focus well and learn from them.

How about impulsivity?

These are inappropriate or thoughtless actions and reactions. These children usually act without thinking of the consequences of what they do. Example is when the ADHD child dashes across the busy street without even looking at the oncoming cars. The impulsive action just suddenly happens for no reason. The child may just shout out things any time or takes something without asking or goes ahead without waiting for his/her turn. These behaviors make other kids shy away from them.

Is the eye problem related?

Doctors have found an interesting link between an eye problem and ADHD. The condition is called convergence insufficiency, the inability of the eyes to focus at close range, which could affect mental focus. While not very common, this has been found in some children with attention deficit hyperactivity disorder and an indication for consultation with an ophthalmologist.

How is ADHD diagnosed?

Simply because one child or person has hyperactivity, inattentiveness, and impulsiveness does not mean it is really ADHD. Some of us show one or all of these behaviors at one time or another. When any of these three signs are inappropriate for the person's age, occur repeatedly, and create a real handicap in at least two areas of the person's life such as in school, at playground, home, in social activities, or in the community. Therefore, someone who exhibits one or more of these three signs, but who is successful in school at work, and in social relationships, does not have ADHD.

What is the treatment for ADHD?

Besides counseling, medications may be needed to manage ADHD. There are stimulant drugs, like ritalin, and more than a dozen others that have been used with good results; but there are drugs that are not stimulants which are now available. They work on the neurotransmitter norepinephrine. The stimulants work on dopamine. More clinical studies are underway, but the evidence to date shows that the new drugs are superior, with more than 70% of children with ADHD showing significant improvement from their symptoms.

Will the children "outgrow" ADHD?

In general, without prompt treatment, no. The earlier the diagnosis is confirmed and the condition is treated, the better for the child. Most of these children are intelligent, smart and skillful, and full of potential. Some of them may even be geniuses. The worst thing parents can do is to reprimand and castigate these children who are "ill with ADHD" and not at fault to begin with. This blind parental reaction will only add insult to injury, and the helpless and unfortunate victim is the pitiful child, who will grow up socially unfit, full of failures and misery. If you suspect your child to have ADHD, promptly consult your family doctor or pediatrician.

Aging and Cholesterol

Why do we age?

Aging is a natural process brought on by the daily wear and tear in our system and bodily function. Each particular species has a maximum life span, determined by our DNA, among others. However, environmental factors do greatly influence the actual longevity, especially among us humans, who are well-known to abuse ourselves.

Medical literature and the Bible have documented man attaining the age of 150 or older. With the advent of modern civilization and the self-abusive lifestyle *Homo sapiens* have developed, man's life span, in spite of today's great advances in medical technology, has been greatly shortened.

While it is naturally possible to stay young longer and maximize our longevity, we humans seem to have placed a lot of barriers (risk factors) ourselves to preclude that natural potential of staying young longer and living to the "ripe old age" of, say, 150 or 180 from happening. These risk factors include high-cholesterol diet, smoking, alcohol excess, sedentary lifestyle, and obesity, etc.

Are we really as old as our arteries?

Yes, we are. If we keep our arteries young, we will look, feel, and remain young longer. Our skin, flesh, tendons, bones, and all other organs and tissues in our body are supplied by arteries that provide the necessary oxygen and nutrition to every cell and tissue of our body. If these arteries are clogged by cholesterol deposits, these tissues and organs (including our skin) receive much less oxygen and nutrition and age much faster. As a result, the elasticity of the skin, for example, is reduced and the skin starts to loosen and sag, wrinkles form, and its youthful appearance disappears. If you look at your friends or relatives, you will observe that those who take good care of their health (and therefore, their arteries) look healthier, much younger, and more active than those who do not.

What is cholesterol?

Cholesterol is a sterol, a complex alcohol constituent of animal fats and oils. This is the substance that forms the plaques which adheres to the inner wall of arteries causing hardening of the arteries and stenoses (blockages), many leading to heart attacks, strokes, or poor leg circulation.

Is there such a thing as "good" cholesterol?

Yes, it is called high-density lipoprotein (HDL), and the bad cholesterol is called the low-density lipoprotein (LDL). For better health, a person should have a high level of the HDL and low level of LDL. These two triglycerides or lipids are important risk variables, hence their serum (blood) levels are also checked, together with total serum cholesterol level.

Where does our body get cholesterol from?

While our liver produces (endogenous) cholesterol, the main source of (exogenous) cholesterol in our body and the blood is from the food we eat. Food that are high in cholesterol include: egg yolk, pork, beef (and other red meats), butter, lard, and other dairy products.

Does milk contain cholesterol?

Yes, but the 2% milk, skim milk, or reduced cholesterol milk have been reconstituted to attain the reduction in cholesterol in them and marketed as such. For young children, skim milk is not recommended, unless they are hyperlipidemic (with high triglyceride level, especially the LDL). Two percent milk is acceptable, but not lower.

How much fat is in our usual diet?

The average US diet contains about 37% total calories as fat Even 37% is too high, and the American Heart Association recommends that this needs to be reduced to 10% to have a major effect in heart attack, stroke, and cancer prevention.

What are the types of dietary fats?

There are three kinds: saturated, monosaturated, and polyunsaturated. Sources of saturated fats are meat, nonskim dairy products, artificially hydrogenated vegetable oils. Monosaturated fats are found in olive oil and canola oil. Polyunsaturated fats are from omega-3 (sea plankton, deep-sea cold-water fatty fish, like salmon, tuna, mackerel), and from omega-6 oils in cultivated vegetable oils (like corn oil).

Is pork white meat?

No, pork is red meat, just like beef is red meat. Both are high in cholesterol and fats. Obviously aimed at confusing the public to promote pork, an old television ad in the United States, featuring actor Robert Mitchum as its spokesman, said "Pork, the other white meat." This is a misrepresentation and a great public disservice.

How about chicken meat?

Chicken breast is white meat, lower in cholesterol compared to pork or beef, but chicken skin is very high in cholesterol. The dark chicken meat (neck, wings, back, legs) is slightly higher in cholesterol compared the breast portion.

Why does the fatty portion of any meat taste good?

The part of the meat that is loaded with fat taste better because the taste of food is in the cholesterol content of the food. If cholesterol is totally removed from beef or pork, these meats will taste like rope fibers . . . flat and tasteless. The higher the cholesterol content of the food, the better it tastes, but the worse it is for our health.

Does fish meat have fats?

It does, but the fat in fish is the good kind, one that is healthy for the heart and blood vessels. They are called Omega-3 oils. Regularly eating only fish (not together with pork, beef, eggs, butter, etc.) has been scientifically shown to lower the incidence or risk of cardiovascular diseases, sudden cardiac death, and even cancer. These oils (eicosapentaenoic acid and decosahexaenoic acid) have also been shown to lower serum triglycerides and "bad cholesterols" and makes blood thinner and less prone to clot, and therefore slows down hardening of the artery.

What is the normal level of serum cholesterol?

The National Cholesterol Education Program (NCEP) defines the normal total cholesterol level as levels less than 200 mg/dL or 5.18 mmol/L. However, new medical studies have shown that this current "normal level" is still too high to be effective in lowering the risk of heart attacks and strokes. The predominant new concept today for desirable level is about 150-160 mg/dL. The level of triglycerides (normal: less than 150 mg/dL) is also very important, if not more, in the maintenance of cardiovascular health. It is wise to have a screening and baseline cholesterol and triglyceride blood tests.

How does one lower his/her cholesterol level?

The initial step, which is quite successful in majority of people, is by not eating red meats or meat products made of pork or beef, non-skim dairy products, eggs (the yolk of which is in itself very high in cholesterol). The diet should consist of fish, vegetables, white chicken meat (no skin), grains, and nuts, and fruits. Indulging a bit in red meats during the holidays is acceptable, except among those whose cholesterol and LDL are very high and the HDL is very low.

If this recommended diet regimen is followed religiously, chances are the cholesterol and triglyceride levels will come down to the desired levels. Medications to lower the cholesterol and triglyceride levels are reserved for those where weeks of strict fish, vegetable, and fruit diet has failed.

Only one out of 500 of these persons has a genetic predisposition to having familial high cholesterol level. While that single individual has an excuse to have elevated serum cholesterol, the 499 of us do not. We simply abuse ourselves to death. There are various medications available today to lower serum cholesterol. Your physician will be a most beneficial partner in planning an effective strategy for you. Equally important, daily regimented physical exercise will go a long way in helping lower the total cholesterol, the bad cholesterol (LDL) and the triglycerides. It also boosts the good cholesterol (HDL). Exercise benefits us in more ways than one.

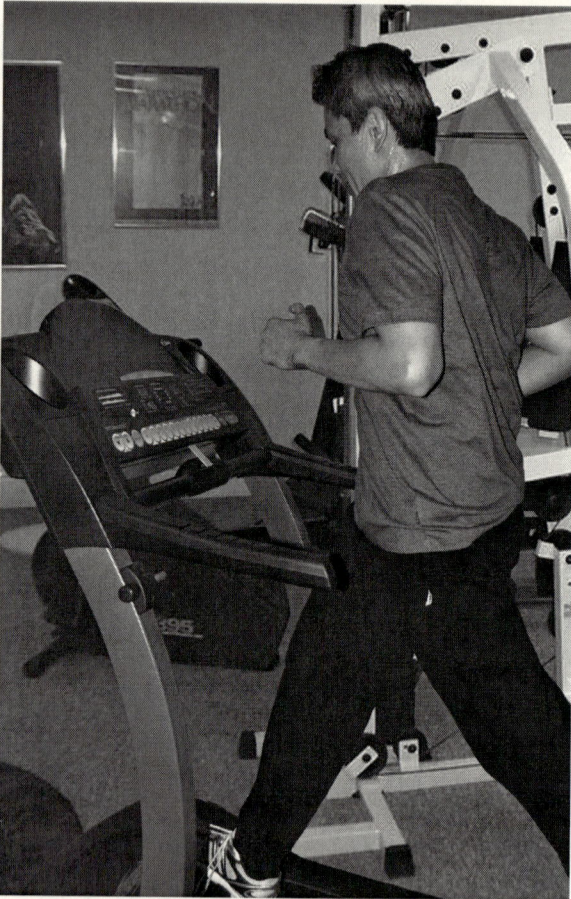

Regular physical exercises for 30 minutes, at least 5 days a week, either using the treadmill, or simple brisk walking, dancing, swimming, tai bo aerobics, provide great health benefits. Exercise boosts immunity, lowers the risk for metabolic diseases like diabetes, osteoporosis, improves cardiovascular health and sexual function. This activity also helps strengthen muscles and balance, and improves neurological and psychological well-being. A bonus: exercise also reduces the cancer risk.

Can aging be delayed?

Why do we age?

Just like machines and engines, our body ages because of the cumulative damages to our cells, tissues, and organs (resulting from daily "wear and tear" and the self-abuse humans are well known for) that exceed our body's ability to repair them. These damages lead to obvious signs of aging: sags, bulges and wrinkles, gray hair, loss of muscle and bone and nerve integrity, impairment of hearing and vision, incompetence of various sphincters (bladder and anal, etc.), lowered immunity and resistance, and increased susceptibility to diseases and infections. The arteries all over the body undergo severe arteriosclerosis (hardening) which leads to circulatory deficits in various organs (brain, heart, glands, legs, etc.) causing stroke, heart attack, reduced libido, and other hormonal deficits.

Can we delay or reverse the aging process?

There have been so many claims made, especially by unscrupulous manufacturers and distributors of "food supplements," that their products can delay or reverse aging and make people 5, 10, or more years younger. There is nothing farther from the truth. Unfortunately, although we are all looking for that "fountain of youth," medical science still has nothing to offer us in this department. Fifty-one top scientists in the world recently refute claims of this "miracle treatment" ad advertised all over the globe and warn the public against this fraud. All the infomercials currently flooding the market and media are bunk, aimed at deceiving the unsuspecting public for a fast buck.

What is the danger of trying some "anti-aging" drugs?

Some of these drugs have adverse side effects that could lead to illnesses. Some may not have bad effects but are simply worthless, useless, ineffective in what they are purported to do. Taking them is like taking an empty capsule or a capsule filled with sugar powder. And they are invariably very expensive. So, if you do not wish to give away your hard-earned money, it is best to stay away from these fraudulent vendors.

How about herbal anti-aging medications?

The same is true with herbs and "natural products" being marketed out there as anti-aging drugs. They are worthless. I would like to underscore the fact that to date, there is nothing, absolutely nothing, that will slow down or reverse the aging process. Simply modifying your lifestyle to a healthier one, which will not entail added expenses (and in many instances even save you money), can make you look and feel younger, safely and wisely.

When is growth hormone used?

Growth hormones are medically prescribed as a part of the treatment regimen for some growth disorders in children. These hormones can "stimulate" the growth of tumors in the body. Additional bad side effects include excess bone growth, kidney problems, diabetes, carpal tunnel syndrome, lung and heart failure, and possible premature death.

Do antioxidants have anti-aging effect?

Unfortunately, they do not. Antioxidants, like vitamin C, E, and A (beta-carotene), are widely advertised to reverse aging and prolong life. Scientists are astounded and angry about this claim by manufacturers and vendors of these and other "food supplement" products, because the claim is unfounded and medically baseless. However, scientists the world over recognize that anti-oxidant-rich foods such as vegetables, nuts, whole grains, and fruits may reduce the risk of illnesses like heart disease, cataracts and macular degeneration, and cancer, and somewhat reduce bodily damages from aging. Megadoses of vitamin E and selenium can cause bleeding that could be fatal, and that of beta-carotene may increase the risk of cancer. Beware: some food supplements on the market may have serious, sometimes even life-threatening, side effects.

How then can we "stay and feel" young?

The process and effects of aging are faster in some individuals, slower in others. To some extent, the changes are within our control. While there is nothing to reverse the aging process, there are things we can do to protect our body, minimize natural wear and tear, and make us feel and look "younger." Putting an end to self-abuse, eating healthy, exercising daily, and the prudent use of protective cosmetic products to ensure proper hygiene and facial skin moisture tones not only our sagging dermal state but our mental and spiritual state as well. In addition, once-a-day multivitamins and minerals plus whatever prescription drugs needed will certainly help us live a healthier life. Taking delicate care of our body by living a healthier lifestyle will most assuredly make us look and feel younger and better.

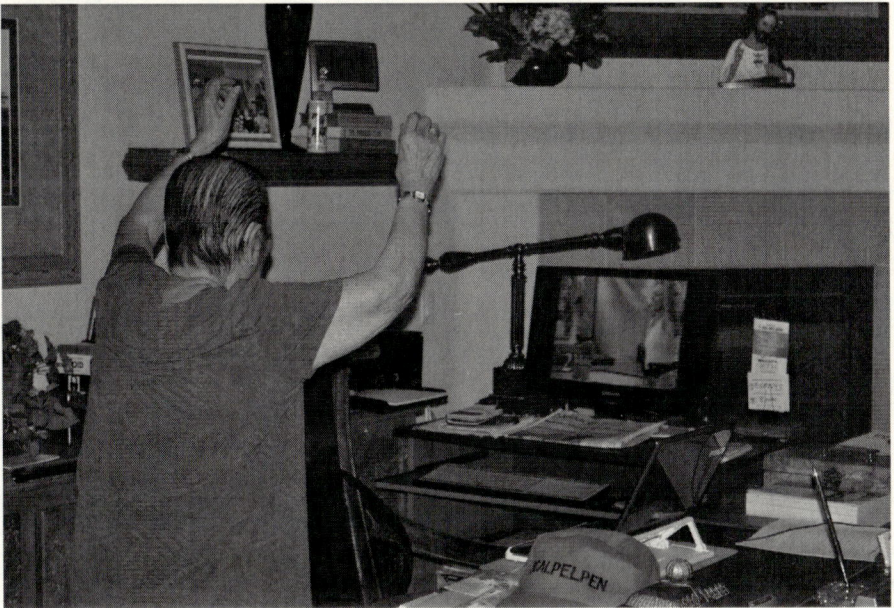

Excerise has no age limit, as shown by this nanogenarian, who is doing video aerobics, using the Leslie Sansone exercise DVD. This activity can be done practically anywhere, even in a small area. Like tai bo, this aerobic exercise can also be performed without the video.

AIDS: A Death Sentence

What is AIDS and what is HIV?

AIDS stands for acquired immune deficiency syndrome and HIV means human immunodeficiency virus, the agent responsible for the disease.

How does the virus cause the disease?

HIV attacks the immune system of the infected person and destroys the CD4 cells (the "generals" in our immune system army), rendering the body's "security force," without its "commanders," weak and defenseless to fight off infections. When the immune system breaks down, opportunistic infections set in, and the person develops serious and deadly infections and cancers. It is not correct to say that someone "died of AIDS," since it is really the infections that cause death.

Can one get AIDS from "contaminated" toilet seats?

No. HIV is a fragile virus that cannot survive outside of the body. Blaming the poor toilet seat is an old wives' tale.

How is AIDS transmitted?

The virus can be transmitted through the following body fluids: blood, pre-ejaculate fluid, semen, vaginal secretions and breast milk. There is no evidence that HIV is transmitted through sweat, tears, urine, or saliva, since the concentration in these body fluids is so small. However, if, say the saliva is contaminated with blood from bleeding gums or a cut in the mouth of an AIDS patient, that saliva can transmit HIV. Kissing, in this situation, is risky.

Can HIV enter the skin?

No, the virus cannot penetrate the skin, unless the skin is cut or broken, in which case transmission becomes possible. Shaking hands with an infected person is safe. The virus cannot be transmitted through the air by sneezing or coughing either. These are the reasons why casual contact with people with HIV infection is absolutely not dangerous. The widespread misinformation and ignorance have led to unnecessary fear in people's mind and the added emotional suffering on the part of victims of AIDS.

How does HIV enter the body?

The virus enters the bloodstream through mucous membranes, like the lining of the rectum, the walls of the vagina, the urethra (passage channel of the penis), nose, mouth, and throat, or by intravenous transfusion of any infected fluid, like blood, plasma, etc., or use of a contaminated needle. The virus must get into the bloodstream to cause AIDS.

Can one get HIV through oral sex?

Most definitely, especially the person giving the oral sex, since she/he is exposed to pre-ejaculate fluid, semen, or vaginal secretions and menstrual blood. If there is dental carries, open sores, cut or abrasions in the mouth or gums, the virus can enter the bloodstream even faster. While the risk in vaginal or anal sex and in giving oral sex is higher than that of receiving oral sex, the latter form of contact is likewise risky and could be as deadly.

Could "finger-sex" cause AIDS?

Just as we have stated above, the HIV cannot penetrate the skin, unless there is a cut or an abrasion. While medical statistics show that this is true, it is obviously prudent, as dictated by common sense alone, that this practice too should be discouraged when dealing with an HIV carrier or a partner with AIDS.

Can a woman transmit HIV to the baby in her womb?

Yes, maternal to fetal transmission is obviously the rule since their individual blood circulation is "connected" with each other.

Does bleach kill the HIV?

Yes, Clorox (bleach), with high concentration of chlorine, kills HIV. This is what "smart" or experienced drug addicts use to "sterilize" their needles and other paraphernalia used in "pushing" narcotics and other illegal drugs. However, there is no guarantee that this practice is 100% effective, since the sterilization technique used could be flawed.

Are condoms effective?

The use of latex condoms has been proven to be effective in the prevention of HIV infection in only about 85% of users. Condoms are known to develop holes or tears during warehousing, transport, rough handling or during the actual sex act, which will then allow HIV transmission. The best practice is not to have sex with someone who could be exposed to HIV or other (STD) sexually transmitted diseases. Those with multiple partners have been shown to be at a greater risk, compared to partners who are both monogamous.

How soon does HIV infection lead to AIDS?

A blood test that is negative for HIV does not guarantee the person exposed to HIV that he/she will not develop AIDS. As a rule, it can take five to seven years or longer (after exposure) before people infected with HIV develop AIDS. This is the reason why everyone must be extra cautious, because AIDS today is indeed a death sentence, one that is preceded by a horrible stage of existence, humiliation, pain, and suffering.

Air Travel: Medical Tips

What common problems do air travelers encounter?

Changes in barometric pressure, decreased oxygen tension, circadian dysrhythmia, psychological stress, and effects of air turbulence are the major problems associated with air traveler.

How is comfort preserved during flight?

Modern aircrafts, including supersonics, maintain a cabin pressure that is equivalent to 5,000 to 8,000 feet above sea level to provide a comfort environment for the people onboard. At such an altitude, free air in the body cavities tends to expand by about 25% and may aggravate certain medical conditions. Most persons with adequately treated chronic illnesses—like high blood pressure, diabetes, or heart conditions that are not severe—can safely tolerate flying, even international flights. However, those with anemia (low blood count), asthma, emphysema, and those already short of breath from other lung problems or heart failure may not be able to tolerate the high altitudes. It is always prudent to check with your physician if you have any concerns about flying

Why do some people get airsickness?

Some people are born with vestibular-labyrinthine apparatus (inner ear structure that helps us balance ourselves) that is very sensitive to motion, more so than average. Stimulation of this apparatus in these people by acceleration and deceleration, or by upward, downward, or swinging movements, cause dizziness or nausea and/or vomiting, which is commonly known as motion sickness, seasickness, airsickness, etc. Oral medications are available for travelers to minimize or prevent motion sickness, seasickness, or airsickness.

What can be done to minimize airsickness?

The night before the trip, have a quiet evening and avoid alcohol and spicy foods, including the morning of the air travel. Wear loose and comfortable clothing for air travel. During flight, eat light and minimize drinking alcoholic beverages, avoid excessive coffee and tea, but ingest about a glass (8 oz) of water for every two hours of the trip to prevent dehydration and its side effects. If nausea occurs, recline your seat, close your eyes, try to relax, and keep your head motionless. If it persists, antiemetic (antinausea/antivomiting) medication may be needed. Some flights have this drug available onboard.

Does biofeedback help?

Yes, biofeedback helps relieve stress and many flight discomforts. While seating back, relaxing your whole body with the eyes closed, think and concentrate hard that your are on a tropical beach, enjoying the white sand and clear sky-blue waters. Breathe normally, nice and easy, punctuated by a deep sigh every now and then. Let your arms and legs and the rest of your body go limp. Meditate, daydream, think good and happy thoughts. This strategy has been found to be very effective, especially on long flights.

Why do young children cry during takeoff and landing?

The changes in the altitude and barometric air pressure during takeoff and landing cause temporary blockage of the Eustachian tube (small channel that connects the nasal passages and the middle ear), and this results in a buildup of pressure that leads to severe pains in the ear, in the head, and/or in the face (sinuses). To relieve the pressure (discomfort of blocked ears), one must swallow with the nose closed or do frequent yawning during takeoff and landing. Filling the mouth with air and blowing hard, with mouth closed and the nose pinched (Valsalva maneuver) may help "pop open" the blocked ears. Babies and young children should be made to suck, drink, or swallow liquid when the plane starts its ascent or decent. For adults and older children, chewing gum or merely swallowing their saliva during takeoff and landing will help prevent the occurrence of the excruciating earaches and/or headaches.

Why the bloating sensation?

The changes in cabin pressure increase the gas production in our guts. As the pressure falls, the air in the intestines expands, causing bloating and discomfort for some people on long flights. Abstinence from alcohol, or drinking in moderation, and eating light, especially on international flights, can minimize or prevent problems during flights and make air travel more enjoyable.

Are upper respiratory infections aggravated by air flights?

Yes, because upper respiratory tract infection and even allergy may obstruct the Eustachian tube, resulting in barotits media (inflammation of middle ear from the increased pressure during flight) or barosinusitis (inflammation of the sinuses in our face around our nose). This is why closed-nose swallowing, frequent yawning, or decongestant nasal spray or antihistamines that reduce clogged nasal passages are helpful in relieving the increased pressure in our middle ear and sinuses during takeoff and landing.

Are patients with a history of collapsed lungs allowed to fly?

People with a history of collapsed lungs (pneumothorax) more than once and not operated on are not allowed to fly because it may recur. If this should happen, especially at high altitudes, the shortness of breath that follows collapse of the lungs will be worse and aggravated to the point that the person might die of suffocation. Those with this condition should undergo a major but fairly simple operation to cut out the portion of the lung that is weak (with very thin wall that balloons out like bubbles) and leaking. Those whose pneumothorax has been corrected by surgery are allowed to fly, but not to pilot a plane.

Are pregnant women allowed to fly?

It is safe for pregnant women to fly on commercial airlines. However, most airlines do not accept passengers who are more than 35 weeks pregnant for obvious safety reasons. Those concerned should check with their airline or immigration office at the country of destination about entry regulations.

Is it safe for heart or lung patients, or diabetics, to fly?

Today's commercial planes are pressurized and generally safe for cardiac, pulmonary, or diabetic patients. Heart patients who are able to climb two flights of stairs (a dozen steps) without chest pains or any difficulty, stable asthmatics or emphysematous patients who can walk a 150-foot distance without breathing problems, controlled diabetics, and high-blood-pressure patients can fly safely. It is strongly recommended that patients carry with them in person their medications. If in doubt, consult your physician.

Why is alcohol bad during flights?

Prudent, moderate consumption of alcohol is generally tolerated by most people on board. Alcohol, just like smoking, increases body fatigue, hypoxia (lowering the oxygen level in our blood), and dehydration. Fatigue and hypoxia, which naturally occur during long flights, explain why some people "do not feel well" following the air travel. Alcohol and/or smoking aggravate these two conditions, together with the severity of circadian dysrhythmia (jet lag).

How does one minimize jetlag and be comfortable on long flights?

Jet lag is a natural physiologic response of the body to traveling to a different time zone, before the individual is able to adjust to a new night/day cycle. During long flights, like international travel, it is best strategy to adjust your sleep cycle starting a couple of days before departure. Avoid eating a heavy meal before a flight. During the flight, eat light, drink a lot of fluids like fruit juices or water (not alcohol or coffee), get up, and walk often and do light aerobic exercise in your seat every couple of hours or so, like foot pumps, ankle circles, knee lifts, neck roll, knee to chest, shoulder roll, and forward body flex exercise. Get enough timely sleep. A mild sleeping pill prescribed by your physician might help in timing your sleep cycle in anticipation of the time zone change in your place of destination.

Melatonin tablets have been effective in reducing jet lag in some people, but reports of possible side effects on the rhythm of the heart on some people have discouraged some physicians from prescribing melatonin. Some people take aspirin or other pain pills to minimize muscle aches and pains. Aspirin also thins the blood and useful during flight to prevent blood clots in the legs due to prolonged sitting. These clots could travel to the lungs and cause serious problems, sometimes fatal. Consult your physician before taking aspirin or any other drugs. The use of lip, facial, and skin moisturizers will also add to your comfort during flight. On arrival, rest for a couple of days and limit your commitments during this first day or so to minimize jet lag and to allow your system to adjust.

Allergies

What is an allergy?

An allergy is a condition where the body overreacts following "contact" with an allergen (dust, molds, pollen, flower, dander, fur, animal protein from hair, perfume, cosmetics, medications applied to skin or swallowed, food, like peanuts, MSG, or drink, etc.). Symptoms could be as trivial as sneezing, rash, or as serious as sudden inability to breathe, shock, and death in severe cases.

What is the incidence of allergies?

About 10% of people have some form of allergies or another. Luckily, most of the allergies people have are mild. If repeated exposures to the same allergen, at the same high dose, are allowed to occur, the symptoms could become more severe.

What triggers the symptoms?

Allergic reaction is triggered and symptoms develop when the body's immune system detects the presence of an allergen. This automatic protective response is aimed at warding off any adverse effects of the "culprit substance" on the body by producing antibodies and mobilizing the "immune soldiers into the battlefield to fight the invading foreign" substance. This is a natural part of the defense mechanism of our body.

What are the symptoms of allergies?

From the mild symptoms to the life-threatening ones, they could be one or a combination of the following: sneezing, nasal congestion, runny nose, red, itchy watery eyes, skin rashes or hives, stomach cramps, nausea, vomiting, tachycardia (fast heartbeat), dyspnea (difficulty breathing), wheezing, hypotension (drop in blood pressure), cardiac arrest (stoppage of heartbeat), and death. While the last three situations are not common, they are nonetheless very significant and still far too many, especially because these are preventable disasters.

Have there been deaths from exposure to animal hair?

Yes, and two such sad and tragic deaths happened to friends of mine—my friend's son and another friend's daughter (both in their twenties), who died within an hour after exposure to horses in a barn.

How about fatal allergy to MSG?

A classmate of mine, a chest surgeon from California, was attending a meeting in Nice, France, a several years ago, when he and his wife decided to eat at a Chinese restaurant after a week of French cuisine. In spite of their instruction to the waiter to make sure the chef would not add MSG (monosodium glutamate, a flavor enhancer) to the food they ordered because he was allergic to it, evidently MSG was used anyway. After ingesting a mouthful, my friend became very short of breath, collapsed, and died from anaphylactic shock within an hour later.

What is anaphylactic shock?

This is a violent allergic reaction, which results in massive swelling and rapid closure of the air passages, precipitous drop in blood pressure, and death by suffocation. In some cases, bee stings have caused anaphylactic shock.

How common is food allergy?

Medical reports have shown that about 2% of adults and about 8% of children have true food allergies. Food allergy is not the same as food intolerance (like stomach aches following ingestion of milk for those with deficiency of lactase, the enzyme that digests lactose in milk and milk products). Food intolerance is due to body metabolism and does not involve the immune system. Some people are allergic to shellfish, peanuts, and a few to chicken. Cow's milk, nuts, soy, wheat, and eggs are common cause of allergies in children. In some cases, children outgrow their allergies, but early peanut allergy can be for life.

What are the signs of an allergic reaction?

Sneezing, skin rashes or hives, runny nose, swelling of the lips or tongue, stomach cramps, vomiting and diarrhea, difficulty in breathing, wheezing, and in more severe cases, anaphylactic shock as described above.

How about allergies to food additives?

Adverse allergic reactions to some food additives have been reported. Among some of them are aspartame (as in Equal, a sweetener), MSG, FD&C Yellow No. 5 (a food color also known as tartrazine), and sulfites (sulfur-based preservatives). Following controlled studies in aspartame, the FDA determined it is not an allergen and that aspartame is safe. Pregnant women with high level of phenylalanine in the blood, some people with a genetic disease called PKU (phenylketonuria), and those with advance liver disease have a problem with aspartame because these people do not metabolize the amino acid called phenylalanine, which is a component of aspartame. High levels of phenylalanine in the body can cause brain damage.

Are sulfite preservatives allergens?

Yes, sulfites, which are antioxidants used to prevent or reduce discoloration of light-colored fruits and vegetables and also to inhibit the growth of bacteria in fermented foods, like wine, are allergens. Although majority of people do not have problems with sulfites, those sensitive to them, especially those with asthma, can develop mild to life-threatening symptoms.

Does maternal smoking cause allergies in children?

Cigarette smoking during pregnancy has been shown to increase the incidence of allergies among the newborns. Rarely, specific allergies can be "inherited" from the parents. Studies have confirmed the assessment that avoidance by the mother of food allergens may reduce the incidence of some food allergies in infants and young children.

How does one manage allergies?

As with any medical condition or illness, prevention is essential. Avoidance of all known allergens is the best regimen in dealing with allergies and asthmatic attacks. Those who have food or drug allergies must read all ingredient labels and be extra cautious before ingesting anything. Fortunately, severe allergic reactions are not very common. Those with more than mild to severe form of allergies must be trained by a physician on the life-saving technique of self-injection of 0.1 ml (one-tenth of a cc) Epipen (unidose syringe of epinephrine or adrenalin) subcutaneously (usually under the skin of the outer thigh) when symptoms first begin to manifest following exposure to known allergens. In this dire situation, every minute counts, and 5 or 10 minutes may spell the difference between life and death. After this initial treatment, the patient must be seen by a physician for diagnostic dermal and blood tests, including immunosorbent assay (ELISA, EIA), and more definitive care.

Is Alcohol Good for You?

Alcoholic drink (ethyl alcohol or ethanol) has gotten an undeserved bad reputation in some segments of society. In the United States, alcoholic beverages were totally banned nationwide between 1920 and 1933 thru the 18th Amendment of its constitution ratified on January 16, 1919, and became effective on January 17, 1920, which ushered in the infamous Prohibition Period (also known as the Noble Experiment), declaring illegal—a federal and state crime—manufacture, transportation, and sale of alcohol in America.

For certain segments of society today, either for moral, religious, psychological, or other reasons, drinking is looked upon with disfavor and, by some, even with disdain. To them, drinking alcoholic beverage, even wine, seems to connote a negative image, a less-than-wholesome habit, even a shameful indulgence. To most of those whose lives were adversely affected by an alcoholic member of the family, the unjustified indictment of alcohol use is even worse and absolute.

Obviously, we are talking about two different things here: alcohol and alcohol abuse. Common sense tells us that abuse of anything—even prescription or over-the-counter drugs, vitamins, aspirin, etc.—is harmful, and potentially fatal. And clearly, alcohol is no exception. It is not the alcohol per se, but the "dosage" of this chemical, as with any drug (since alcohol is a drug), that will determine what ultimate effects (beneficial or harmful) it will confer upon the body.

Good News for Those Who Imbibe

When taken with discipline and in moderation by those without medical contraindications, like pregnant women, persons allergic to alcohol, etc., drinking alcoholic beverage as described below has been found to be good for health, cardiovascular and otherwise.

In 1995, when the US federal government declared that drinking alcoholic beverage may be good for the heart, there was wide public dissention. In this information age, when practically everyone has instant access to almost any data, including medical statistics, and since people are more health-conscious today, the new dietary guidelines from the US FDA, which includes alcoholic beverage in its food pyramid, following the Mediterranean food pyramid, is received by most with an open mind, reassurance for some, and joy for others.

The Science behind the New Guidelines

A most convincing body of evidence is derived from more than 50 independent clinical researches that revealed "moderate drinkers live longer than teetotalers and are less likely to have heart disease."

The 42 studies reviewed by Harvard investigators in 1999, published in the *British Medical Journal*, "concluded that regularly consuming 30 grams of alcohol—the equivalent of about three drinks a day—increased good HDL cholesterol (high-density lipoproteins) and reduced factors in the blood that lead to clotting, which translates to a whopping 24.7% reduction in heart-disease risk."

Considered the world's greatest wine connoisseurs, the French, a year earlier, presented a 5-year study that showed "people who drank two to five glasses of wine a day had up to 31% less risk of death from any cause than nondrinkers."

Researchers at Howard University Hospital in Washington, DC, reported that "the benefits may go beyond the heart; moderate drinkers are 14% less likely than nondrinkers to develop age-related *macular degeneration*, a disease of the retina that can cause blindness."

A glass of wine or beer with a meal daily may also lower the risk of diabetes. A 6-year study in Harvard on 41,000 health professionals published in the *British Medical Journal* revealed that "the moderate drinkers were almost half as likely to develop the disease (diabetes) as nondrinkers."

Alcohol Does Not Benefit Young People

The Harvard Nurses Study reported in the *New England Journal of Medicine* that "alcohol cut heart-disease risk almost in half and lowered overall death rates by 14%, but mostly for women over 50." Those who were in their 20s and 30s did not benefit from alcoholic drinks. On the contrary, irresponsible drinking has caused a significant number of deaths from accidents among young people.

Alcohol abuse has the opposite effect at any age. It raises the risk for heart disease, heartbeat irregularity, high blood pressure, stroke, and cirrhosis of the liver. The caffeinated alcoholic "energy" drinks (containing between 50 and 500 mg of caffeine and between 5 and 12% alcohol), popular among students, are unsafe, deadly in some cases. More than 100,000 people die each year from alcohol-related causes.

One Drink a Day

As far as health benefits from alcohol are concerned, the essential question is, how much is the right "dose"?

A study published in the *Journal of American College of Cardiology* showed that "the risk of certain cancers may begin to outweigh the heart benefits after only two drinks a day." Playing it safe, the US federal guidelines recommend no more than one drink a day and emphasize that alcohol has been proven to confer health benefits only to those (starting) in the middle-age group.

While a glass of red wine, especially Pinot Noir, which contains the highest amount of resveratrol (a potent cardio-protective antioxidant), is a popular choice, a can or glass of beer, or one glass of mixed drinks, or a shot of liquor, have also been deemed healthy for a "daily dose" of not more than one.

Although I truly savor a glass of Beefeater's Martini or Pinot Noir every now and then, especially at parties, it has not been a daily routine for me. As a cardiovascular surgeon, I do not recommend for those who do not enjoy alcoholic beverages to start "therapeutic drinking" for the potential health benefits. For those "qualified" ones who do, science is on your side.

Since alcohol is a drug, it is highly advisable for those interested to use it as a part of their health regimen to seek appropriate medical consultation first to make sure alcohol is right and safe for their particular situation.

In the meantime, here's to your health—Cheers!

Prevent Alzheimer's

Alzheimer's, a severely devastating disease of the brain that, in an instant, totally robs and erases the person's memory, is a nightmare everyone fears. When it occurs, it happens so fast like transforming a well-lit room into total darkness with a flip of a switch. The entire memory bank is emptied, turning even a great, talented mind and a charismatic communicator, like the late president Ronald Reagan, one of the best presidents the United States has ever had, into a confused, nonverbal, totally dependent, and helpless stranger, oblivious of his environment, his loved ones, and even of his own self.

The single greatest fear of most Americans over age 55 is memory loss. Reason: there are more than 4 million people in the United States who are afflicted with Alzheimer's disease, and the Alzheimer's Foundation projected this to quadruple by 2050.

The postmortem pathology found among Alzheimer's patients is the abnormal and extensive buildup of beta-amyloid plaque in the brain, which damages the nerve cells and their connections, resulting in memory loss.

EGCG From Green Tea

A new study from the University of South Florida (USF), which came out September 2005, published in the *Journal of Neuroscience*, reported that high doses of an antioxidant ingredient in green tea, called epigallocatechin-3-gallate (EGCG), significantly reduced the formation of beta-amyloid proteins by 54% in the brain of laboratory mice that were first genetically induced to develop Alzheimer's for this particular experiment, and then treated with high doses of EGCG.

This substance is among antioxidants called flavonoids found in plants. Abstinence from red meat and eating a diet that is rich in vegetables and fruits are known to protect active people against heart attack, stroke, and cancer.

Drinking Green Tea Not Enough

There are a variety of antioxidants in green tea, and some of these have been found to decrease the ability of EGCG to reduce beta-amyloid production. So drinking green tea alone is definitely not enough to ward off Alzheimer's. There is obviously a need to selectively concentrate the EGCG antioxidant to override the negative effects of the other flavonoids in green tea.

More extensive studies in the laboratory are needed to confirm the efficacy and safety of EGCG, followed by clinical studies in humans, before we get the final word on this issue. But certainly, green tea is a healthier beverage compared to the colas, alcoholic drinks, and to the so-called "energy drinks" that are now flooding the market and are potentially dangerous to health, with their irresponsible and baseless claims.

Fatty Acids from Plants Show Promise

A fatty acid in safflower, corn, and sunflower oils may help prevent Alzheimer's in some people, according to Sara M. Debanne, PhD, professor of epidemiology and biostatistics at Case Western Reserve University School of Medicine in Cleveland.

"In people who did not have the inherited Alzheimer's risk factor gene (ApoEe4), eating a diet rich in linoleic acids reduced the risk of developing Alzheimer's disease by about 50%. But in those who carried the disease-causing gene, linoleic acids appeared to raise the risk of developing the mind-robbing disease even further," says the researcher.

Brain Exercise

As physical exercise is good for our muscles and the cardiovascular system, brain exercise, as a part of an overall regimen for a healthy lifestyle, is an effective weapon against dementia or Alzheimer's. Doing metal calisthenics (doing cross word puzzle, computer works, reading, solving math or science problems, etc.) strengthens the integrity of the brain cells and helps lessen the risk for the development of Alzheimer's disease.

Statins Against Alzheimer's

Debanne says she suspects "the fatty acids' cholesterol-lowering properties account for their protective effect in some people, since several studies have shown that the cholesterol-lowering statin drugs appear to ward off the disease."

This research finding may be a good reason for people to get tested to find out if they carry the ApoEe4 gene.

Fish Fat Fights Alzheimer's

New studies from the Louisiana State University's Neuroscience Center of Excellence revealed that decosahexaenoic (DHA), an omega-3 fatty acids found in fish like herring, mackerel, and salmon, etc., might help prevent Alzheimer's. The DHA helps the brain cells by (1) minimizing the production of beta-amyloid proteins, and (2) increasing the production of another protein called NPD1 which helps the brain cells stay alive.

Previous researches have shown that people who eat fish at least 4 times a week, or those who take refined omega-3 from fish oil in gelcaps twice daily, reduce their risk of developing this dreaded disease, compared to those who hardly eat fish. A healthy lifestyle—daily exercise, abstinence from tobacco, moderation in alcohol ingestion, a low-fat and low-carb diet, like eating vegetables, nuts, and grains, and fish *instead of* (not together with) red meats—significantly lowers the risk, not only for Alzheimer's, but also for cardiovascular diseases and cancer.

Amebiasis

What is amebiasis?

Also known as entamebiasis, this protozoal infection of the colon is caused by *Entamoeba histolytica*, a one-celled parasite, and is usually asymptomatic (no symptoms). When clinical manifestations are present, they may range from mild diarrhea to severe dysentery to complications involving some vital organs.

What is *Entamoeba dispar*?

This is another form of amebiasis, and is caused by *E. dispar*, about 10 times more common than the infection with *E. histolytica*, but very mild and mostly asymptomatic. Many times, those patients (mis) diagnosed to have *E. histolytica infection,* but who have no symptoms whatsoever, are actually infected with *E. dispar.*

How is the infection transmitted?

The infection may be transmitted directly from person to person (through amoeba cysts) or indirectly through contaminated water or food from infected food handlers or lack of personal hygiene among them. Most often, the infection occurs when a person ingests food or water contaminated with feces from an infected individual or by touching a surface that has amoeba cysts and putting the fingers in the mouth. The onset of the illness starts within 1 to 4 weeks, but could be longer or shorter, depending on the "dose of contamination" and the person's body resistance.

Who are the usual victims?

Anyone (including the rich and famous) can get amebiasis, but the most usual victims are people in developing countries who have poor sanitary conditions, living in crowded dwellings with contaminated water sources. They are obviously also common among traveling immigrants from these third world nations.

Is amebiasis a sexually-transmitted disease?

Yes, among those who indulge in anal sex. The feces that contain amoeba cysts are the source of infection. Unlike the trophozoite form of the *E. histolytica,* which dies fast outside the body, the cysts are resistant to the external environment and survive even on the surface of furniture, etc.

How do the amoebae cause injury?

The amoebae stick to the inner wall of the colon and kill the lining epithelial cells, leading to severe diarrhea with mucus and blood. The protozoa also secrete proteases that destroy the extracellular matrix of the colon and allow invasion into the bowel wall and beyond. Amoebae can also invade the portal (liver) circulation and cause liver abscesses. This infection then spreads from the liver to the adjacent organs or through the blood circulation to the lungs, brain, and other organs.

What are the signs and symptoms?

The majority of people are asymptomatic. They have the infection and continue to excrete amoeba cysts in their stools but appear as normal as can be. When the cysts and their enzymes invade the tissues, intermittent diarrhea, flatulence, constipation, abdominal cramps develop. The feces may have mucus and blood, and the area over the liver and ascending (right) colon may be tender. Other symptoms will depend on the other organs affected.

What is amebic dysentery?

This is the severe acute form of the infection, where there are episodes of frequent diarrhea of semiliquid stools containing mucus, blood, and live trophozoites. There is high fever, dehydration, and toxic symptoms, mild tenderness to frank abdominal pains, enlarged and painful liver. There may be relapses, emaciation, and anemia.

What is the chronic form of amebiasis?

The chronic or long-standing form shows diarrhea with mucus, abdominal cramps, flatulence, and weight loss. There may also be palpable tender masses in the ascending colon or cecum (part of the colon connected to the small intestine), which could feel like cancer masses, but they are actually amoebomas (benign tumor caused by the chronic irritation, inflammatory changes, and scar formation in the colon).

How is the diagnosis made?

The diagnosis does not come easy. The milder nondysenteric form of amebiasis is commonly confused with irritable bowel syndrome, diverticultis, or regional enteritis, ulcerative colitis, etc. Hepatic (liver) amebiasis and amebic abscess must also be distinguished from other liver ailments. Several stool samples from different days may be needed for examination. The presence of trophozoites in the stools or biopsied recto-sigmoid part of the colon clinches the diagnosis. Extraintestinal form of this infection is harder to diagnose.

Any other tests?

Yes, greater than 80% of those with amebic dysentery and almost 100% of those with amebic liver abscess have positive serologic tests. Among those without symptoms, only about 10% are positive. The most sensitive tests available are the indirect hemagglutination and the enzyme-linked immunosorbent assays (ELISA). The antibody titers following infection could remain positive for months or years. Radioisotopic liver scan or CT scan may show the location and size of the liver abscess. Ultrasound will also demonstrate the fluid present in the abscess cavity. Needle aspiration is done for lesions that are larger than 10 cm, those suspected to have imminent liver rupture, and those who do not respond after five days of drug treatment.

How can one prevent amebiasis?

Personal hygiene and any practice to preclude contamination of water and food with human feces will prevent amebiasis. Thorough hand washing after using the toilet, after changing baby diapers, and each time before eating are effective means of preventing the infections. Maintaining and cleaning the home (especially the bathrooms, kitchen, and dining area) properly every day are also helpful. The normal level of chlorine in the water which kills bacteria will not kill the *E. histolytica* cysts. Boiling or treating water with tetracycline hydroperiodide tablets will kill the cysts.

What is the treatment for amebiasis?

The treatment varies and is tailored to the type of amebic infection. The basic regimen includes relief of symptoms, blood replacement where needed, correction of fluid and electrolytes. Some of the drugs used depending on the form, severity of the infection, and presence of spread to other organs are diloxanide flurate, iodoquinol, metronidazole, emetine or dehydroemetine, choloquine. Since these drugs could potentially have serious toxic side-effects, consultation with and supervision by a physician is mandatory during the entire course of therapy.

How does one prevent it while traveling?

When traveling to developing countries or to any area where sanitation is suspect, drink only commercially distributed bottled water or water boiled for at least 1 minute or carbonated pop beverages. Filtering water yourself using "absolute 1 micron or less filter" and dissolving iodine tablets to the filtered water will render water safe for drinking. These could be found in camping and outdoor supply stores. Also, do not eat fresh fruits and vegetables that you did not prepare yourself, and do not drink milk nor eat cheese or dairy products, which may not have been pasteurized. Stay away from food or drinks sold by street vendors.

Androgen and Pimples

Three out of four, or 75%, of young people ages 11 to 30 develop acne. There are approximately 17 million Americans who have acne at any given time, according to Brown University, USA. Also known as pimples, this skin condition affects all races and practically all ages. There are individuals in their fifties who get pimples. While both young males and females are prone to acne formation, men tend to suffer from pimples worse and for a longer period, because of the high level of testosterone in men.

What is acne?

Acne is a skin disease caused by blocked follicles, which are tiny canals that connect the oil glands of the skin to the pores (small holes), through which sebum (oily liquid, which carries dead skin cells) exits the skin. When the follicles are plugged, sebum is trapped and get infected, causing acne or pimples develop when the plug starts to break down. The areas most commonly affected are the face, back, shoulders, and neck.

What are the types of acne?

There are six varieties: whiteheads, which are small and confined under the skin; blackheads, which are obvious, black in color, and appear on the skin; papules, usually small pink bumps on the skin; pustules, red at their base and have pus at the top; nodules, which are large, solid pimples, embedded deep in the skin and are painful; and cysts, painful, filled with liquid pus, and prone to cause scarring.

What causes pimples?

This is an unsettled medical question. Scientists think a rise in the level of a class of hormone, called androgen, which naturally happens during adolescence, induces the oil glands under the skin to grow and produce more oil. This leads to a greater amount of sebum produced, which break down the cell walls in the skin pores. This ultimately becomes a fertile medium for bacteria to grow, causing infection. Genetic predisposition to acne formation is also suspected to play a role. Medications (containing androgen and lithium) and greasy cosmetics may also cause pimples to form. Because of hormonal changes, pregnant women may also be prone to develop acne. Poor personal hygiene promotes bacterial infection.

Does masturbation cause pimples?

No. This common perception is a myth. Increase in androgen (testosterone) increases the sex urge among adolescents and also induces pimple formation as explained earlier. Their similar prevalence in this age group is purely coincidental, both being hormonal. While ejaculation or orgasm releases the hormonal "tension," it does not lower the hormonal level; and it does not minimize, lessen, or make the pimples less severe.

Does application of alcohol help?

While alcohol is a disinfectant, it is also harsh to the skin, besides causing severe dryness, especially of the face. The use of alcohol itself, off the shelf, is discouraged. And so with the use of early morning baby urine, tea, vinegar, wine, or fruit juices, laundry/kitchen detergents—all a myth, without any scientific basis, ineffective, and may even be harmful.

What can aggravate acne?

The following factors make acne worse: poor hygiene, eating, stress and anxiety, squeezing acne, oil-based makeup, menstrual cycle, use of greasy hair products (cocoa or coconut butter), and hot and humid environments.

What can one do to treat acne?

A healthy, low-fat, low-cholesterol diet greatly helps. Personal hygiene is an important weapon against pimples. Daily shower and frequent hand washing are essential habits. Since hands and fingers have bacteria most of the time, not touching or scratching the face and not squeezing the pimples will minimize infection and scarring. The face should be washed with mild soap at least twice a day. Do not scrub the face or areas with pimples. Hair must be shampooed to remove sebum and skin residue. Eyeglasses should be cleaned regularly. For makeup, use only nonacnegenic (nonceomedogenic), and do not go to bed with makeup on.

Most of the people with acne have the mild form, which can be initially managed with over-the-counter topical medications for acne applied to the areas involved.

What are these OTC antiacne drugs?

Majority of these topical medications prescribed by physicians for acne contain any of the following active ingredients in the forms of cream, gels, pads, lotion, or soaps:

Resorcinol—a crystalline phenol that is also used for treating psoriasis, eczema, and dandruff. It breaks down whiteheads and blackheads.

Benzoyl Peroxide—a white crystalline peroxide used in bleaching flour, fats, or oils, which works as peeling agent, stimulating new skin formation, cleaning the pores, thus cutting down the bacterial count.

Salicylic Acid—also used as fungicide, antidandruff in shampoos, and in making aspirin, perfumes, and dyes, this white crystalline substance stimulates the epidermis to shed skin more easily, preventing pores from getting plugged and stimulating new cells to grow.

Sulfur—with an action not well understood, elemental sulfur is known to oxidize slowly to sulfurous acid which has a mild reducing and antibacterial actions. It helps break down whiteheads and blackheads.

Retin-A—containing an acid form of Vitamin A, called tretinoin or all-trans retinoic acid (ATRA), this drug "combats" aging of the skin and also acts as a chemical peel. Tretinoin is also used in the treatment of acute promyelocytic leukemia.

Azelaic Acid—a saturated dicarboxylic acid naturally present in barley, wheat, and rye, this acid cleans up free radicals, fortifies cells that line the follicles, stops oil eruptions, slows down bacterial proliferation, and lessens inflammation. This is also good for dark skin patches on the face called melasma.

Some oral contraceptives, which control the overactive oil glands of the skin, have been found to be effective for women with acne.

When is a dermatologist needed?

Use of any of those medications listed may cause skin irritation, redness, and burning. It is best to use the lowest strength. The side effects usually cease after continued applications. If they persist or if the trial with OTC drugs does not show improvement after a couple of weeks, or if the acne is very severe to begin with, consultation with a dermatologist is recommended. The skin specialist may additionally prescribe oral or topical antibiotics, like erythromycin and tetracycline, clindamycin, or sulfacetamide to reduce the population of Propionibacterium acne, the bug commonly found in blocked follicles of the skin where the pimples are.

Angina Pectoris

What is angina pectoris?

Angina pectoris is the medical term for chest pains, more specifically pains emanating from and involving the heart. It is most common for people to associate chest pains with impending or insipient heart attack. The same is true within the medical community: chest pains, especially by the breastbone, are considered angina pectoris till proven otherwise.

Why do physicians think this way?

Since heart attack is treacherous and potentially fatal, it is safer for the attending doctor to put this condition at the top of the list of his probable diagnoses when dealing with a person with chest pains. The physician's high index of suspicion is most essential for patient safety and effective health management. In 1997, the cost of treating heart disease in the United States was a staggering sum of 58 billion dollars, followed by expenditures for cancer and trauma.

What are the other causes of chest pains?

There are a variety of other causes of chest pains. Some of them are a pinched nerve in the neck, viral inflammation of the rib and cartilage, diseases of the ribs, the lungs (pneumonia, other infections, cancer, etc.) and their covering (pleurisy and cancer), diseases of the breathing pipe, diseases of the esophagus (food pipe), chest muscle spasm, muscle contusion or injury, arthritis of the spine or almost any joints in the chest area, diseases of the diaphragm (muscular "tent" that divides the chest cavity from the abdominal cavity into two separate airtight compartments), and referred pains from intra-abdominal pathology.

What is the cause of angina pectoris?

Just like any muscle in the body, the myocardium (heart muscles) need oxygen and nutrition in order to "feel" comfortable, remain healthy, and function well. The oxygen and nutrition are carried by blood that is circulating inside the arteries that supply all muscles, other tissues, and organs throughout the body. If any of these arteries are blocked for any reason, the blood supply to the intended areas is diminished or totally cut off. The heart muscles are supplied by the coronary arteries. If these coronary arteries are blocked, the heart muscles are deprived of blood and suffer from "asphyxiation" from lack of oxygen, and go into severe spasm, causing the angina pectoris, much like leg muscle pains and spasms when the leg artery is blocked.

How are these arteries blocked?

Blockages in the arteries in our body is caused by arteriosclerosis (hardening of the arteries) brought on and/or aggravated by several health risk factors. The main culprit ingredient is cholesterol, which mostly comes from saturated fats from the red meat and eggs we eat. These food items thicken the blood consistency, which leads to thick cholesterol deposits on the inside walls of our tiny coronary arteries. This situation is like using thick paint applied layer after layer, every second, day after day, year after year, onto the inner walls of these tiny pipes. Just like the sewer or drain pipes in our homes, this cholesterol "junk" could clog up our coronary arteries.

Is thicker blood therefore unhealthy?

In essence, and simplistically put, yes. The body maintains a normal consistency of our blood, not too thick to cause clots, and not too thin to cause spontaneous bleeding. Our body does that normally as a natural inherent protective mechanism. Any one or a combination of any of the following risk factors can upset this healthy natural balance, causing blood to thicken which leads to arteriosclerosis and cholesterol blockages: smoking, ingestion of the high-cholesterol foods we listed above, sedentary life (absence or lack of daily exercise), presence of diabetes and/or hypertension (high blood pressure), aging, stress, worry, fear, and to some extent, heredity or genetic predisposition.

When does a heart attack occur?

Myocardial infarction (heart attack) occurs when the heart muscles are deprived of the amount of blood they need to maintain normal tissue oxygenation and nutrition. Since this blood supply to the heart muscles is provided by the coronary arteries, heart attack will result when the coronary arteries are severely blocked due to the reasons and causes explained above. Since muscles are flesh, they start rotting when blood supply is cut off for more than a few minutes, resulting in muscle damage. The actual acute heart attacks occurs when the very narrowed artery is totally blocked by a clot.

How could the clot be prevented?

The prudent thing to do discuss a strategy with your physician for such an eventuality. Most likely, unless there is a contraindication, he/she will recommend that you take four 81-mg low-dose aspirin when severe chest pains occur, and rush to the emergency room for proper diagnosis and care.

How do we minimize these risk factors?

The most effective way to minimize these risk factors is by living a healthy lifestyle, which includes the following: (1) abstinence from tobacco; (2) eating fish, vegetables, whole grain foods, nuts and fruits (high-fiber foods); (3) staying away from eggs and red meat (pork, beef, and anything made of them), fried foods, lard, butter, excessive dairy products; (4) excess alcohol is poison, but drinking a glass or two of red wine with meals is good for the heart so long as your physician does not find any contraindication in your case; (5) doing daily exercises (walking, ballroom dancing, etc.); (6) fish oil supplement and low-dose aspirin as prescribed by your physicians; (7) savoring life and managing stress with meditation, yoga, soothing music, frequent mini-vacations or breaks, and doing other activities that give you joy and personal satisfaction.

How is blockage of the arteries diagnosed?

To show coronary artery stenosis (blockage), a practically painless dye test called coronary arteriogram or angiogram (also known as heart catheterization) is the best way to find out if there are any stenoses in the coronary arteries.

If blockages are found, then what?

To prevent heart attack, the blocked artery should either be opened with balloon angioplasty and stent placement, if it is still amenable to this simpler and less invasive procedure. However, if the blockages are multiple and severe and not manageable with angioplasty, then the next prudent option to ward off heart attack is to do coronary bypass surgery. Thanks to modern technology today, these wonderful life-saving procedures are available, performed by super specialists in invasive and noninvasive cardiology and cardiac surgeons trained in standard cardiovascular surgery and in minimally invasive beating-heart surgery.

Anti-cancer foods

The new television show in the USA, "Food Revolution," hosted by passionate health advocate Jamie Oliver of Essex, England, has pointed out glaringly how junk foods (loaded with fats, cholesterol, additives, processed meats) have significantly contributed to the "pandemic" of obesity, hypertension, heart disease, stroke, diabetes, cancer, etc., and premature deaths among peoples of the western hemisphere.

In man's fight against all those diseases mentioned above, medical studies have data to suggest that phytochemicals in natural foods help ward off or minimize the risk for the development of those illnesses, including cancer. However, this protective health benefit has not been found in the pills or potion being sold as phytochemicals or antioxidants.

Science unceasingly searches for the truth, and when new data or evidences are discovered, it accepts the invalidity of any disproven past theories and corrects itself.

There was a time when drinking milk (to counteract the acids) was a part of the accepted treatment for stomach ulcer, until it was proven to be causing acid rebound, making the situation worse. Whole milk and eggs were supposed to be healthy foods, until science discovered evidences the high fat contents of regular milk and the saturated fats in egg yolk were deleterious to health. Vitamin E, beta carotene (Vitamin A), and selenium supplements were favorite recommendations, but today people are discouraged from using them. However, those same nutrients derived from food are considered safe and good.

One basic fact remains valid and lasting over the centuries and even before the dawn of civilization: unadulterated natural food sources, foods of plant origin, like vegetables, nuts, whole grains, and fruits, are man's best friend in his quest for health and longevity. This truth appears to be self-evident and constant to this day.

In our battle against cancer, here are eight food items, among the twelve superfoods we have written about before, that are readily available to help us minimize our risk for the development of malignancies and also aid us in preventing most diseases afflicting man today.

Tomatoes

While fresh tomatoes have lycopene, the higher concentration is found in cooked or processed tomatoes (juice, paste, ketchup, stewed) together with other unidentified beneficial substances which have been shown to lower the risk of prostate cancer. Whether it is the lycopene itself or any of the other substances in processed tomatoes which protects men from prostatic cancer is not clear. In the experimental lab, lycopene has been shown to stop the growth of other forms of cancer, including inner lining of the uterus, breast, and lungs. Lycopene may also be found in red bell peppers, watermelon, and pink grapefruit.

Garlic

Garlic fights bacteria, including *H. pylori*, which causes stomach ulcers, lowers the risk of colon cancer formation, and may also enhance DNA repair. Suggestion: peel and chop garlic cloves for 15 minutes before cooking to maximize the chemical benefits from its enzymes and protective sulfur-compounds. Other studies suggest that "garlic is the powerhouse of the allium family, but onions, leeks, chives, and scallions might also protect against stomach cancer."

Broccoli

Broccoli and other cruciferous vegetables (cauliflower, kale, and cabbage), when chewed, release phytochemicals called glucosinolates, which produce protective enzymes, like sulfuraphane (highest in broccoli and broccoli sprouts). This compound detoxifies toxic substances (smoke, smog, air pollutants) and "are most protective against cancers of the mouth, esophagus, and stomach," according to a review of hundreds of clinical studies conducted for the World Cancer Research Fund and the American Institute for Cancer Research.

Berries

Strawberries are loaded with natural antioxidants that are a good weapon against heart disease, Alzheimer's, and cancer. Black raspberry and strawberry extracts were found to slow down cancer cell growth, especially in colon cancer. The ellagic acid in berries appears to have anticancer, and the flavanoids in these fruits suppress an enzyme (linked to lung cancer) that damages DNA. The other berries packed with flavanoids and anthocyanins (with anti-inflammation effect) are blueberries, cranberries, blackberries.

Carrots

Carrots contain beta-carotene, which protects cell membranes from toxin and retards cancer-cell growth. It also contains phytochemicals that ward off cancers of the mouth, esophagus (food pipe), stomach, and cervix (mouth of the womb) by destroying HPV (human papillomavirus). Carrots also have falcarinol, a natural pesticide. Cooked carrots confer more protective benefits (with higher level of antioxidants) than raw.

Spinach

Also dubbed super carotenoid, spinach contains lutein, which is essential for the eyes. It also provides fiber and folate, both anticancer agents. Spinach is likewise packed with zeaxanthin, which eliminates free radicals from the body before they do any damage. Spinach and other green leafy vegetables are said to help in reducing the risk for the development of cancer of the mouth, esophagus, stomach, ovaries, uterus, lungs, and colon and rectum. Romaine lettuce, kale, collard greens, and Swiss chard are excellent substitutes.

Whole Grains and Nuts

Besides providing a lot of fiber, whole grains are also rich anticancer substances, like lignans (antioxidants) and sapponins (prevent cancer cells from multiplying). "100% whole wheat" bread sprinkled with sesame or flax seeds contains the most level of lignans. Oats and barley are two of the best cereals. Whole grains also reduced the risk for type 2 diabetes. Nuts, which has polyunsaturated (good nonanimal) fats, are antioxidant and high fiber-food items.

Dark Chocolate

Dark chocolates have been very popular the past few years because of its polyphenol content, which has been shown to lower the blood pressure and is considered cardioprotective. They also have flavanoids (epicathechin and quercetin) which have anticancer effects.

If you think about it, these health foods are no different from regular foods available for us. The problem is that many of us have taken them for granted and do not eat enough of them. Nature has blessed us with these wonderful foods that prevent cancer and other diseases. All we need to do is to learn to love and enjoy them, together with daily physical exercise.

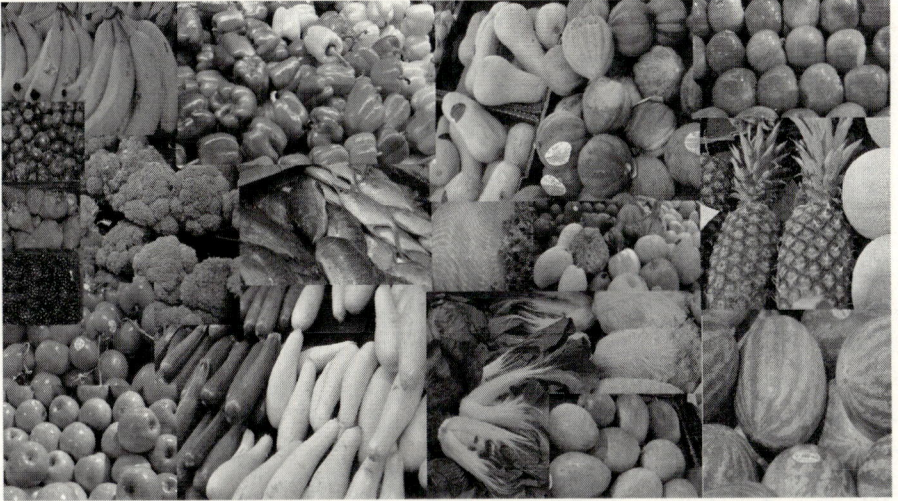

Fish, vegetables, and fruits are essential parts of a healthy diet. They are nutritious and loaded with antioxidants and fiber.

Anxiety/Panic Attack

What is anxiety?

Anxiety is an unpleasant emotional state of heightened feeling of fear, worry, or concern. All of us experience fear and anxiety at one time or another. It is normal for anyone to feel anxious, to some degree, about certain things or events. As long as that feeling is proportional to the problem or situation at hand, it is not abnormal.

Why do we have anxiety?

Anxiety is an "alarm system" of our mind, a protective and defense mechanism that prepares our entire body, alerting us to danger, for "fight or flight." When a visibly angry person comes toward you with a knife, your heart beats faster, your breathing more intense, your palms and forehead get cold sweats, and your mind races. In this instance, adaptive anxiety is not only normal but is a beneficial and helpful reaction, allowing you to make a split-second decision and a swift response to the danger that lies before you. When one is busy and has a handful, anxiety can provide the will and energy to finish the job or get things done more efficiently. Medical science still does not fully know the causes of anxiety.

What is an anxiety attack?

An anxiety attack is an abnormal and exaggerated degree of worry over trivial incidents or things, or for no reason at all. Here, anxiety is out of control and disproportional, leaving the individual with an overwhelming and incapacitating sense of fear and dread for justifiable reason. This maladaptive anxiety disrupts life, happiness, and peace of mind. Panic attacks are a type of anxiety disorder, which is related to some specific trigger object or situation (example: a woman scared of mice may panic when she sees a mouse). Some of the symptoms are similar to those of generalized anxiety plus the following: choking, chest pains, fear of dying, fear of losing control or going crazy, chills and flushes, sweating, shortness of breath, numbness and tingling sensation, feelings of detachment from environment, strangeness and unreality (like being in a dream). They also fear that they might have a serious heart or lung disease or a brain tumor and go to the emergency room or to their physician for urgent care.

What is a phobia?

Phobia is an abnormal and extreme fear and anxiety as a reaction to specific situation, event, or objects. Example: fear of bridges, snakes, crowds, heights, spiders, open places, or fear of social gatherings. All of us have a certain degree of normal phobias. It becomes a problem only if it disrupts normal life. Posttraumatic stress disorder follows a severely traumatic physical or emotional experience. Example: serving in the military during an active war; assault or rape; surviving a plane crash, torture, or tornado, or a serious car accident. These individuals relive the traumatic events thru flashbacks, memories, or dreams.

How does one handle anxiety?

1. Take control of your worry by picking a place, a specific time period to do your worrying. Spend a few minutes analyzing your concerns and think of what you can do about them, and don't dwell on what might happen, but on what is happening and of the rational way to resolve them.

2. Learn how to relax, listening to soft music, doing yoga, meditation, biofeedback, deep breathing, dancing, and enjoying time with friends and/or family members, etc.

3. Exercise regularly to decrease your anxiety.

4. Try to sleep at least 8 hours a day.

5. Confront the things that have made you anxious before in order to get used to handling them and be more comfortable doing it.

6. Stay away from cigarettes, alcohol or drugs.

7. Avoid coffee, soft drinks with caffeine (colas), tea, and chocolate, since all of these tend to increase anxiety.

8. Consult with your physician. Most of these conditions respond well to proper medical care, which might include simple advice and reassurance, psychotherapy, and/or medications.

Recognizing and accepting the fact that there is a medical problem and taking action to resolve it promptly is the first step toward healing. Modern medicine has so much to offer today, thanks to the mind-boggling, cutting-edge technology in health and sciences.

Antioxidants: Are they harmful?

In a separate clinical investigation published in 2009, 47 independent studies assessing antioxidant supplementation "found a slight increase in deaths among people who took beta-carotene, vitamin E, or vitamin A supplements."

"There is little evidence of a benefit for antioxidant supplementation and mounting evidence of potential harm," according to Christian Gluud, MD, who coauthored the analysis.

The unfounded idea that we can prevent diseases by simply taking supplements, without exerting any effort, is mostly the result of brilliantly crafted infomercials and marketing gimmicks that the $6-billion-a-year industry has flooded all the media with.

The illusion of a modern medical fountain of youth and health has become almost too real to resist in our quest for a convenient and instant potion, lotion, or pill to make us look and/or feel good without sweat.

But reality is something else. To attain good health, we must work at it and for it. Medical science is not enough. Since the start of civilization, it has been recognized that a healthy mind and body comes from good nutrition, physically active body, adequate rest, and healthy habits. While this awareness was expressed in its simplistic and archaic term then, its principle, wisdom, and basis in science had faithfully served countless generations and have remained pertinent even today.

Good Free Radicals?

The same investigator, Dr. Gluud, and colleague Goran Bjelakovic, who are both with Copenhagen University Hospital, wrote a fascinating editorial about their hypothesis that free radicals may not be all that bad after all.

The current popular view is that antioxidant vitamins protect people against diseases, like heart disease and cancer, "by reducing the free radicals that are thought to promote these conditions through oxidative stress."

Gluud and Bjelakovic theorize that "free radicals may do some good by targeting and killing harmful cells, such as those that cause cancer to grow."

"Antioxidant supplements (which decrease free radicals) may actually cause some harm," says the editorial. "Our diets typically contain safe levels of vitamins, but high-level antioxidant supplements could potentially upset an important physiologic balance."

If this theory is, in fact, found to be valid and true in the future, it will radically revolutionize the medical thinking on vitamins and antioxidant supplements.

More extensive studies are, of course, required to prove or disprove this most interesting hypothesis.

Back to Basic

While scientific studies around the world continue to unravel medical mysteries to help humankind prevent or cure diseases, one caveat remains constant and clear: unless we, as individuals, learn to love our body enough to actively protect it by living a healthy lifestyle, no matter how much sacrifice it entails, no amount of advances in medical science and technology can save us from ailments and diseases, preventable morbidities and premature death, especially those illnesses resulting from our self-abuse.

Aphrodisiacs

What are Aphrodisiacs?

Aphrodisiacs are pro-sexual drugs or substances that will heighten libido (sexual desire), orgasm (ecstasy and pleasure), and performance in males and females, not partner specific.

Are these substances new?

No, the cultural quest for aphrodisiacs has been the obsession of man, from ancient to modern times. Natural substances such as belladona, datura, and henbane were key ingredients in the sexual orgies of ancient fertility cults.

What is this popular drug Yohimbine?

Yohimbine is an alkaloid derivative found in the bark of yohimbehe tree which has long been used by the natives of Africa to enhance their sexual prowess.

Is Viagra an aphrodisiac?

No, not in this strict medical sense. Viagra does not directly increase the libido (sexual desire) or orgasm (sexual pleasure), although it improves sexual performance of the male with erectile dysfunction (inability to maintain erection). Indirectly, it enhances sexual performance and adds to sexual pleasure. If there is no sexual desire between the partners, Viagra does not help. Aphrodisiacs, on the other hand, are substances that make a person want to have sex, almost an uncontrollable sexual desire with practically any person.

What medications or food items have an "aphrodisiac effect"?

Ginseng, oysters, mandrake plants in medieval Europe, L-dopa and pergolide mesylate (two drugs used for the treatment of Parkinson's disease), Quaalude, Apomorphine, Nomifensine and Bupropion (antidepression drugs), Bethanechol, Afrodex (combination of Yohimbine, testosterone and strychnine), Clomipiramine, Fluoxetine, Chinese Chan Su, "Love Stone," "Hard Rock," "Stud 100" are some claimed to have aphrodisiac effect.

What are causes of impotence?

There are a variety of causes of impotence. It could be psychogenic (stress or psychological problem), neurogenic (nerve injury), vascular (poor circulation), medication related (as those patients taking high blood pressure pills), or anatomical (severe deformity of the organ), and, of course, aging (which normally reduces libido and the ability to maintain erection).

Is there any aphrodisiac that is effective and safe?

Medical research and studies on aphrodisiacs have been ongoing for centuries. The Food and Drug Administration in the United States has not approved any drug as an aphrodisiac per se. Drugs for the treatment of some illnesses, with "aphrodisiac-effect," as mentioned earlier, have not been officially approved and recommended for use as aphrodisiacs. Most of the reports on their effectiveness are anecdotal.

The main problem to date, even in the case of yohimbine, is the absence of a definite and convincing medical proof of the consistency in its efficacy and safety of this substance. Some people have tried some of the "aphrodisiac" drugs and substances mentioned above (like Chinese Chan Su, Hard Rock, Chinese Love Stone, Stud 100). Some people have died from them. We are not aware of any safe and effective "legitimate" aphrodisiacs to date.

What then can enhance the mood for a romantic encounter?

Feelings, situation, and atmosphere are important, especially among females, in setting the mood for a romantic sexual rendezvous. There must be mutual liking and desire, and both partners must be in a happy frame of mind. And remember, protection, when needed, is very important for the peace of mind for both parties.

The ambiance must provide security, privacy, and serenity, preferably with romantic music in the background. The bedroom encounter must be at least 3 to 4 hours after a meal and perhaps following a glass of wine or an after-dinner drink for a more relaxed mind, if desired. Partners must try to be as natural and as spontaneous as can be. Some form of communication and body contact must be maintained after the act, so the partner does not feel abandoned "after use." This, today, might be the safest "aphrodisiac."

What Controls Appetite?

What trigger hunger and satiety?

The urge to eat (hungry or not) is, to a large extent, controlled by hormones in our body. And these hormones fluctuate depending on how much sleep we get, what types of food we eat and how much calories we take in, and on how much physical activities we indulge in daily. Scientific researchers are focusing on four specific substances they call "fat hormones," which our own endocrine glands in the body produce. There are hormones that make one eat, and there are also hormones that signal the brain to tell the person to stop eating. These substances control hunger and satiety.

Which is the "hunger hormone"?

The hunger hormone is ghrelin, which is secreted by our guts (stomach and intestines). When its level goes up, we feel hungry and have the urge to eat. The level of ghrelin goes up when we get less sleep or not enough sleep. This is the reason why those who are trying to lose weight should get adequate amount (about 8 hours) of sleep. An imbalanced meal and stress also elevate the ghrelin level. Food deprivation obviously increases the ghrelin level, hence it is better to keep the level of this hormone on an even keel and not fluctuate too much by eating regularly (or even more than 3 times a day) but at a controlled total calorie ceiling, to maintain health and body weight. So starving oneself is not a good way to lose weight, since this will lead to a ghrelin "boomerang" in the latter part of the day.

Which is the "satiety hormone"?

The opposite or counterhormone, which is called leptin, signals the brain when to stop eating. It controls the appetite. This "satiety hormone" is produced by fat cells in the body. When a person loses weight, the leptin level in the bloodstream also goes down. As a result, there is a "rebound" weight gain. The best strategy in losing and maintaining a desired weight level is to lose in a slow and steady pace, about one to two pounds a week, and not more. In this manner, there will still be an effective level of leptin in the body to control the urge to eat.

What's the effect of imbalance meals?

High-carbohydrate diet (rice, bread, sugar, pop drinks, ice cream, and other sweets) leads to a faster metabolism of these food items that have high glycemic indices and floods the bloodstream with high glucose level. This is why those who eat a lot of these food items (rice is a great culprit!) are feared to have a higher risk of developing type 2 diabetes. Personally, much as I loved rice (a 3-meal rice addict), I had decided to give it up following all the convincing scientific evidence today of its link to diabetes.

How about emotional stress?

When one is high on stress and low on energy, the body tries to compensate by producing more cortisol hormone. This substance mobilizes the blood sugar transformation (glycogen into glucose) and increases the blood sugar level to provide energy. But it makes the person hungry. And so the person eats more. The connection between cortisol level and obesity is not a settled question yet. Physical stress, like regimented physical exercises daily, is another story. This has a positive effect on our body in more ways than one. While it also raises the cortisol level and increases blood sugar, exercise burns calories and also helps put our body hormones in good balance. As a matter of fact those who do daily exercises have lower risk of developing heart attack, stroke, diabetes, and cancer.

What is obestatin?

This is a hormone recently identified by researchers at Stanford. This substance has been shown to slow down the digestive process. While the studies on obestatin are still ongoing, it is postulated that this hormone, like the first three above, could be held in check by adequate sleep, balanced diet, physical exercise, and minimizing stress.

Are appetite suppressants Safe?

Most appetite-control pills, juices, solutions, and powders on the market are not physiological and unnatural way to suppress (by force) the appetite for weight control. While they are readily available and very popular, they have potential adverse side effects on the heart, liver, kidneys, and brain in the long haul. Some serious complications, and even deaths, have been reported from the use of these diet substances. Since greater calorie intake than output is the cause of increase in body weight, the safest, most natural, strategy is to eat less and burn more calories with physical exercises, making the output of calories (energy) greater than the intake of calories (food). The use of appetite suppressants could be dangerous. Consult with your physician before using any of them.

Arthritis Breakthrough

What is arthritis?

Arthritis or osteoarthritis is a degenerative disease of the joints and is the leading cause of disability in the world today. It is twice more common among women. Forty million Americans (about 15% of the population of the United States) have some form of arthritis in 1995, and by year 2020, this is predicted to go up to 59 million or 18% of the population. In general, 50% of those above 50 years olds have some form of osteoarthritis.

What is the cause of osteoarthritis?

Osteoarthritis (*osteo* means "bone," *arthro* means *joint*, and *itis* means "inflammation") is caused by daily wear and tear of aging, or of repeated trauma (as in sports), and is characterized by a general breakdown of the cartilage (collagen cushion) in the joints, leading to pain and stiffness. One theory implicates the immune system. As a person gets older, he/she loses some of the joints' proteoglycans (which makes the cartilage more resilient to pressure and weight-bearing). The cartilage deteriorates and thins out, reducing the shock-absorbing protection for the joints so the joints get eroded. The inflammatory component is minor, compared to that in rheumatoid arthritis. Majority of arthritis we hear about is osteoarthritis. Other causes include metabolic diseases, infection, immune system malfunction, arterial blood supply deficit, etc. Most mammals suffer from arthritis in old age.

What is cartilage?

Cartilage is a connective tissue that holds joints together like a biological glue. It is made of about 70-80% water, 10-15% collagen fibers, 5-10% proteoglycans (glycosaminoglycans), and other proteins.

The glycosaminoglycans are made up of chains of chondroitin-sulfate disaccharides. The cartilage acts a cushion, a shock absorber between two bones, thus preventing them from grinding against each other and wearing down faster. The proteoglycans gives it the ability to withstand heavy loads, compression under heavy weight, and reexpansion to its original dimension when the load is removed. Just like shock absorbers in vehicles!

Is osteoarthritis the same as osteoporosis?

No. Osteoarthritis involves the joints (where two bones meet, with a cartilage in between), like the elbows, knees, and fingers. Osteoporosis is thinning of the bones as a result of a loss of calcium and other minerals that make up the bones. It is not infrequent to see patients, especially women, suffering from both ailments.

Which joints are usually afflicted?

The knees, hips, and spine are the most commonly involved joints. Next are the finger joints, the joint at the base of the thumb, and the joint at the base of the big toe. Other joints, like the neck joint, may also be affected.

Do high-heeled shoes contribute to osteoarthritis?

Yes, it has been shown that wearing high-heeled shoes can cause osteoarthritis. High-heeled shoes alter the forces at the knees, thigh bones, and hips and predispose the joints to osteoarthritis. Any trauma to any joints can cause osteoarthritis.

What is this "revolutionary" arthritis pill?

The latest drug combination (in one pill) for osteoarthritis is glucosamine sulfate with chondroitin sulfate (GS-CS). This drug duo has been getting a lot of attention in the press and in the medical literature for its effectiveness. Many rheumatologists today prescribe it. Glucosamine is a natural substance normally found in our body, which stimulates the biosynthesis of some proteoglycans and restores damaged chondrocytes (cartilage cells). Chondroitin stimulates the production of collagen and proteoglycans and also inhibits the enzyme that degrades proteoglycans. Aging and joint trauma cause the normal levels of these two substances in our body to decrease, leading to the onset of osteoarthritis.

How effective is the GS-CS pill?

One third of arthritis patients taking the GS-CS pill obtain moderate to significant relief from the pains and stiffness of arthritis, another 33% get slight improvement, and a third without relief. So about 66% are helped by this drug combination, which is certainly more effective than aspirin preparations, NSAIDs (nonsteroidal anti-inflammatory drugs, like ibuprofen and naproxen). Some patients require both GS-CS and NSAIDs to obtain relief.

What is the concern about NSAIDs?

Like aspirin, even the enteric-coated or buffered aspirin, NSAIDs cause a lot of gastric irritation. Some patients have developed stomach ulcers, with and without bleeding, from the use of aspirin or NSAIDs, glucosamine, and chondroitin. Minor and temporary side effects of gastric upset and nausea and rare allergic reaction have been reported.

Can diabetics or pregnant women take GS-CS?

The usual recommended dose of GS-CS for osteoarthritis is 500 mg three times a day, and the glucose molecule in GS-CS pills is quite low so that it may be taken by diabetics, so long as it is under medical supervision. No studies on the effects of GS-CS among pregnant women have been published, so we do not recommend this treatment for those in the family way.

Do vitamins and minerals help in osteoarthritis?

Yes, a study in Boston University Medical Center showed that vitamins C, B, and D are of benefit in the treatment of osteoarthritis and that antioxidants (as the flavonoids and carotenoids in fruits, vegetables, grains, legumes, etc.) inhibit the progression of the disease. The roles of minerals in osteoarthritis are not clear, but it is safe to say that taking multivitamins with minerals daily is a healthy practice.

How can we prevent osteoarthritis?

We cannot totally prevent osteoarthritis until we have the ability to stop aging, but we can take some measures to minimize or slow down the process of wear and tear of our joints. Among these are: (1) Eating a healthy diet, with a lot of fish, vegetables, nuts, whole grains, and fruits, (2) Taking multivitamins with minerals daily, (3) Quitting tobacco, (4) Doing daily physical exercises, (5) Maintaining a normal body weight, (6) Assuming a good posture at all times, (7) Avoiding repetitive activities that will overburden the joints in the body, and (8) Consulting with your physician as needed.

Aspirin and colon cancer

One medication present in almost every household around the world is a wonder drug called acetylsalicylic acid, popularly known as aspirin.

Besides acting as a mild blood thinner taken by millions to help minimize the risk of blood clot formation in heart arteries and the chances of a heart attack, aspirin has been found to help lower the risk of the development of cancer of the colon, as previously reported by *Medical Oncology*, stating that "aspirin and other related nonsteroidal anti-inflammatory drugs might exert a chemo-preventive effect."

Previous randomized placebo-controlled trials have revealed that the use of aspirin, or of its "relatives" celecoxib and rofecoxib, significantly reduced the risk for the formation of adenoma (precancerous lesion) among patients at high risk for colorectal cancer.

And now, adding to its amazing versatility, newer studies revealed that aspirin taken regularly by those who have already been diagnosed to have primary cancer of the colon, specifically the type with the so-called "high COX-2 expression," even in stage 2 and 3, lowers the mortality rate and prolongs life, compared to those colon cancer patients not taking aspirin. A fabulous drug, indeed!

The improvement in the survival rate was reported in an article in the *Journal of the American Medical Association* on August 12, 2009, which stated that "the overall 5-year survival for patients using aspirin regularly was 88%, compared with 83% for those who did not, and the ten-year survival rates were 74% for regular aspirin users and 69% for those who were not."

Taking aspirin as a part of a regimen to lower the risk of colon cancer is, at this stage, still not an official medical recommendation nor a standard of care.

"These results are observational and, in the absence of a clinical trial, we can't make a clinical recommendation," according to Andrew Chan, MD, MPH, assistant professor of medicine at Harvard Medical School in Boston, Massachusetts, who authored the study.

Dr. Chan further stated that the most encouraging results of this study provides a very compelling justification to do randomized controlled trials, in a much larger patient population, in order to confirm and validate the impressive initial clinical observations.

Aspirin Caution

Aspirin (acetylsalicylic acid), an inexpensive popular household item once relegated to the role of analgesic (for pain), antipyretic (for fever), and anti-inflammatory (for arthritis), has been proven to be a sophisticated, versatile, and a most beneficial drug for a variety of other conditions.

Leroux of France first discovered a substance called salicin, an active ingredient in willow bark. In 1838, Piria produced salicylic acid from salicin, but it was Dreser in 1899 who introduced aspirin into medicine.

In the United States alone, millions of people are taking aspirin daily, and more than 20 tons of this wonder drug is consumed annually.

How versatile is aspirin?

Besides being used as an analgesic for pain of various causes (headaches, body aches, arthritis, dysmenorrhea, neuralgia, gout, etc.), and for febrile states, aspirin is also useful in the treatment of rheumatic heart disease, as an antiplatelet (to thin the blood and prevent blood clots) in coronary (heart) artery and in the deep veins in the legs and pelvis. Aspirin has also been found to reduce the incidence of colon cancer and melanoma. Many physicians and patients today take low-dose aspirin (81 mg once daily) to reduce the chances of getting a heart attack and a form of stroke.

Where else is it used for?

Aspirin is also prescribed alone or in combination with other drugs for some patients with atrial fibrillation (irregular heart rhythm) and for those who have undergone coronary angioplasty and stenting.

Aspirin has also been used with success in the treatment of children with Bartter's syndrome and also in enhancing the closure of patent ductus arteriosus, an abnormal connection between the aorta (main artery connected to the heart) and the pulmonary artery (to the lungs) in the newborn.

Can aspirin cause allergy?

Yes, but, fortunately, aspirin intolerance or hypersensitivity, which leads to severe toxicity or fatality, is uncommon. There have been reports of aspirin-induced bronchial asthma and aspirin-induced nasal polyp (tumor) formation. The more common side effect of aspirin ingestion is stomach irritation and heartburn, sometimes causing stomach ulcers and bleeding. Enteric-coated aspirin helps reduce stomach irritation.

What is the danger of aspirin in children?

Pediatricians all over the world have discontinued prescribing aspirin for children for pain and fever, because aspirin has been implicated in the occurrence of Reye's syndrome in children following a viral (upper respiratory or gastrointestinal) infection, which syndrome could be fatal. For fever or pain, physicians now prefer to prescribe acetaminophen (like Tylenol, Paracetamol, and other brands). However, for some specific illnesses (like Kawasaki disease, juvenile rheumatoid arthritis, etc.) aspirin is still being used effectively under the strict care of pediatricians.

What is low-dose aspirin therapy?

Low-dose aspirin, using 81 mg of aspirin (same dose as the formerly available "baby aspirin"), is a popularly prescribed regimen today to prevent heart attack and the embolic-type (clot-related) stroke. For aches and pains, adults usually take two tablets of regular aspirin (325 mg per tablet), so this preventive mini dose of 81 mg is about 1/8 of that full dose of 650 mg. The idea is to use the smallest dose of aspirin possible, just effective enough to prevent blood clot, and at the same time minimizing its side effects of gastrointestinal bleeding. Other medications usually taken with low-dose aspirin is omega-3 (fish oil), which should be factored in since fish oil is also a blood thinner.

Should we carry aspirin with us?

Many physicians, myself included, carry 81-mg tablets of aspirin with them every day. The idea is to take 4 tablets (½ the dose for a headache) when severe chest pains occur to prevent a heart attack, and rush to the emergency room. Talk to your physician about this safety precaution because not everyone is a candidate for this regimen.

What are the dangers of aspirin therapy?

The more common side effect of aspirin, even in low-dose of 81 mg several times a week, is upper gastrointestinal bleeding. While the goal is to thin the blood so it does not thicken and form clots which could block arteries to cause heart attack or stroke, in some persons the blood could become too thin and lead to bleeding in the stomach, in the nose, under the skin (ecchymosis), in the urinary bladder, or even in the brain. Although a double-edged sword, low-dose aspirin therapy provides life-saving benefits which outweigh the risk.

Who may be on low-dose aspirin therapy?

Those individuals who had a heart attack or stroke should continue with their low-dose therapy. Men who are 45 to 79, with increased risk of heart attack may be on daily lose-dose aspirin. Women, who are 55 to 79 years of age and in danger of having a stroke from blood clot, are candidates for low-dose aspirin treatment. All the regimen above should be used only under a physician's supervision.

Who should not be on this regimen?

Persons who are 80 years and older have a higher risk of gastrointestinal bleeding and should, therefore, not be on aspirin therapy. Men who are under 45 and women 55 and younger, in general, are not candidates for aspirin therapy because their risk for heart attack and stroke is lower, and the risk of bleeding outweighs the potential cardiovascular benefit. The physician needs to also consider other factors, like family history, in these age groups and customize his/her recommendation.

Who would benefit most from aspirin therapy?

The more risk factors the individuals have (like high blood pressure, diabetes, high cholesterol, family history of heart attack or stroke) the more likely they will benefit from taking low-dose aspirin. In properly selected patients, low-dose aspirin therapy, as an adjunct to a healthy lifestyle, is a boon to the prevention of heart attack and stroke. Most recently, a study show that taking aspirin for at least 5 years can significantly lower the risk of the development of a deadly skin cancer called Melanoma. Aspirin is truly a wonder drug.

Athletic Heart Syndrome

What is athletic heart syndrome?

This is a condition among athletes who show a constellation of physiologic adaptations in the body system, especially in the heart, in persons trained to perform endurance exercise.

What are these changes?

One of them is the so-called resting bradycardia (heart rate below 60 beats per minute). The usual normal heart rate at rest is between 60 and 80, and goes higher with activities. Among conditioned athletes, the heart rate could be as low as 36 or 40, and they feel well. Among non-athletes, a heart rate this slow, which the body is not used to, could lead to dizziness and weakness, or shortness of breath.

What are the other changes?

The others are the presence of a heart murmur, 3rd and 4th heart sounds, a variety of EKG abnormalities, heart enlargement on chest X-ray. Even the muscles of the heart is thicker (hypetrophied), and the four chambers of the heart dilated—all these increase the pumping capability of the heart and increase oxygen delivery to all tissues by increasing stroke volume.

How about their blood count?

The total hemoglobin and blood volume of endurance-trained athletes are also increased, further improving oxygen transport to tissues. In trained athletes, the pressures inside the heart chambers are normal and so with the heart ventricular function.

Do the changes disappear when endurance training is stopped?

Yes, heart enlargement and bradycardia (slow heart rate) regress when the endurance training is stopped.

Do these athletes have abnormal heart rhythm?

Many of them do have atrial and ventricular arrhythmias, or irregularity of heart rhythm. However, while these could cause symptoms in nonathletes, these abnormal rhythm among trained athletes do not cause any symptoms in most of them and may even disappear with exercise. Those with perisistent arrhythmias should be monitored by a physician.

Is strenuous activity harmful to the cardiovascular function?

There is no evidence in the medical literature to suggest that even the most strenuous physical activity is deleterious to the nonathletic person who has normal heart rate and rhythm, and in good physical condition. However, we advise everyone to consult with his/her physician before indulging in strenuous physical activities.

How about sudden deaths in athletes?

Sudden deaths occasionally occur among athletes, both at rest or during exertion, due to the heart (ventricular) rhythm disturbances. In most of these sudden deaths, they were due to undetected arteriosclerotic coronary artery disease, hypertrophic cardiomyopathy, myocarditis (inflammation of the heart), aortic valve abnormality, congenital coronary anomalies, or Brugada's Syndrome as described somewhere in this book. This is the very reason why it is advisable for everyone to consult with his/her physician to get medical clearance before undertaking strenuous physical activity or endurance training.

Do these sudden deaths occur only in older people?

No. There are reports of sudden deaths even among college, high school, or even elementary-grade students. One of the less common illnesses also causing sudden death is a heart rhythm disturbances due to some inherited trait or genetic makeup.

Does this mean sports and exercise should be avoided?

Of course not. These physical activities (sports, exercises) are good to keep both the body and the mind healthy. As long as a medical clearance is obtained and the activities are done in moderation and are reasonable, aerobic exercises, ballroom dancing, sports, etc., are healthy habits to maintain. The advantages and benefits from them outweigh whatever little risk they may pose. Your physician should be able to guide you accordingly in this regard.

Bacteria in Ground Beef

The all-American fast food, the hamburger, has been killing about 60 people a year in the United States alone. And we are not talking about the cardiovascular death toll (one person dies every 60 seconds in the USA) from heart attack and stroke, etc., from a high-saturated-fat-and-cholesterol diet. We are talking about bacteria-contaminated ground beef, and "E. coli burger" is one culprit.

More than 70,000 people get sick every year (2,000 are so ill to require hospitalization) from burger-borne E. coli bacterial gastrointestinal disease, whose incubation period is about 10 days after ingestion.

A study by the US Center for Disease Control and Prevention in 2008 showed that "one in every 200 samples of ground beef was contaminated by E. coli," a bacteria that comes from feces (excreta). Obviously, some meat handlers did not wash their hands (well) after going to the toilet, or other modes of contamination played a role.

Since it is not practical to test each and every ounce of meat because a minute E. coli contamination is enough to make people sick, one way to virtually kill all bugs "is by radiation of the meat, the closest high tech magic bullet" for prevention, say the experts. Numerous studies have confirmed that irradiation of meat is safe and effective, in spite of public doubts. The USADA, which has approved this "magic bullet," needs to counter all myths and campaign to reassure the public once more and save the 70,000 yearly victims of E. coli burger contamination.

In the meantime, we suggest that burgers be cooked "well done" at 160 degrees heat, which kills most bacteria, at burger stands or at home.

Chlorine Dioxide for Bad Breath

What is halitosis?

Halitosis is the medical term for bad breath. Dental reports in the United States say there are about 40 million Americans who have bad breath. This is a rough guesstimate; and the figure, of course, varies in different subgroups in the community. Halitosis, as a general rule, is less among those who live in the city (compared to rural areas); those who are more affluent, higher in socioeconomic status; those who are more educated or professional; and those in the younger generation. Obviously, the financially handicapped could ill afford the luxury of toothpaste, dental floss, mouthwash, regular dental checkup, and proper dental care. They may also be not as well-nourished and as healthy as those who can afford. But realistically, just about anyone, in any profession or walk of life, may have annoying bad breath, persistently or occasionally.

What causes halitosis?

There are a variety of causes of bad breath. Eating food that causes foul breath (like garlic, onion, etc.), poor dental hygiene, decayed tooth or infection of the gums or oral cavity, diseases like diabetes, esophageal diverticulum, esophageal reflux, sinusitis, emphysema, etc. But the commonest underlying cause is poor dental hygiene where care of the teeth and mouth is neglected. There are people who do not brush their teeth at all and go to bed at night with food particles stuck in between their teeth. They may gargle and rinse their mouth with water (or water and salt) after each meal or even use mouthwash, but the food caught in between their teeth (especially meat and fish) rot and stink. This is putrefaction and the foul-smelling odor is from the volatile sulfur compounds (VSC) produced by the decaying meat, which usually results in gram-negative (anaerobic) bacterial infection (and more bad odor), and this makes for a vicious cycle.

Does the tongue harbor bacteria?

Yes, as a matter of fact, the tongue is a major culprit in the causation of bad breath. Bacteria hide in the furrows of the tongue, especially in the back (base) of the tongue. Hence, the regular use of tongue scraper or brushing all the way back to the base of the tongue (till you feel like gagging) at least twice a day is essential.

Can mouthwash eliminate bad breath?

Mouthwash alone cannot do the trick. First, the food particles that can rot must be removed from in-between the teeth immediately after each meal (by dental flossing, since tooth pick alone will not do the job). Then, brushing the teeth using toothpaste (that contains fluoride and other ingredients like poly [methylvinylether maleic acid], copolymer, and triclosan) for added tooth protection, is essential at least 3 times a day, after each meal. Mouthwash (with stabilized chlorine dioxide) can be added to the regimen. A study made on 15 mouthwashes showed that most masked the bad breath for a few minutes; only a few were still effective after a few hours. Those with stabilized chlorine dioxide are impressively effective.

Can mouth containing alcohol cause cancer?

Yes, according to a 1991 study in the *Journal of the American Dental Association*, which stated that mouthwashes "containing more than 25% alcohol could increase the risk of oral and pharyngeal (throat) cancer by 50%." Fortunately, most, if not all, mouthwashes in the market today contain less than 15% alcohol. The safety of chlorine dioxide "has been confirmed by Richardson et al in an extensive study of the reaction of chlorine dioxide with water borne organics by the EPA (Environ. Sci. Technol., 1994;28:592)."

How effective are breath fresheners, sprays, and gums?

If used as a part of the comprehensive regimen we have outlined here, these various forms of breath fresheners could be of help, in between flossing, teeth brushing, and rinsing with stabilized chlorine dioxide mouthwash. Chewing parsley, cilantro, basil, or mint also helps maintain a fresh breath. In general, the incidence of halitosis is less among vegetarians.

Do people know they have bad breath?

It is odd, but most people with chronic halitosis do not know they have it. Their own sense of smell is so conditioned to the bad breath in their mouth to the point that they do not even perceive or know they have halitosis. And their friends and relatives (including most spouses) would not even tell them "to spare" them the embarrassment (which actually leads to more widespread embarrassment because of the persistence of this very offensive but treatable problem, one which can ruin one's reputation, business, and social life.) One trick to find out is by licking your forearm and smelling it. The next time you see your lover or a close friend or relative, beg them to be brutally candid with you and tell you if you have bad breath. This honesty will show them you care and are considerate. This might even change your reputation and love life forever, for the better.

What causes the rotten egg smell?

The rotten egg or decaying meat smell in the breath, brought on by neglected or poor dental and oral care, is caused by hydrogen sulfide, methyl mercaptan, and other volatile sulfur compounds (VSCs) produced by anaerobic bacteria, mostly thriving at the (airless) base of the papillae of the tongue, from front to back, in between the teeth, and in the crevices missed by the toothbrush and dental floss.

What factors lead to halitosis?

The main one is poor dental hygiene and oral (tongue) care. The other factors include thick saliva and dry mouth (from inadequate fluid intake), excess mucus (food for bacteria) in the throat, hormonal changes in women, some medications (for blood pressure pills, decongestants, antihistamines, tetracyclines, sulfas, or antidepressants, etc.), smoking, alcohol (in drinks or in mouthwashes), any gum, sinus or tonsil infection, diet high in proteins (red meat, eggs, dairy products, etc.), or even ketosis (especially when fasting where the body breaks down stored fats to produce energy).

Is drinking milk before bedtime a good practice?

The preference is a personal one and should be followed by tooth-brushing before going to sleep. Except for plain water, nothing else should be taken after one brushes/flosses teeth and scrapes the tongue, before going to bed. Any residual food particles from left in the mouth will "rot" overnight and cause bad breath. Sweets, pop drinks are not only bad for our teeth but aggravate bad breath day or night.

What is the treatment for halitosis?

A visit to the dentist at least every six months, for "preventive maintenance" and cleaning, is vital. Brushing, flossing, and using a tongue scraper after each meal eliminate a lot of the foul-smelling VSCs. Tongue scraping is a *must*. Chewing sugarless gum helps hydrate the mouth, but it is not the solution. Toothpicks are bad for our gums and teeth. Using an effective mouth wash is very important.

Today, there are 3 or 4 truly proven-effective "anti-VSC" mouth rinses, sprays, and toothpastes. The main ingredient in them is stabilized chlorine dioxide. These do not contain alcohol or zinc. Using them 3 times or more a day kills the harmful anaerobic bacteria that irritate the gums and teeth besides causing halitosis. Unlike the common mouthwashes that mask or cover up the bad breath temporarily or not at all, these "anti-VSC" mouth rinses neutralize the effects of the odor-causing volatile sulfur compounds and thus eliminate halitosis almost instantly after gargling for a minute or two. These "new" mouthwashes are indeed one of the wonders in oral care today, when used in conjunction with good regular oral-dental hygiene.

Baldness: Is It a Health Risk?

Baldness, often a subject of jokes and also popularly considered by some women as a symbol of virility, appears to have a more serious implication as far as health risks are concerned.

In a study on more than 22, 000 men ages 40 to 84, published in the *Archives of Internal Medicine*, the findings suggest that "men with male-pattern baldness may be at increased risk for heart disease."

"Compared to men with no hair loss, those with severe vertex baldness (balding at the crown of the head) had a 36% increased risk of heart disease; men with moderate crown balding had a 32% increased risk, while mild balding on the crown carried a 23% increased risk . . . Men with frontal baldness had a 9% increased risk."

The correlation was especially evident in men with vertex baldness whose cholesterol level or blood pressure was high. Baldness is a nonmodifiable health risk, unlike smoking or eating high-fat diet; so hair-loss remedies, like Rogaine or Propecia, might improve the look but won't reduce the risk to heart disease.

Another health risk related to baldness is the increased risk for cancer of the prostate, according to the US National Cancer Institute of the National Institute of Health Division of Cancer Epidemiology. Their study on 4,421 men with male-pattern baldness (ages 25 to 75) without history of cancer of prostate revealed that the risk for prostatic cancer was significantly elevated among these men, compared to their peers with abundant hair.

Physicians now use male-pattern baldness as an early clinical marker or indicator of susceptibility to heart disease and prostatic cancer.

How common is baldness?

Baldness affects approximately 40 million men and 20 million women in the United States. Male-pattern baldness is recession of the hairline from the forehead upward and back, thinning or fallout from the crown of the head, leaving a horseshoe-shaped hair mass around the sides and back of the head. Female-pattern baldness is a diffuse hair loss throughout the scalp. Even Julius Caesar, according to legend, used the ceremonial wreath of laurel leaves as a crown to hide his baldness.

What causes baldness?

About 95% of hair loss is caused by a hereditary condition called androgenetic alopecia. DHT is dihydrotestosterone, which comes from a male hormone called androgen, which circulates in the bloodstream. Androgen is converted to DHT by an enzyme called 5-alpha reductase. Those with more reductase activity have more DHT binding to the hair follicle receptors, which adversely affects hair follicles, until the follicles wither away.

How does one know if he/she will have baldness?

All men have to do is to look at their father's hair, and the women, at their mother's hair, since baldness or thinning hair is strongly hereditary. Of course, there are some other medical conditions that could affect the future of one's hair besides genetics.

Does baldness mean premature aging?

No, there are many bald men who could perhaps look younger with a set of hair on them; but physiologically, they are as young or as old as their chronological age. Their life span is normal also.

What is the normal rate of hair loss?

Normally, we lose about 100 hairs a day, and they regenerate, unless a person has a tendency to baldness or has an illness that affects hair growth.

What is alopecia areata?

This is a condition due to autoimmune disease of unknown cause, where inflammatory cells attack the bulbs of the hair follicles under the scalp, resulting in hairless patches or areas of baldness, hence "areata." While baldness only hurts one's psyche, some of the causes of hair loss may signal a health problem, like alopecia areata. This is why consulting with one's physician is essential.

Could hair fall out from the entire head at once?

Yes, in more serious cases, which luckily is not very common, hair may actually fall out of the entire head, eyebrows and beard included, and hair from the rest of the body. In many cases, though, hair spontaneously regrows.

What medical conditions can cause hair loss?

Severe malnutrition, childbirth, thyroid problems, a form of lupus, and, more popularly, total hair loss can be seen among cancer patients following chemotherapy.

Can pigtails or cornrows cause hair loss?

Yes, if worn too long, pigtails or cornrows can lead to hair loss due to the stress to the hair shaft.

Can mental stress lead to hair loss?

Psychological stress has been reported to have caused hair loss but only at times of extreme emotional trauma. The medical community doubts the role of emotional stress as a significant factor in the causation of baldness. Sudden appearance of spots or areas of premature gray hair in some people who were under severe personal stress is not uncommon.

Does using hair dryers/blowers cause hair loss?

No, not if you do it with the normal care. If you use too much heat and for prolonged periods, it could damage the hair and even burn the scalp.

How about hair coloring?

There is no medical evidence to show that coloring hair with commercial hair dyes available in the market causes baldness. Even the previous theory that using hair coloring caused cancer has not been scientifically proven.

Do herbal potions or lotions help prevent hair loss?

No, there is no known cream or ointment, lotion, or potion, mousses, gel, volumizers, or shampoo that can prevent baldness, much less cure them. The US Food and Drug Administration has banned all these over-the-counter salves in 1989. The only two things that will surely grow when you use these costly preparations are your expenses and the bank accounts of the manufacturers and dealers.

Do multivitamins and minerals prevent hair loss?

No, except in very rare instances where multivitamin/mineral deficiencies are severe and aggravating the malnutrition present. In general, we believe that daily multivitamin/mineral supplements are good for health maintenance and general well-being.

What can be done then?

The FDA approved medication Rogaine (minoxidil-based) has been claimed to have led to moderate hair regrowth after four months in 26% of men between 18 and 49. An additional 39% had some regrowth. In women, about 20% had moderate regrowth among those 18 and 45 years of age plus an additional 40% with minimal regrowth. Hair (micro or minigraft) transplantation and the use of hairpieces (toupees and wigs) are the two other options. State-of-the-art hair transplant centers have had great successes with most natural-looking hair growths. Synthetic hair transplant has been legally banned by the FDA because of the attendant complications and dangers. In today's society, baldness is well-accepted and so is the use of hairpieces or hair transplants.

How about the related health risks mentioned above?

The prudent way is to minimize all modifiable health risks, like cigarette smoking, excess alcohol intake, high-cholesterol and high-fat diet, a sedentary lifestyle, and unmanaged stress. This strategy for a healthier lifestyle will also help counter the increased risk for heart disease and prostate cancer among all individuals, including those men with male-pattern baldness.

Ballroom Dancing

Is ballroom dancing good for everyone?

For the majority of people who love to dance, ballroom dancing is one of the best exercises for cardiovascular fitness. Only those with medical or physical impairment that disable them to dance will not benefit from it. While walking on the treadmill or doing rowing exercises makes one feel he/she is engaging in a boring "forced labor," dancing provides the exercise with much more fun and social enjoyment that one even loses, not only calories, but track of time.

Who should not indulge in ballroom dancing?

Anyone with physical disability or medical condition (heart disease, untreated or uncontrolled high blood pressure, severe emphysema, dizziness, etc.) that would make one severely short of breath and/ or have chest pains or simply feeling not well after a couple of minutes of physical activities should not indulge in ballroom dancing. The most prudent to do, if you have an illness or if have any doubt, is to have a good medical checkup and clearance by your physician before going ballroom dancing.

How much calories does one lose doing ballroom dancing?

Energy dissipated or calories lost during any physical activity is a function of time, how much one weighs, how vigorous one performs the activity, and the environmental temperature. Medical research shows that, on the average situation, one loses about 200 calories doing fast dancing (for instance the swing or boogie) nonstop for 30 minutes. Medium aerobics for half an hour burn about 197.4 calories. Walking (4 mph) for half an hour consumes about 155 calories. Foreplay and actual sex burns a total of 90 calories. For total cardiovascular fitness, one should have a daily regimen of aerobics and/or walking and/or ballroom dancing.

Is ballroom dancing better than jogging?

Yes, most definitely. In the '60s and early '80s, the experts recommended jogging as "the best exercise for cardiovascular fitness." Following enough experience in this form of activity—which showed attendant injuries to bones, joints, etc., in the feet, legs and hips and spine—the experts changed to a new recommendation: ambulation, the simple, unadulterated old-fashioned exercise, walking, the benefits of which were well-known to our parents, grandparents, and even to our great-grandparents. Common sense dictates this, and yet we had to go through extensive medical studies to find out and convince ourselves about something that was obvious. Jogging 5.5 mph for 30 minutes burns 294 calories,

or ten calories a minute.

Is there an age limit for people to do ballroom dancing?

No. The oldest couple I know is in their 80s now who are still actively doing ballroom dancing, using it as their "cardiac rehabilitation exercise." Age is, indeed, a matter of mind and not of time. As long as one is feeling well and able to do activities, like ballroom dancing or fast walking, and has no medical contraindication, one should continue to do so, not only for cardiovascular fitness but also for social and mental health.

Bariatric Surgery

More than a 33% of Americans are overweight or obese. This has transformed a surgical procedure that was once reserved for a handful of dangerously obese patients to a very popular operation the past few years. In 2005 alone, there were about 200,000 surgical weight-loss procedures that were performed. In the United States, gastric bypass has been the most popular one. Some surgeons now claim that gastric "banding" is a safer, just as effective, and has lesser side effects and complications as gastric bypass. The least favored procedure is called bilio-pancreatic diversion/duodenal switch, an operation even much more complicated than its name sounds.

What is bariatric surgery?

Stated simply, bariatric surgery is the general term used for operative procedures performed on the stomach and the small intestine to enable the obese patient to lose weight more expeditiously and maintain as normal a weight as possible long-term for better health.

What is done in gastric bypass?

There are two basic things done in this procedure: (1) stapling the stomach to make a small stomach pouch (reduced to about 5% surface area), thus reducing the stomach volume by 95%, so the absorbing area is 95% less, allowing only 5% of the food absorbed; and (2) bypassing a small part of the upper intestinal tract. These two procedures make the patient feel full faster and with a small amount of food in that small pouch. This also reduces the appetite, besides reducing the calories absorbed. The procedure carries a 1.5%-2% death rate. About 75% to 80% of all bariatric surgeries in the USA involve gastric bypass.

How effective is gastric bypass?

The Roux-en-Y gastric bypass procedure is very effective, allowing the patient to lose 65% to 75% of the excess weight. Eating more calories than the prescribed diet will obviously negate or reduce the effectiveness of the surgery.

What is gastric banding?

The second most common (15%-20%) slim-down surgery in the United States is called gastric banding, also known as "lap band" and "adjustable gastric band." This is a surgical procedure where a hollow silicone "band" is placed over the top of the stomach and inflated with saline (salt) solution to compress that part of the stomach to restrict the amount of food that can get in and pass thru the stomach. In Europe, this is the procedure of choice. Unlike gastric bypass or other weight-loss surgeries, gastric banding is fully reversible (the band can be removed) and has the lowest mortality (death) rate of one-tenth of 1%. The only downside is that adjustments are needed to maintain its effectiveness, and the band can erode into the stomach over time. Also, the weight loss is achieved over a longer period of time, because it does not include a bypass component. It will take banding four to five years to achieve what gastric bypass can do in a year. However, some physicians, especially in Europe, think this is a more "physiological and safer" way to lose weight.

What is bilio-pancreatic diversion/duodenal switch?

The least common of the 3 procedures, this diversion-switch procedure has the highest mortality (2.5% to 5%) and the riskiest as far and malnutrition and death are concerned. This slim-down surgery results in 60% to 80% loss of excess weight in one year.

Who are candidates for bariatric surgery?

Not all people who have excess weight or who would like to have a slimmer body are candidates for weight-loss surgery. The sequelae (aftermaths) and possible complications are too significant a price to pay for aesthetic vanity. The appropriate medical indication is reserved for persons who have a BMI (body mass index) of 40, or a BMI OF over 35 only among those patients with weight-related diseases, like diabetes or high blood pressure.

What are the possible complications of weight-loss surgeries?

Bariatric surgery alters the natural body physiology of food transit and absorption and as such has attendant side effects and possible complications.

Foremost among them are gas, abdominal pain, diarrhea, and reduced appetite, and in some cases, nausea and vomiting, leading to malnutrition and deficiency in minerals and vitamins, like calcium, iron, B1, B12, etc. Osteoporosis is a possible complication. Severe thiamine (B-1) deficiency could lead to Wernicke's encephalopathy, a brain dysfunction syndrome that was often hard to diagnosis among these patients before. With greater experience with these procedures, the index of suspicion is much higher today on this syndrome. The symptoms may include mental confusion, abnormal eye movement, muscle weakness, and movement incoordination, which could result in permanent disability. Hearing loss from vitamin deficiency has also been reported as a possible complication.

How do we avoid this surgery?

While some obesity may be hormonal in nature, majority of overweight problems are due to self-abuse, too much food—especially carbs, like rice, pop beverages, and sweets—and too little or no exercise at all. If we take full control of our lifestyle to safeguard our health, eat just enough to maintain our normal weight, and do daily regimented exercises, we will not need any of these painful and expensive surgeries.

OPCAB: Beating Heart Surgery

What is OPCAB?

OPCAB stands for off-pump coronary artery bypass surgery, which is the most popular minimally invasive heart bypass operation today, one that is done on a beating heart. Conventionally, coronary bypass is done on an arrested heart (chemically induced cardiac arrest to allow for a quiet field) with the patient connected to a heart-lung machine (pump) that temporarily takes over the oxygenation (lung function) and circulation (heart function) of the patient while the surgery is going on.

Is OPCAB better?

If at all possible, OPCAB, or beating heart surgery, is preferred. Doing the coronary bypass on a beating (non-arrested) heart precludes the use of the heart-lung machine. This pump has the potential of destroying some blood cells, of wasting some essential clotting factors in the blood, and of forming blood clots or air bubbles that could cause stroke, albeit very rare. So not using the heart-lung machine is a definite advantage, much less invasive and stressful for the patient. As a result, OPCAB patients recover a lot faster, go home much sooner, usually after 3-4 days after surgery. However, OPCAB is not for everyone.

How is the heart stilled?

With the patient connected to the pump, the heart is arrested by lowering the body temperature (thru blood cooling using a special cooler machine connected to the pump) down to about 28-30 degrees centigrade and by giving the patient a high dose of potassium chloride which stops the heartbeat in a relaxed (flabby) muscular state. This allows the cardiac surgeon to make tiny (2 mm-4 mm) anastomoses (suturing together two arteries or a vein and an artery of the heart, like sewing a sleeve to the shirt, an end-to-side or T-connection) using a magnifying surgical loop (special eyeglasses for an enlarged view) on a nonbeating heart.

How are blockages diagnosed?

The stenoses (narrowing) or occlusion (total blockage) of the coronary arteries are diagnosed with the aid of coronary angiogram (also referred to as cardiac catheterization), where a spaghetti-sized catheter is inserted into the femoral (groin) artery under local anesthesia and its tip directed to the opening of the left and right main coronary arteries. Dye is injected into the coronary arteries and the whole procedure is recorded in a video movie. This will show the dye in motion, the diameter and integrity of the lumen (inner channel) of the arteries, and whether there are blockages or none.

Why not do this test on everyone?

While cardiac catheterization is a safe procedure done daily in various heart centers around the world, it has potential complications like transient irregular heart rhythm, blood clots, arterial leak, disruption in the wall of the artery, bleeding at the puncture site in the groin. While these are rare, there is a golden rule in medicine that says tests, in general, must only be done if there is an clinical indication (justification). If a person has no symptoms or strong family history of heart disease, cardiac catheterization is not recommended. Just about the only exceptions could be an employer required executive check-up, or airline mandated test for commercial pilots. Besides, this is an expensive procedure and insurance companies do not consider this to be a reimbursable prophylactic test.

How is OPCAB done?

With the patient under general anesthesia, the chest is split in the middle, from the base of the neck down to about the tail of the sternum (breastbone), same as in the conventional technique. With OPCAB, the patient is not connected to a heart lung machine. There is a special instrument (cardiac stabilizer) that minimizes the heart action in the area of the artery to be bypassed. The rest of the heart continues to beat. This stabilizer restricts the contraction of the heart in the target area, allowing the cardiac surgeon to do his suturing, aided by a surgical loop for magnified (3-4 times) view. With beating heart surgery, the patient does not feel so zapped, rundown, and tired compared to the standard procedure where heart lung machine and cardiac arrest are used.

Does every heart surgeon do OPCAB?

No. Only those who had additional training on this particular technique perform beating-heart surgery. It is a more tedious procedure and more difficult for the surgeon but much easier on the patient. Putting sutures on tiny arteries while the heart is beating is just like "shooting a tiny moving target." A surgeon has to "retrain" his mind and hands and get used to this cutting-edge technology to be able to do OPCAB. I had to undergo such hands-on OPCAB surgical training at the Boston University Hospital in Massachusetts, under Dr. R. Cohn, the inventor of the genzyme cardiac stabilizer. My team and I did our first OPCAB on a 68-year-old man from California on June 8, 1999. Only a little more than 60% of heart surgeons today perform OPCAB procedures.

Is the conventional bypass obsolete?

Most definitely not. There are still a large number of patients who could be better served with the conventional on-pump heart bypass. As I stated earlier, OPCAB is not for everyone. But the trend shows more and more coronary bypass procedures are being done on beating hearts today. It stands to reason that OPCAB is here to stay.

Big-breakfast Myth

Eating a big breakfast will help people lose weight—fact or fiction?

It is a common belief that eating a full breakfast aids in calorie and weight control, and that it is a healthy practice.

A recent German study disproved the notion that ingesting a large meal in the morning staves off hunger longer and reduces caloric intake during lunch and dinner and helps in weight control. The findings showed that eating a huge breakfast only increases the total caloric intake for the day and did not reduce intake during lunch and dinner.

Eating a cup of oatmeal or other high-fiber, low-sugar bran cereals, with a serving of fruit and a glass or two of water, instead of rice or bread with eggs and meats (bacon, ham, or sausage), is healthier breakfast that is within 400 calories.

For those who are overweight trying to control their intake, a glass of milk and/or coffee plus a couple of glasses of water for breakfast can work wonders, so long as they do not compensate in the next two meals and go beyond their total daily caloric limit. Diabetics must likewise be within their prescribed diet.

A healthy lifestyle, which confers a superior quality of life and longevity, requires a lot of discipline and determination. But the great dividend is all worth it.

What Causes BO?

Body odor, medically termed bromhidrosis, ozopchrotia, and osmidrosis, is very common. This embarrassing condition is gives off an unpleasant scent of foul-smelling sweat.

The offensive smell is caused by the bacterial breakdown of body protein into propionic acid or isovaleric acid. We have bacteria all over our body. Frequent shower/washings reduce their presence. Under normal condition, we have a certain bacterial count on our skin, especially in the armpits, mouth and tongue, genital area, groin, behind the ear, eyelids, nose, breasts, belly button, feet, etc. Those who are obese or are diabetics are more prone to body odor. Of course, those with poor hygiene are harbinger of severe body odor.

Normally, we have our individual body odor from our natural pheromones. This gives us our sexually stimulating scent to the opposite sex and affect how we react to each other. It is when bacterial breakdown takes place due to hygienic reason, genetic predisposition to sweating, or for health reasons that offensive body odor (mostly sweat from the apocrine glands of our body) results.

Personal cleanliness, including daily complete shower, total facial hygiene (mouth, tongue, teeth, ear, nose), keeping feet clean and dry, and perhaps the use of antiperspirant/deodorant are the mainstay of preventive regimen against BO. Those with resistant and persistent offensive body odor should seek medical advice for any underlying medical condition causing the problem.

Dangers of Body Art

What is body art?

Body Art is a popular fad among adolescents and young adults, which includes tattooing or body-part piercing. The tattoos are usually on the chest, arms, belly, butts, ankles, or on just about any area of the body. They come in different shapes, design, color, and various objects, like a girl, snake, flag, heart, words of protest, or love messages. It is estimated that 10% to 25% of young adults (25 and under) have at least one tattoo.

What is body piercing?

Piercing the septum of the nose, the eyebrow, jaw, lips, upper part of the ears, the skin of the arm or leg, or the skin of the belly button to wear a dangling piece of jewelry. Physicians have attended to infected pierced skin of the genitalia with a custom diamond stud.

How prevalent is body art?

A survey in one university involving 454 students (236 females and 218 males), which was 14% of the total enrollment, revealed that 23% (106) of them had one to three tattoos. This could well mirror the prevalence in other schools and universities in the country, perhaps higher in big cities, compared to the conservative communities. The most popular sites were the back among women and the arms and hands among men. One hundred twenty-nine (51%) of those surveyed had a least one body piercing, 90% of men having had ears pierced, and 54% of the females had pierced navel, 49% ears and 27%, the tongue. Some of both the males and females had pierced nipples, eyebrows, and genitalia.

What complications can arise from body art?

Infection of the tattooed or pierced skin, transmission of hepatitis B and C, and HIV (AIDS) with either procedure. Allergic reaction, besides pain, swelling, and bleeding, are potential complications of tattooing or body piercing. Keloid and scar formation is another. Infection is common because the needle and instruments used for tattooing or body piercing are mostly not medically sterile. A significant number of patients with hepatitis subsequently develop hepatoma, cancer of the liver, which is deadly.

When are these sequelae noted?

The allergic reaction can be observed after exposure to the sun, which leads to severe itching, redness and swelling. Some people are allergic to the dye used in tattooing. Infection takes at least a couple of days before becoming evident.

How is infection of pierced body parts treated?

Infection of pierced body part is managed by removing the foreign body irritant (jewelry, etc.) inside the pierced area, washing the part well with water and perhaps disinfectant, and application of topical triple-antibiotic ointment to the infected hole. For severe infection, wound debridement (cutting out rotting tissues) and oral or IV antibiotics may be needed.

Are stick-on "tattoos" safer?

Yes, most definitely. Stick-on "tattoos" are work of art in themselves. They are colorful, beautifully designed, and fairly inexpensive. For those who want to wear "tattoos" for special occasions, because of peer pressure or simply to impress a friend, using the stick-on body art is a lot safer and healthier. Besides, you can wash and peel them off fast anytime you wish.

Body weight and calories

Today, more than ever, people are more health conscious; and since food greatly impacts our health, we are also interested to know how much calories are contained in a certain portion of each food items we choose to eat. It's just like watching our budget for our financial health.

Calorie is the amount of energy in food/drink we ingest and also the energy consumed or lost with any bodily activity. The more we eat, the more calories we absorbed into our body. The more we exercise we perform, the more we burn or lose calories. The balance in the calorie intake and output determines whether we maintain, lose or gain weight.

To find out how much one's total calorie requirement (TCR) is, one must compute his/her ideal body weight (IBW). The Tannhauser formula will give us the answer. IBW (in kg) = (height in cm minus 100) less 10%. Example: If a person is 5 foot 2 inches, the height in centimeter is (62 inches x 2.54) or 157.48 cm. So 157.48 minus 100 = 57.48. And 57.48 minus 10% (or 5.748) equals to 51.73 or about 52 kg is the IBW.

Now that we know the IBW, we must find out the level of physical activity of the person. Using the Krause formula, the standard average calories burned are as follows: sedentary, just sitting behind the desk, 30 calories; average housewife chores, 40; carpenter, 45.

To find out the TCR, multiply the IBW with the physical activity, say, sedentary. So TCR in this example will be 52 kg x 30, or 1560 calories per day. This energy is what is required to maintain the body weight, no loss, no gain. In general, the average calorie requirement per day ranges between 1,500 and 2,000.

Eating 500 calories more a day (in excess of the total calorie requirement) will make a person gain one pound in a week, and conversely, eating 500 calories less than the TCR per day will reduce one pound from the person's body weight in a week.

The average calories burned in 30-minute of any of these activities are as follows: sleeping, 35; typing on computer, 50; ironing, 63; cooking, 86; light housework, 115; mopping floor,119; lovemaking, 90; shopping, 102; fishing, 119; climbing hills (no load), 232; walking slowly, 106; walking briskly, 120; running slowly, 280; running fast, 384; jogging, 215; cycling, 123; swimming, 311; ballroom dancing, 98; aerobic dancing, 198; volleyball, 96; football, 253; basketball, 265; golf, 140; tennis, 209; and, badminton, 186.

As the above data show, it takes a lot of work, a lot of physical exercise, to lose even a pound, and so much easier, so fast, to gain weight. Calorie awareness is essential to good health.

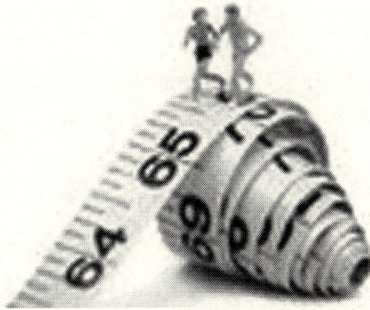

Brain Aneurysm

One of the most treacherous and challenging medical conditions is brain aneurysm, especially the leaking or ruptured variety.

What is a brain aneurysm?

The medical word *aneurysm* means ballooning out of an artery, causing the affected wall of the artery to stretch (from the high pressure inside it) to form a "bubble," whose wall is thinner (and weaker) than normal. So brain aneurysm, also called intracerebral or intracranial aneurysm, is a medical condition where the cerebral artery in the brain has formed such "bubble." This can happen to any artery in the brain, but usually the arteries that cross between the base of the skull and the undersurface of the brain are the ones involved.

What causes it?

Majority of brain aneurysms are congenital, an inborn genetic predisposition which makes them prone to such arterial wall weakness and "bubble" formation in the brain artery, which is riskier among those with high blood pressure. The out pouching or ballooning usually forms at the site where the artery branches off. Brain aneurysms are more prevalent among those with genetic illnesses, like connective tissue disorders, polycystic kidneys, and arteriovenous malformations. Other causes include infection in the wall of the artery, trauma, tumors, hardening of the arteries, cigarette smoking, drug abuse, and the use of oral contraceptives have been suspected to increase the risk of development of cerebral aneurysms.

How common is it?

Cerebral aneurysm is not uncommon. Up to about 4% of autopsies revealed the present of cerebral aneurysm, and about 5% of people will have brain aneurysm during their life. Ten percent of them will have a rupture (aneurysm bursting). A rough estimate reports that annually between 25,000 and 50,000 people in the United States will have a brain hemorrhage due to ruptured brain aneurysm. The incidence is higher among women and among African-Americans.

What are the symptoms?

Quite often a brain aneurysm goes undetected, without causing any problem, without any symptoms. The first sign shows when the aneurysm ruptures, usually a sudden severe headache, the worst the individual has ever experienced in the past. Some other symptoms might include nausea, dizziness, sensitivity to light, neck pains, fainting, seizures, and in some cases, patients lapse into comma. Thirty percent to 50% of patients suffer minor bleeds (called "warning leaks") which later eventually lead to a massive brain hemorrhage a few days after the episodes.

What is the "peak age" for rupture?

Statistically, the highest incidence of rupture is found among persons in their middle age (in their 40s and 50s), but it could happen at any age, even among teenagers with cerebral aneurysm.

What condition can mimic brain aneurysm?

A congenital vascular defect known as arteriovenous (AV) malformation is a condition that could mimic brain aneurysm. It can also lead to vascular rupture and cause brain hemorrhage. However, the pathology here is an abnormal connection between an artery and a vein in the brain. Normally, there is no connection between an artery and a vein, except at their terminal endings. The clinical presentation in AV malformation is very similar to brain aneurysm.

How does one prevent a disaster?

The way to reduce the danger from an aneurysm requires prompt diagnosis and surgical or minimally-invasive intervention. The following would be helpful: living a healthy lifestyle, no smoking, moderation in alcohol intake, avoidance of heavy exertions, and effective treatment of high blood pressure, if present. Persons with recurrent headaches should seek prompt medical checkup, and those with high blood pressure should be treated promptly and continuously.

When does one seek medical consultation?

When brain aneurysm is suspected, the best thing to do is to seek immediate medical treatment. If the diagnosis is confirmed and surgery is deemed feasible, it is the best option to take. Two procedures used to stop the bleeding include microvascular clipping (where the leaking artery is clipped during surgery) and an alternative to surgery, a less invasive procedure called endovascular embolization, where a coil is inserted into the leaking artery to cause clotting within the artery, thereby stopping the hemorrhage.

What's the prognosis?

Unfortunately, the outcome is not very certain. When the cerebral artery bursts and causes brain hemorrhage, sudden death can result. The mortality rate following a rupture is about 40%, and another 25% die from complications. Prognostication in this condition is medically difficult since many variable factors come into play. When a window of opportunity presents itself to allow institution of prompt medical treatment, the prognosis becomes better. Once definitive treatment, either with clipping or embolization, is initiated, the outlook significantly improves. A healthy lifestyle, together with vigilance about health, is fundamental.

Minimally Invasive Brain Surgery

The trend in surgery today is toward minimally invasive techniques, all geared for patient comfort, lesser blood loss, lesser pain, lesser morbidity, shorter hospital stay, faster recovery, with much less obvious scars. In neurosurgery, a revolutionary endoscopic approach also enhances a surgeon's ability to reach critical areas of the brain and spine. Minimally invasive surgery must still be "maximally effective" to attain its major purpose. These procedures are performed by surgeons specially trained in minimally invasive surgery.

Our guest consultant today is Dr. Jeremy D. W. Greenlee, MD, assistant professor in neurosurgery, University of Iowa Hospitals and Clinics, a specialist in minimally invasive neurosurgery, who provided us the answers to these most frequently asked questions below:

What are the goals of minimally invasive surgery?

In minimally invasive neurosurgery, the goals are the same as those of any traditional brain and spine surgery, such as to completely remove a tumor or relieve pressure on a pinched nerve, or drain an infection, but with the added goals of minimizing postoperative pain, shortening hospital stay, expediting return to normal lifestyle, and achieving excellent cosmetic results.

Are all minimally invasive surgeries the same?

No. For example, in cases of very large blood clots over the surface of the brain from trauma, or large tumors near the surface of the brain, it is not possible to safely and effectively achieve the main goal of the operation (complete removal) through tiny incisions. A long skin incision can still be considered a minimally invasive surgery if the incision that is used is the shortest possible incision that allows the safe completion of the operation and the least amount of normal tissue disruption, or "collateral damage" in the process.

What are examples of minimally invasive neurosurgeries?

An example is the removal of tumors at the base of the brain (like pituitary tumors) by working through the nose (endonasal surgery), therefore avoiding any skin incision at all. Another example is using a small camera (endoscope) for removal of tumors or cysts within the brain using only a tiny (1/2 inch) opening in the skull. Yet another example is operating on the spine through tubular retractor systems so that only 1 1/2 inch or shorter incisions are necessary to successfully remove herniated disks, relieve pinched nerves, or fuse vertebrae together.

What other advantages does "minimally invasive" offer?

The conventional practice requires shaving of hair prior to undergoing brain surgery. Studies have shown that "shaveless" surgery does not increase a patient's risk of infection compared to shaving large areas of hair around incisions. Minimally invasive technique use dissolving skin stitches or skin glue to repair the skin incision so that no stitches or staples have to be taken out once the skin is healed. This lets the patient avoid a trip to the doctor's office and the slight discomfort of the removal. Another advantage is the use of intraoperative "guidance" or "navigation" systems, which are used by surgeons during procedures to allow the mapping of brain tumors prior to starting surgery. These "GPS-like" systems can serve as roadmaps to know exactly where tumors sit relative to the scalp and therefore facilitate planning the smallest-possible skin incision and bony opening (craniotomy) necessary for tumor removal. While these are technical considerations, they nonetheless provide better quality of care and comfort for the patient.

Is a minimally invasive surgery more risky than a traditional surgery?

Minimally invasive surgery should not be performed at the expense of achieving the main goal of the procedure and should not add any risk to the patient if done properly. In fact, some minimally invasive surgeries have been shown to *reduce* risks compared to the traditional techniques. Overall, it is much less invasive, as the name suggests.

Are there surgeons that specialize in minimally invasive surgery?

Yes. Some surgeons spend significant time training to learn these special techniques. As with any surgery, experience with the technique is important so that the surgeon's movements are refined and both the surgeon and assistants are familiar with the special instruments that are needed for minimally invasive procedures.

How can I find a surgeon that performs these procedures?

There are several ways. The best is probably simply asking around your area—family, friends, your regular doctors, nurses in their office, etc., who may have first-hand experience with a particular surgeon. Another way would be to do online Internet searches. Patient support groups can be found for almost any diagnosis. Talking with other patients that have already "gone through it" can be comforting to newly diagnosed patients in need of surgery. Keep in mind that is there very good information available on the Internet as well as incorrect information too.

Will my insurance cover minimally invasive surgery?

Insurance coverage should not be any different than for traditional techniques. However, it is always a good idea to discuss the surgery, as well as preoperative and postoperative care with your plan provider. In addition, it is recommended, and in most plans required, to get preauthorization as coverage plans can vary widely.

What other questions should I ask my surgeon?

Patients should always understand the risks and benefits of their medical treatments, whether it is a drug prescribed to them or a surgery recommended to them. Ask enough questions so that the goals of surgery are clear, expectations are realistic, and possible complications are reviewed. Ask if the surgeon incorporates minimally invasive techniques or if a minimally invasive alternative exists for that procedure.

Is there surgery for Parkinson's disease?

One of the recent advances in the management of Parkinson's disease is a minimally invasive procedure called deep brain stimulation (DBS). DBS is also being used for other movement disorders such as essential tremor and dystonia. Two electrodes are implanted, one on each side of the brain, and these are connected to a battery pack (like a cardiac pacemaker) placed under the skin in the upper chest. A handheld magnetic device is used to adjust the settings until an optimal balance is achieved to effectively control the tremors. DBS can be a life-changing treatment, transforming a helpless person with such severe tremor that they cannot feed themselves or drink into an independent, self-sufficient person. This dramatic change occurs within seconds of activating the DBS unit. In some cases, no tremor is even visible! As a result, patients can be more hopeful and positive. While the patient needs to continue taking their medications, DBS is a great solution for now until the final cure for these conditions are found. Currently, DBS is being investigated for possible use in the treatment of depression, obesity, Alzheimer's, and epilepsy. Indeed, the future holds a lot of promise in almost every facet of our life.

Breastfeeding and Its Magic

One of the wonders of nature is the inherent ability of the mother after giving birth to produce milk and sustain her young by breastfeeding. Interestingly, in human and among other mammals, the newborn comes with the instinct of sucking and searching for the nipple; and the mother's breasts at that point in time, through a most sophisticated postpartum hormonal physiology, are generally ready to manufacture milk for the baby. All this happens so naturally and so efficiently coordinated that we might deduce that breastfeeding not only provides nutrition for daily sustenance but more essential ingredients for long-term survival of the species.

Evidently, the ancient history of breastfeeding in early humans (among *Homo sapiens* or extinct species of hominids more than 2.4 million years ago) started with the very first baby of the very first couple on earth. They had undoubtedly observed various animals around them breastfeeding their young.

During those times, when the mother died during childbirth or from disease or accident, the baby was left to die, unless the prevailing social dynamics at the area allowed "group nursing," breastfeeding by other lactating women within the same tribe. Wet nursing, where only one woman feeds the baby, was and is practiced even today in many cultures. In the absence of lactating women, the motherless infant was fed animal milk. Apparently "formula feeding" started then too and is not a modern invention.

It was in the 1800 when physicians and scientists started studies to find out the best baby-food mixes, and in 1867, the first commercial baby food created by Justus von Liebig came out. Since then many other brands and types have been marketed.

The convenience of the formula, hyped up to be modern and better, attracted mothers who eventually chose them over breastfeeding. As a result, more than 50% of the babies were fed baby formula by 1950. Twenty years later, better-informed and more health-conscious women decided to "go back to the basic." Breastfeeding became popular once again, especially among the educated mothers.

The concepts and practices in feeding the baby have changed since the first newborn. However, one fundamental scientific principle remains: breastfeeding for at least two years, as recommended by the World Health Organization, or *at least* 12 months as practiced in the United States, confers great benefits to the child.

Tons and years of research have shown that mother's breast milk is best. It is the perfect food for her baby. No commercial or animal's milk can equal the quality of breast milk, the only one which contains valuable ingredients that boost the baby's immune system, providing it antibodies that fight diseases, and is nonallergenic and less expensive. Breastfeeding also strengthens the mother-child bonding, which studies have shown results in more secure children with 30% less behavioral and social problems when they start school.

Bottle Feeding Boosts Obesity Risk

Infants who are still bottle-fed at age two have increased risk of being obese by the time they reach 5, according to a new research involving 6,750 children in the Early Childhood Longitudinal Study, Birth Cohort, which included children born in 2001 in the United States.

Twenty-three percent of children who were still feeding off from a bottle at age 2 were obese by age 5 ½, while only 16% of those who stopped using a bottle by age two were severely overweight. Obviously, the bottle encouraged more uncontrolled calorie intake as reported in this study in *The Journal of Pediatrics*.

Authorities in nutrition for children suggest weaning them from the bottle around age 12 to 14 months, which will also avoid tooth decay from putting the child to bed with a bottle, besides iron-deficiency anemia.

Solid Foods

Babies are introduced to solid foods at age 4 to 6 months, which will eventually be the main source of nutrition for the baby. A one-year-old will usually require about 10 to 16 ounces of whole milk a day, supplemented by a variety of healthy table foods, like fish, vegetables, and fruits. Vegetable and fruit juices should be limited to 4 ounces a day, and the rest of the liquid should be filtered water. If fish, vegetables, and fruits are well-tolerated, red meat is not a necessity.

For parents who have problems with weaning a child from the bottle, consultation with their pediatrician is recommended. A transition from a bottle to a cup might help staging the withdrawal.

The ultimate goal

The surgeon general of the United States in 2010 set the following goal: 75% of the babies breastfed when they leave the hospital, 50% of babies still on breast milk at 6 months of age, and 25% of babies still being breastfed *after* 1 year of age.

The American Academy of Pediatrics in 1997 advocated breastfeeding "for at *least* 12 months and *thereafter* as mutually desired."

Hopefully, all mothers will breastfeed their baby up at least age 6 months, preferably to age one, or even age two.

The countless benefits children derived from breastfeeding during those months of significant growth in their brain and all other organs in their body are immeasurable and priceless.

The powerful magic ingredients in the mother's milk cannot be found in any supermarket or pharmacy at any cost.

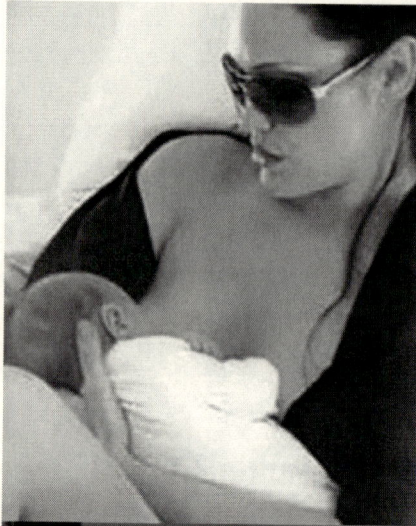

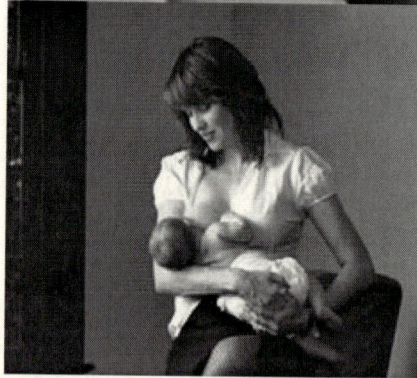

Breastfeeding babies confers more than just a superior healthy nutrition for the infant, a boost to its developing immune system and bonding between mother and child. There is more it provides the young than what today's science is able to determine. Breastfeeding is very popular, even among celebrities like Angelina Jolie, Catherine Zeta-Jones, Sophia Loren, Celine Dion, Christie Brinkley, Demi Moore, Diane Lane, Uma Thurman, Jodie Foster, Kate Winslet, Diane Sawyer, Princess Di, Hilary Clinton, Queen Elizabeth II, Eleanor Roosevelt.

Brown Rice: A Healthier Choice

Misinformed rice lovers eat white rice and consider brown rice as food for the peasants, the poor, and for animals. How very wrong they are! Modern-day science and health food experts have proven that brown rice is far better and the healthier rice. Brown rice is the most balanced of all cereal grains. In 1897, it was discovered that eating white rice caused beri-beri, a potentially fatal disease due to lack of thiamin (vitamin B1), because this essential vitamin was stripped out of the rice in the processing. Since then, following governmental regulations, white rice was enriched with the naturally occurring vitamins. Unfortunately, these vitamins are markedly reduced by washing prior to cooking. Also, rice manufacturers could not put back the all-important fiber and valuable nutrients known as phytochemicals which are cholesterol-lowering, heart-disease-fighting, and cancer-fighting ingredients. That's why brown rice is far superior to white rice. Indeed, brown rice is fit for royalty and the affluent.

What are phytochemicals?

Phytochemicals are healthy and protective biochemicals naturally found in plants, including brown rice, vegetables, fruits, nuts, and grains. These antioxidant substances protect plants and their fruits and all animals, including humans, from the health-damaging effects of oxidation on our cell structures, especially DNA. Phytochemicals, when ingested, serve as our biochemical defenses against bacteria, fungi, viruses, and cancer. Throughout civilization, mothers have coerced, intimidated, or bribed their children to eat vegetables and fruits, nuts, and grains, because "they are good for you, with all those nutrients, vitamins, and fiber." Obviously, even then, mothers knew best, well ahead of today's science and technology, which have proven and confirmed what mother knew for centuries.

Origin of Rice

History books show that rice originated in China as far back as 2500 BC. This staple food has fed more generations of people all over the globe, over a longer period of time in history, than any other crop. From China, the tradition spread throughout Sri Lanka, India, and surrounding regions, then to Greece and the Mediterranean. It then passed on throughout Southern Europe and North America and reached the New World. It was brought to Brazil from Portugal and from Spain to South and Central America. In many parts of the world, brown rice and wild rice are preferred.

The Brown Rice Advantage

Contrary to the popular belief that rice is nothing but carbohydrate, rice in general, especially brown rice, contains carbohydrates, protein, fats, vitamins, and minerals. The unpolished brown rice has higher content of protein, minerals, fiber, flavor, and the antioxidant phytochemicals than white rice, which is mostly starch. Other whole grains that are healthy like brown rice, containing those essential ingredients and phytochemicals are oats, barley, rye, wheat, buckwheat, corn, quinoa, millet, and wheat berries. White rice is certainly quite inferior to brown rice and to all these grains when it comes to nutrition and health benefits they provide.

Does White Rice Contribute to Diabetes

Yes, eating too much rice increases the risk for diabetes. Worldwide, there are about 180 million type 2 diabetics and 18 million type 1. In China, there are 21 million people who are diabetics. About 2.7 million of Filipinos have diabetes. Ninety percent of all diabetic worldwide are type 2, or adult-onset noninsulin dependent diabetes mellitus (NIDDM). The pathology here is the inadequate insulin production by the beta cells in the Islets of Langerhans in the pancreas, and/or the cells' inability to use the insulin produced. This leads to persistently high blood glucose (sugar) level, called diabetes mellitus. Some of the risk factors in the development of diabetes are obesity, high-fat and high-simple-carbohydrate diet, smoking, and lack of exercises.

A Comparison of Contents

There is a stark difference in the nutritional value between unenriched and unprocessed brown rice and enriched fortified white rice. Brown rice has 4% more calories because it has more fat, 19% more protein, 219% more magnesium, 203% more vitamin K, 185% more vitamin B6, 86% more B2, 33% more B3, 144% more folacin, 147% more phosphorus, 139% more potassium, 37% more elenium, 25% more zinc, and 349% more dietary fiber. Because white rice is enriched, it has 21% more vitamin B1, unless it has been prewashed off before cooking. The bran in brown rice contains essential oils and fibers, which is useful in the prevention of gastrointestinal and heart disease, rheumatoid arthritis, etc. The vast difference in the nutritional and health value of brown rice is obvious.

The Glycemic Index

The glycemic index indicates how fast a certain food raises the blood sugar level after ingestion. The lower the glycemic index, the healthier it is. Brown rice has a low glycemic index (55), compared to white rice, which is 70, which even goes up to 87 with parboiling. A donut has 76, practically pure sugar that elevates the blood glucose rapidly. The occurrence of diabetes later in life (type 2, NIDDM) has been associated with extra high consumption of foods with high glycemic index, like cakes and other pastries, nondiet soft drinks, regular bread, white rice, and other carbohydrates. Examples of other foods and their glycemic Index: most vegetables, beans, etc. (30-40); bran (51); soy milk (31); yogurt (14); grapefruit (25); orange (43); papaya (58); banana (56); oatmeal (48); wheat (67); corn flakes (83); corn Chex cereals (83); and Cheerios (74). Intravenous glucose has a Glycemic Index of 100, because when administered, it raises blood glucose or sugar level 100% instantly. This gives a comparative basis for all the Glycemic Index for the various foods on the list above. For better health, weight control and daily nutrition, we would prefer foods with low glycemic index. Brown rice is one of them.

Brugada Syndrome

(Unexplained Cardiac Arrest)

What is Brugada syndrome?

Brugada syndrome is a baffling condition where a person who appears to be healthy unexpectedly develops cardiac arrest for no apparent reason. Most victims do not survive the episode. This condition is now believed to be responsible for countless sudden deaths among young people—athletes, students, etc.,—who suddenly dropped dead.

Did the victims have any prior symptoms?

No, majority of victims did not have any prior symptoms. They were "in good health" when suddenly they collapsed, went into coma, and later died, or instantly died on the spot. There were some individuals who were lucky enough to have responded to prompt cardiopulmonary resuscitation. Patients like these, with aborted cardiac arrest and death, inspired the three doctors Brugada (R, P, and J) and their colleagues at the Unitat d'Aritmies, Hospital Clinic, in Barcelona, Spain, to pioneer in the study of this baffling condition and became the first to describe the syndrome in the medical literature as a functional cardiac disorder with unique EKG findings. To honor them for this astute discovery, their peers around the world named the entity Brugada syndrome.

What were their findings?

The study conducted by the doctors Brugada in 1992 included 8 patients with a history of aborted sudden death with a distinct and specific EKG tracings that were abnormal (in medical lingo, there were right bundle branch block, ST segment elevation in the right precordial leads, and prolonged QT interval), in the absence of any structural or anatomical heart defect. The physical and clinical examination, biochemical tests, echocardiographic and angiographic tests among these patients yielded normal findings. In 4 of them, a family history of unexplained sudden cardiac arrest was present. The occurrence of ventricular fibrillation (beginning cardiac arrest) in the absence of any structural defect classifies this as a "primary electrical disease." These specific and characteristic EKG findings among these patients discovered by the doctors Brugada, together with the family history of unexplained cardiac arrest, are today the paradigms for the diagnosis of the Brugada Syndrome.

When was this syndrome first discovered?

In science, it is usually hard to accurately date the very first actual discovery of anything, because many scientists/physicians/researchers work simultaneously all around the world. Many of them do not even report their findings right away. But the first officially reported EKG findings, which later was to be known as Brugada syndrome, was made in the late 1980 by other physicians, where 6 patients with sudden cardiac arrest were resuscitated successfully and found to have these characteristic and unique EKG tracings to be described in 1992 by the doctors Brugada as a distinct disease entity, which heretofore was undiscovered and unexplained.

How many cases of this syndrome are there?

This entity is increasingly recognized. The doctors Brugada reported 63 cases by 1998, and a Japanese multicenter reported an additional 63. The past few years, another 163 cases were discovered that satisfy the Brugada criteria, 76 (73%) of whom had actual cardiac arrest and 28 (27%) with syncope (unconsciousness). Ninety five (58%) of them were Asians, with mean age from 22-65. In 36 of them (22%) had a strong family history of syncope, cardiac arrest, or sudden death, without prior symptoms or apparent illness. In some cases, the typical abnormal Brugada EKG findings were noted during a routine screening medical exam performed because of a family history of sudden death.

How does one prevent Brugada Syndrome?

Since this disease entity has now been "described," which makes diagnosis of this entity possible, everyone, especially those with a family history of unexplained sudden cardiac arrest, should be tested, starting with an EKG and some "provocative" tests (with disopyramide, flecainide, ajmaline, procainamide) done to reproduce the characteristic Brugada EKG findings.

Can genetic testing help?

Since this disease is secondary to a mutation of SCN5A gene of chromosome 3 that has a dominant autosomic transmission pattern, with genetic defect in the alpha subunit of the sodium channel, genetic testing may be in order. However, 30% to 80% of patients will have negative (normal) gene screening in spite of overt or latent clinical Brugada syndrome.

What's the treatment for Brugada Syndrome?

If one is diagnosed to have Brugada syndrome, an automatic implantable cardiac-pacemaker defibrillator (AICD) may be implanted, which will pace the heart and increase the rate if the rate goes down (awake or when asleep, 24/7) and shocks and jolts the heart back to normal rhythm, when the heart goes to ventricular fibrillation. Hundreds of thousands of people worldwide have AICD to prevent sudden death. None of the available drugs today are effective against Brugada syndrome.

Bypass Better Than Plasty

Patients with two or more blocked arteries to the heart live longer if they have coronary bypass surgery instead of angioplasty (dilating open the narrowed arteries) and stenting (inserting a wire-mesh coil to prop open the dilated arteries to minimize reclosure), reports a major clinical study.

The research, which was done on 60,000 patients managed from 1997 to 2000, provides clinicians the first long-term comparison of death rates for the two procedures. Edward Hannan and his colleagues at the State University of New York in Albany stated that "patients were 33% to 56% more likely to die after angioplasty and stenting than after bypass surgery."

As a cardiac surgeon, I would like to qualify and explain this statement in layman's term, because the way the medical result above was presented, people may get the wrong idea that a person who undergoes angioplasty and stenting has a 33%-56% risk of dying from the procedure. No, that is not what the researchers meant. What the findings showed was, in the long run, say in 3 years or more following the procedure, 33% to 56% more deaths have been noted among those who had angioplasty and stenting than among those who had coronary bypass surgery. The actual risk of angioplasty and stenting is 1% or less and coronary bypass, being a surgical procedure, between 1% and 3%. What the research findings suggest is that bypass surgery procedure is longer lasting in protecting the patient's heart and in prolonging life, compared to angioplasty/stenting (a much less invasive procedure.)

Hannan said, "The analysis suggests that in just three years, there were up to 540 'excess deaths' that might have been avoided if angioplasty and stent patients had had bypass surgery instead."

The results of this clinical study were published in the *New England Journal of Medicine* May 2005 and "reflect real-life experience and not tightly controlled clinical trials . . . only four prior studies compared the relative outcomes for the two procedures, and they yielded mixed results."

The journal reported that "Hannan's team analyzed the data from 37,212 heart bypass patients and 22,102 angioplasty/stent patients in the New York heart registries. Within the years of the procedure, patients who had angioplasty along with insertion of a stent consistently had higher death rates than those who had bypass surgery. In the sickest group of patients, the death rate was 15.6% for those who had angioplasty versus 10.7% for those who had bypass surgery."

This clinical study "could have a profound implications for heart patients because twice as many now have angioplasty to avoid the trauma of surgery, and the new findings will have a dramatic reversal from just a decade ago," according to many physicians.

"What is new is the impressive advantage of heart bypass surgery over angioplasty," goes the editorial in the journal, authored by Bernard Gersh and Robert Frye of the Mayo Clinic in Rochester, Minnesota. They further stated that "bypass surgery may be superior in a larger group of patients than initially considered," which means, if the analysis had included all the patients who had angioplasty and those who has bypass surgery since the mid-1960s—the past 45 years—the overall advantage and superiority of bypass surgery over angioplasty/stenting would have been even more overwhelmingly dramatic.

In the year 2006 alone, cardiologists in the United States performed 1.3 million angioplasties, about half with stent; and cardiac surgeons did about 800,000 coronary bypass surgeries. With these significant new research findings, those statistics will surely change the biases and mind-set among patients and the medical community alike. This is a natural part of therapeutic evolution and medical progress.

Cancer

What is cancer?

Cancer, or carcinoma, is a vicious uncontrolled growth of tissues that is characterized by the loss of cell control. Normally, each cell in the body regulates how large and how fast it should grow, die and regenerate, in every organ (stomach, lung, kidneys, etc). Carcinogens (cancer causing agents) that invade the organ in the body takes away that cell control. This results in a rapid abnormal and excessive growth of the cells way beyond their normal size leading to the formation of a malignant tumor in the particular organ it grows in, with propensity to spread to adjacent tissues and to distant organs (example: cancer of the lungs spreading to the brain, or cancer of the breast metastasizing to the liver or bones).

What causes cancer?

The basic underlying cause is the constant, repeated irritation or injury to body parts or organs, leading to changes in the DNA and loss of cell controls. Examples: cigarette smoking as the cancer-causing irritant to the breathing apparatus including the trachea, breathing pipes and the lungs, urinary bladder, kidneys, pancreas. Another irritant is animal (saturated) fat from the red meat we eat, causing cancer of the colon, breast and uterus. Alcohol is linked to cancer of the digestive tract, breast and liver. More than 75% of all cancers are associated with only 3 factors, diet, tobacco and alcohol. There are theories that implicate virus, weakened immune system, radiation, chemicals, etc. as the probable cause of cancers, but there is no doubt that the 3 factors mentioned above are associated with more than three quarters of all cancers in man. If we can control those 3, we can prevent most cancers known to man.

Are cancers preventable?

Most of the cancers are preventable with a healthy lifestyle. Examples of these are cancer of the lungs, esophagus, pancreas, kidney, urinary bladder and throat among those who smoke, melanoma (cancer of the skin from chronic and prolonged exposure to sunlight), mesothelioma (cancer of the inner lining of the chest wall from exposure to asbestos), cancer of the mouth and throat from chewing betel nut, etc. If we think about it, there are many things we can do to prevent cancer, and that many cancers have been caused by unhealthy practices people did to themselves. Smokers, for instance, know that tobacco cause a variety of deadly cancers, and yet they continue to smoke.

Are there cancers that are curable?

Most cancers detected at an early stage (before it has spread) are potentially curable. This is the reason why one should report to his/her physician any lumps or bumps, sores or non-healing wounds, or abnormal bleeding or discharge, unexplained cough or weight loss. A prompt medical check-up in this situation is essential, if early diagnosis is to be made. Better than this is to have a yearly medical check-up, which should include, among others tests, chest-ray, breast (Mammography), vaginal (Pap Smear) and rectal examination among females, chest-ray, prostate, and rectal examination among males. Majority of the "cancer cures" were among patients who sought preventive medical care annually and were diagnosed and treated early. Early detection is the key in the fight against cancer.

Can self-examination help detect cancers?

Yes, a significant number of malignant growths were first discovered by the patient himself/herself or by the spouse or a family member. Self-examination (breasts among females; testicles among males; for sores, discharges, or lumps and bumps in the neck, armpit or groin or anywhere in the body) is a good habit one should practice and do about once a week. As you feel your body parts frequently, you will be familiar with their normal appearance, consistency and size, and discern more easily when changes or abnormalities take place.

How about the role of geography?

In Japan, the incidence of breast and colon cancer is low, but the incidence among Japanese immigrants to the United States is higher and approximates that of the native Americans, obviously from diet and lifestyle changes. Eating red meat, smoking cigarettes, and lack of exercise are the significant factors in the role of geography in the causation of cancers.

Does eating red meat increase cancer risk?

Yes. There is no question that eating animal fat, especially from red meat, is a significant factor which increases the risk of people developing cancer (colon, breast, uterus, etc.). One third (33%) of the 500,000 cancer deaths each year in the United States is due to this dietary factor. This is well documented in medical literature. Now, what medical science does not know at the present is who among those who eat animal fat would develop cancer, and who would not. The same thing with smoking. This is why physicians recommend avoidance of red meat, cigarettes, and moderation in alcohol intake

What are chemical carcinogens?

Chemical carcinogens include exposure to arsenic, chromates, asbestos (lung cancer), aromatic amines (bladder cancer), benzene (leukemia), nickel (lung and nasal sinus cancer), vinyl chloride (liver cancer), alcohol (esophageal and oropharyngeal cancer), tobacco (lung, esophageal, urinary bladder, head and neck cancer), betel nuts (oropharyngeal cancer), and, ionizing radiation (lymphomas, aplastic anemia, multiple myeloma, thyroid cancers).

What are the available treatments for cancer?

There are various treatment modalities available, depending on the organ and cell-types of the different cancers. In brief, among them are chemotherapy, radiotherapy, hormonal therapy, whole body irradiation, combined therapy and surgery. The management of cancer has greatly advanced the past two decades. Those interested in the details of each regimen should discuss this with their family physician or oncologist.

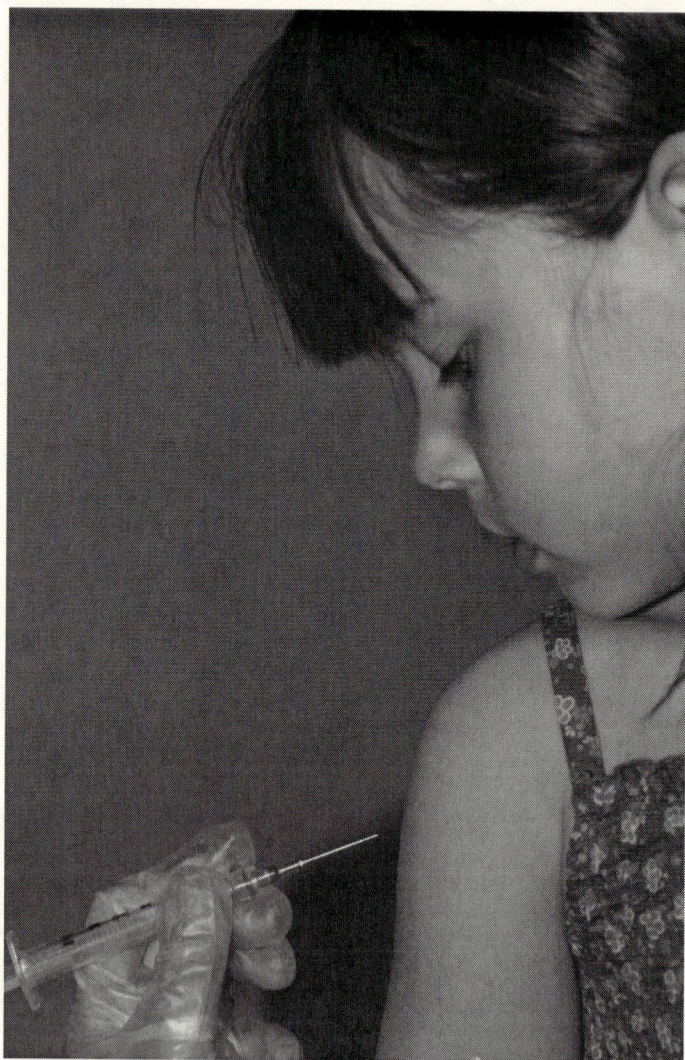

Vaccines can prevent major diseases, including cancer of the cervix.

Caffeine + Alcohol: Deadly Combo

In my newspaper column on April 26, 2010, we warned the public about the dangers of caffeinated energy drink plus alcohol, with the following article:

Combining alcoholic beverage with caffeine energy drink is a popular cocktail today. This mix has been found to be dangerous, leading to higher state of drunkenness and severely impaired driving, compared to drinking alcoholic drink alone. "There's a very common misconception that if you drink caffeine with an alcoholic beverage the stimulant effect of the caffeine counteracts the depressant effect of the alcohol, and that is not true," says Bruce Goldberger, director of toxicology in the University of Florida College of Medicine. Being wide awake and drunk can lead to dangerous, if not deadly, behaviors.

FDA bans energy drinks

Recently, following reports of several deaths and dozens of hospitalizations among young adults who ingested the caffeinated alcoholic energy drink, the US Food and Drug Administration decided to ban the sales of these beverages. New York Sen. Charles Schumer supported the ban on the drinks marketed as Four Loko and Joose, and stated that "the Federal Trade Commission planned to notify manufacturers that they are engaged in the potential illegal marketing of unsafe alcoholic drinks."

The super caffeinated beverage, which contains anywhere between 50 and 500 mg of caffeine and between 5 and 12% alcohol, has been deemed unsafe by the FDA.

The drinks are very popular among college students and young children. The US Centers for Disease Control and Prevention estimated that the concoctions "are consumed by 31% of 12—to 17-year olds and 34 percent of 18—to 24-year olds."

Individuals who drink these energy drinks are 3 times more likely to lead to binge drinking, compared to those who consume alcoholic drinks only. The caffeine in the energy drink appears to "keep the drinker less sedated," masking the feeling of drunkenness from the initial effect of the alcohol and prolong the drinking session. Then, after a few hours, the cumulative effects of the high dose of caffeine and the high alcohol level in the blood take their toll. These energy drinks also make it easier for people to develop alcohol addiction.

Unsafe, premixed or not

New studies revealed that drinking caffeine and alcohol, even not pre-mixed and ingested separately but one after the other, almost simultaneously, poses the same danger and risk to health. Another finding reported by *Health.com* showed that "college students who consume nonalcoholic energy drinks such as Red Bull at least once a week are more than twice as likely as their peers to show signs of alcohol dependence, including withdrawal symptoms and an inability to cut back on drinking, according to the study." This was published in the journal *Alcoholism: Clinical & Experimental Research.*

The common scenario describes students who party the whole night and have to cram for an exam the following day. They then resort to energy drinks with alcohol during the party, and drink non-alcoholic drink like Red Bull in the morning to shake hangover and keep them awake for the test. The amount of caffeine in Red Bull has the adverse effects of nervousness, anxiety, headache, rapid heart rate, palpitation, and insomnia. Other energy drinks include Rockstar, Monster, Burn, Full Throttle, and Amp, which, led by Red Bull, the market leader, had around $5 billion sales in the United States in 2008.

Cocaine controversy

There were reports in April and June 2009 that Red Bull cola drinks imported from Austria were found to contain between 0.1 and 0.3 microgram of cocaine per liter, according to Hong Kong officials. Importing cocaine is illegal and carries life imprisonment or death. Out of 16 German states, 11 have already banned the energy drinks as of May 25, 2009.

An article in *The Daily Telegraph* on February 3, 2000, reported, "Red Bull may have triggered heart condition that killed the 21-year-old woman who died after drinking four cans of Red Bull and alcohol."

Synthetic Marijuana

Another teenagers' new drug of choice is synthetic marijuana, sold under the names K2 and Mr. Nice Guy. A death claimed to be due to this substance has brought it under scrutiny by the FDA, the media, and the public. These items, peddled on the streets and some stores discreetly, are cheaper than genuine marijuana and are not detectable by standard lab exam. This synthetic drug causes paranoia, hallucination, vertigo, mental confusion, and exacerbate schizophrenia. Driving under the influence of this drug could kill not only the driver but other drivers, passengers, and pedestrians.

Calcium and Vitamin D3

Calcium and vitamin D3 were on the spotlight in the fall of 2010. The report from the Institute of Medicine (IOM) released in Washington on November 30th that year sets the new official dietary guidelines on calcium and vitamin D "to maintain health and avoid risk associated with excess."

With the hype on megadose vitamins and "super" beverages and pills claiming to have health benefits and "cures for dozens of all diseases, including cancer," the food supplement industry is propelled by the billions of dollars it rakes in annually.

The dangerous public misinformation majority of the various companies use in the marketing of their "wonder" products has resulted in countless hospitalizations and deaths around the world. Since these products are exempt from the scrutiny of drug, food, and health agencies, they are available to the public in general, without prescription. Most of these companies are taking advantage of the consumers' ignorance, gullibility, and obsessive search for the illusive fountain of youth.

The New Guidelines

According to the Institute of Medicine, "most Americans and Canadians up to age 70 need no more than 600 international units (IUs) of vitamin D3 per day to maintain health, and those 71 and older may need as much as 800 IUs. The amount of calcium needed ranges, based on age, from 700 to 1,300 milligrams per day, according to the IOM report, which updates the nutritional reference values known as Dietary Reference Intakes (DRIs) for these interrelated nutrients."

These new guidelines from the IOM were based on recommendations based on almost 1,000 independent "published studies and testimony from scientists and stakeholders." The investigation was sponsored by the United States Department of Health and Human Services, US Department of Agriculture, US Department of Defense, and Health Canada. "Established in 1970 under the charter of the National Academy of Sciences, the Institute of Medicine provides independent, objective, evidence-based advice to policymakers, health professionals, the private sector, and the public."

Evidence-based Rationale

The following are segments of the IOM report: A large amount of evidence, which formed the basis of the new intake values, confirms the roles of calcium and vitamin D3 in promoting skeletal growth and maintenance and the amounts needed to avoid poor bone health. The committee that wrote the report also reviewed hundreds of studies and reports on other possible health effects of vitamin D3, such as protection against cancer, heart disease, autoimmune diseases, and diabetes. While these studies point to possibilities that warrant further investigation, they have yielded conflicting and mixed results and do not offer the evidence needed to confirm that vitamin D3 has these effects. Rigorous trials that yield consistent results are vital for reaching conclusions, as past experiences have shown. Vitamin E, for example, was believed to protect against heart disease a decade ago, but further studies disproved it.

"There is abundant science to confidently state how much vitamin D and calcium people need," said committee chair Catharine Ross, professor, and Dorothy Foehr Huck, chair, Department of Nutritional Sciences, Pennsylvania State University, University Park. "We scrutinized the evidence, looking for indications of beneficial effects at all levels of intake. Amounts higher than those specified in this report are not necessary to maintain bone health."

Meeting the Needs

The science on calcium's role in bone health shows that 700 milligrams per day meets the needs of almost all children ages 1 through

3, and 1,000 milligrams daily is appropriate for almost all children ages 4 through 8. Adolescents ages 9 through 18 require no more than 1,300 milligrams per day. For practically all adults ages 19 through 50 and for men until age 71, 1,000 milligrams covers daily calcium needs. Women starting at age 51 and both men and women age 71 and older need no more than 1,200 milligrams per day.

As for vitamin D, 600 IUs daily meets the needs of almost everyone in the United States and Canada, although people 71 and older may require as much as 800 IUs per day because of potential physical and behavioral changes related to aging. Vitamin D3 is the preferred form of D for supplement.

Risks of Abuse, Upper Safe Limit

Excessive calcium from dietary supplements, beyond the recommended dose, has been associated with kidney stones; and ingesting too much vitamin D can damage the heart and the kidneys.

In view of this, the IOM thoroughly studied the upper *safe* limit for vitamin D3 and calcium to educate and warn the consumers to stay away from the dangerous levels, with the following data: "Upper intake levels represent the upper safe boundary and should not be misunderstood as amounts people need or should strive to consume. The upper intake levels for vitamin D3 are 2,500 IUs per day for children ages 1 through 3; 3,000 IUs daily for children 4 through 8 years old; and 4,000 IUs daily for all others. The upper intake levels for calcium are 2,500 milligrams per day from age 1 through 8; 3,000 milligrams daily from age 9 through 18; 2,500 milligrams daily from age 19 through 50; and 2,000 milligrams per day for all other age groups."

The new guidelines for the Daily Reference Intakes (DRI) today are based on a lot more updated information and more sophisticated studies compared to those available when the DRIs for calcium and vitamin D were originally set in 1997.

Both calcium and vitamin D3 supplements have vital roles in the maintenance of health and prevention of illnesses for all of us. Taken in the recommended dosage, these two nutrients and genuine multivitamins, in general, confer upon our body physical and physiological integrity as they boost our immune system. As long as we do not abuse them, they will remain our friends and protector.

Can CT Scan, mammogram cause cancer?

Computerized tomography (CT) scans is one of the greatest advances in medicine in the last century, which expedites early diagnosis and with more accuracy, not easily possible before its introduction.

However, whenever a test involves X-rays, concerns about radiation exposure and the risks it poses are seriously monitored and researched by the medical community. Besides the usual evaluation of the cost-benefit equation, the risk-benefit ratio is likewise examined under the microscope.

Recent studies, published in the *Archives of Internal Medicine* December 14, 2009, stated that radiation from CT scans "may cause cancer decades later," estimating "about 29,000 future malignancies would occur in the US because of CT scans done in 2007."

CT scans are done for the head, chest, heart, blood vessels, abdominal organs, etc. If the strict medical indication for CT scan is followed to the letter, there will be a lot less CT scans done around the globe. Patients' demand for a CT scan, if without medical justification, should be ignored by the physician, for their own safety.

The radiation a CT scan delivers is equivalent to about 100 to 200 times those of conventional chest X-ray. If your doctor says, "We will do 100 to 200 chest X-rays on you today," you will surely be scared and question its safety, if not refuse altogether. But practically everybody accepts CT scan without care.

Majority of the predicted CT scan victims of cancer are women, and about 33% of these cancers are projected to happen to those who were 35 to 54 years of age when they had the CT scan, based on an estimated 72 million CT scans performed in 2007, a triple increase in the number of CT scans since 1993. About 30% of CT scans done are deemed unnecessary, not medically justifiable.

"We know that there are great medical benefits to CT scans, but they also involve small risks of cancer because of radiation exposure," said Amy Berrington de Gonzalez, the lead researcher at the National Cancer Institute in Bethesda, Maryland. "For an individual, the risks are small. So if the scan is clinically justified, then the benefits should outweigh the risks."

The researcher pointed out that "the overall risk for any individual is small and depends on the type of scan given and a person's age . . . A 70-year-old who has a CT scan of the head would have a 1 in 10,000 chance of developing cancer from the test, while a baby who had a chest CT scan would have a 1 in 200 chance."

Type of Cancers

The prediction is that lung cancer, followed by colon cancer and leukemia, will be the most common radiation-related cancer. Fifty percent of those predicted 29,000 people who may develop cancer from CT scan in 2007 will die, according to the study.

This published research also pointed out that if the use of CT scan remains at its present number or higher, "eventually 29,000 cancers every year could be due to past CT scan use." This translates to about 2% of the 1.4 million cancers diagnosed in the United States annually.

"There's a risk with anything we do, whether it's taking antibiotics or crossing the street," stated Donald Frush, chairman of the American College of Radiology's Pediatric Imaging Commission and chief of the division of pediatric radiology at Duke Medical Center in Durham, North Carolina. "We can't lose what the benefits of CT scanning are. The benefits are that CT scans save tens of thousands of lives each year in the United States and really helps the medical community diagnose things. CT is one of the most invaluable medical advancements in the last 100 years," Dr. Frush added.

One unfortunate mistake that has complicated the CT scan issue is that of a wrongly programmed CT scan which apparently has happened in Cedars Sinai Hospital in Los Angeles, where patients undergoing CT scan of the head were reportedly exposed to excess radiation. This news has directed the spotlight on the risk of radiation from CT scan. In view of this, the US Food and Drug Administration on December 7, 2009, issued interim regulations requiring closer monitoring of CT scans after more than 250 cases of exposure to excess radiation were reported since October 2009.

Mammography and Breast Cancer

On another front, a report from the annual meeting of the Radiological Society of North America "verified that annual mammography screenings may be responsible for causing breast cancer in women predisposed to the disease."

The study included high-risk women and showed that low-dose mammography radiation "increased these women's risk of developing breast cancer by 150% .... women under 209 who have had at least five mammograms are 2.5 times more likely to develop breast cancer than high-risk women who have never undergone low-dose mammography screenings."

University Medical Center Groningen in the Netherlands' epidemiologist Marijke C. Jansen-van der Weide cautions physicians when screening younger women, especially those under age 30. The researcher suggested alternative screening tests like ultrasounds, MRIs, and heat thermography, where no radiation is involved.

Clearing the Air

I realize how much fear and confusion this issue has caused the public. The truth of the matter is even the medical community has been impacted by this. After all, the CT scan has been a most reliable diagnostic tool in the physician's armamentarium for the benefit of his patients.

The debate on this matter is far from over. More studies are surely to be conducted to verify these initial findings.

In the meantime, one thing is clear: where medically indicated, CT scan, which saves millions of lives every year, is a precious tool in competent hands. Unless a superior and safer substitute comes along, CT scan will be with us for some time in man's fight against diseases, especially cancer.

Early Cancer Detection

The ideal strategy against any form of cancer is prevention. To complement this, one must be armed with current information, most of which are available on the Internet, for the early detection of the malignancy before it develops into a more serious stage or becomes incurable.

Periodic medical examination for those 20 and older should include exam for cancers of the skin, oral cavity, thyroid, ovaries, testes, and lymph nodes and other tests for noncancerous illnesses.

The following helpful guidelines were developed by the American Cancer Society for the various common cancers, which can aid the public in the early detection of these cancers. We are presenting them hereunder:

Breast Cancer

1. Annual mammogram starting at age 40 and yearly thereafter

2. Breast examination by a physician every 3 years for women in their 20s and 30s, or sooner if concerned, and every year for women who are age 40 and older.

3. Every woman must feel and look at their breast infront of a mirror regularly and be familiar with their breasts so that when a change or an abnormality in shape, size, color, is noted, she can promptly report it to her healthcare provider. Breast self-exam is an initial option for women in their 20s.

Those women with a family history of breast cancer, a genetic tendency, or other factors are advised by the American Cancer Society to have screening by MRI on top of a mammogram. This subset of women is less than 2% of all women in the United States.

Colorectal Cancer and Polyps

The following testing schedules are recommended for both men and women beginning age 50 by the American Cancer Society:

Tests that find polyps and cancer

- flexible sigmoidoscopy every 5 years*
- colonoscopy every 10 years
- double contrast barium enema every 5 years*
- CT colonography (virtual colonoscopy) every 5 years*
  Tests that mainly find cancer
- fecal occult blood test (FOBT) every year*,**
- fecal immunochemical test (FIT) every year*,**
- stool DNA test (sDNA), interval uncertain*

*Colonoscopy should be done if test results are positive.
**For FOBT or FIT used as a screening test, the take-home multiple sample method should be used. A FOBT or FIT done during a digital rectal exam in the doctor's office is not adequate for screening.

Those with any of the following colorectal cancer risk factors (as listed by the American Cancer Society) should confer with their physician about having colorectal cancer screening earlier or having it more often:

- a personal history of colorectal cancer or adenomatous polyps

- a personal history of chronic inflammatory bowel disease (Crohn's disease or ulcerative colitis)
- a strong family history of colorectal cancer or polyps (cancer or polyps in a first-degree relative [parent, sibling, or child] younger than 60 or in 2 or more first-degree relatives of any age)
- a known family history of hereditary colorectal cancer syndromes such as familial adenomatous polyposis (FAP) or hereditary nonpolyposis colon cancer (HNPCC).

Cervical cancer

- All women should begin cervical cancer screening about 3 years after they begin having vaginal intercourse, but no later than when they are 21 years old. Screening should be done every year with the regular Pap test or every 2 years using the newer liquid-based Pap test.
- Beginning at age 30, women who have had 3 normal Pap test results in a row may get screened every 2 to 3 years. Another reasonable option for women over 30 is to get screened every 3 years (but not more frequently) with either the conventional or liquid-based Pap test, plus the HPV DNA test. Women who have certain risk factors such as diethylstilbestrol (DES) exposure before birth, HIV infection, or a weakened immune system due to organ transplant, chemotherapy, or chronic steroid use should continue to be screened annually.
- Women 70 years of age or older who have had 3 or more normal Pap tests in a row and no abnormal Pap test results in the last 10 years may choose to stop having cervical cancer screening. Women with a history of cervical cancer, DES exposure before birth, HIV infection, or a weakened immune system should continue to have screening as long as they are in good health.
- Women who have had a total hysterectomy (removal of the uterus and cervix) may also choose to stop having cervical cancer screening, unless the surgery was done as a treatment for cervical cancer or precancer. Women who have had a hysterectomy without removal of the cervix should continue to follow the guidelines above.

Endometrial (Uterine) Cancer

The American Cancer Society recommends that at the time of menopause, all women should be informed about the risks and symptoms of endometrial cancer and strongly encouraged to report any unexpected bleeding or spotting to their doctors. For women with or at high risk for hereditary nonpolyposis colon cancer (HNPCC), annual screening should be offered for endometrial cancer with endometrial biopsy beginning at age 35.

Prostate cancer

The American Cancer Society (ACS) does not support routine testing for prostate cancer at this time. ACS does believe that health care professionals should discuss the potential benefits and limitations of prostate cancer early detection testing with men before any testing begins. This discussion should include an *offer* for testing with the prostate-specific antigen (PSA), blood test and digital rectal exam (DRE) yearly beginning at age 50, to men who are at average risk of prostate cancer and have at least a 10-year life expectancy. Following this discussion, those men who favor testing should be tested. Men should actively take part in this decision by learning about prostate cancer and the pros and cons of early detection and treatment of prostate cancer.

This discussion should take place starting at age 45 for men at high risk of developing prostate cancer. This includes African American men and men who have a first-degree relative (father, brother, or son) diagnosed with prostate cancer at an early age (younger than age 65).

This discussion should take place at age 40 for men at even higher risk (those with several first-degree relatives who had prostate cancer at an early age).

Remember, if cancer "sneaks in" in spite of preventive measures through healthy lifestyle, early detection can lead to a possible cure.

Will you get cancer?

While science today still does not have a practical and fool-proof test to determine who among us will develop cancer, there are some medical facts and statistics now available that can tell us who among us are more prone or at a higher risk for the development of cancer of which organs.

How Cancer Develops

Cancer forms when cells of tissues, which compose the various organs of our body, are repeatedly subjected to an irritant, be it chemical (ingested, inhaled, or applied), radiation (solar, natural, or man-made), electromagnetic, or even repeated physical trauma. As years of exposure to any of these insults continues, the cells, which normally are well-regulated and healthy, are transformed to wild, aggressive, uncontrollable "monster" cells that grow without "order and discipline," destroying the organ involved and spreading to and ravaging other organs. The cancer cells even enter the blood or lymph channel and invade distant vital organs all over the body, causing them to malfunction as well.

The culprits

The more common etiologic agents include cigarettes, unhealthy diet of saturated fats and cholesterol, alcoholic beverages, certain drugs, prolonged sun exposure, and deficiency in vegetables, whole grain, nuts, fresh fruits, and physical exercises. Pregnant mothers who smoke or drinks alcoholic beverages or take unprescribed drugs infuse these poisonous agents to their baby in utero. Any of these can cause damage to the child's DNA, mental deficiency, physical deformities, and even certain rare form of cancer.

The best strategy

In dealing with a treacherous and deadly disease, the two key proactive strategies we have are prevention and early detection. A healthy lifestyle that includes discipline and good habits is a significant armor against cancer. And if with this first line of defense, cancer still manages to slip thru, prompt diagnosis becomes a vital necessity. Most cancers are curable when detected early, in their precancerous or localized stage.

The Common Cancers

PROSTATE CANCER—The risk of getting prostate cancer goes up with age. Two out of 3 men over the age of 65 develop prostate cancer. A diet high in saturated animal fats predisposes the individuals to this malignancy. Heredity is also a factor. A blood test called PSA (prostate-specific antigen) and DRE (digital rectal examination) starting age 50 can help detect prostatic cancer early. When diagnosed early, this cancer can be cured.

BREAST CANCER—Except for skin cancer, cancer of the breast is the most common malignancy among American women. A little less than 1 in 8 (12%) of women will develop invasive breast cancer sometime in their life. The American Cancer Society estimated about 207,090 breast cancers and 39,840 would die from it in 2010. Worldwide, the annual incidence is about 1.15 million. The ACS recommends yearly mammogram starting age 40 and clinical breast exam every 3 years for women in their 20s and 30s and annually for those 40 and over. Women should also be familiar with their breast as to their size, shape, consistency, color, appearance of their nipples, and do SBE (self—breast exam) at least once a week. Those with strong family history of breast cancer are advised to have MRI on top of the mammogram.

LUNG CANCER—is the leading killer among all cancers, and 90% of lung cancers are caused by smoking. A smaller number of lung cancers are related to exposure to asbestos and radon. People who smoke are 23 times more likely to get cancer of the lungs. The annual death rate from lung cancer is about 130,000. This is one disease that is preventable in most cases. Tobacco maims and kills, even thru secondhand smokes. Staying away from this poison is the only smart option.

CERVICAL CANCER—In the United States, 30 women are found to have cancer of the cervix (mouth of the woman's womb) every 24 hours, and eleven die from it daily. These are preventable deaths. There is a vaccine today that prevents cervical cancer. About 3 years after the woman starts having sexual intercourse (but no later than age 21), she should have a cervical cancer screening every year with regular Pap test or every 2 years using the newer liquid-based Pap test. Starting age 30, those with 3 normal consecutive Pap tests, may be screened every 2 to 3 years. Those older than 30 may have it (plus HPV test for human papiloma virus, which causes cervical cancer) done every 3 years. Women 70 or older who have had normal Pap test in 3 consecutive tests in ten years may opt not to have any more Pap tests, like those with noncancer total hysterectomy. Those with hysterectomy, leaving behind the cervix, need to Pap test screening as above.

UTERINE CANCER—Endometrial cancer is a risk among those with menopause. Any spotting or bleeding requires prompt medical consultation. In some cases, endometrial biopsies may be needed, depending on the medical history of the woman. In 2010 alone, there were 43,470 cases of endometrial cancer in the United States, with a death toll of 7,950. As with any other malignancy, early diagnosis is vital here.

COLON CANCER—is the second leading cause of cancer deaths in the USA. The American Cancer Society estimated about 146,970 new cases of colon cancer with a death rate of 49,920 in 2009. Around 72% are in the colon and about 28% arise from the rectum. More than 90% of cases survive for more than 5 years when detected during its local (confined) stage. Starting at age 50, a yearly fecal (stool) occult blood test (FOBT) or annual fecal immunochemical test (FIT) is recommended. Every 5 years sigmoidoscopy and double contrast barium enema, and every ten years colonoscopy are recommended. If the occult blood is positive, or if there are signs or symptoms of gastrointestinal problem, colonoscopy may be done at that point.

SKIN CANCER—People who are sun lovers and exposed to the sun a lot, especially between 10:00 a.m. and 4:00 p.m., are at a high risk of developing skin cancer. Those with family history of melanoma (a form of very malignant skin cancer) and those who suffered severe sun burns early in life, are also much more prone to get cancer of the skin. The incidence of melanoma has risen from 1 out of 1,500 in 1935 to 1 out of 75 in year 2000, with a mortality of almost 33%. Wearing a hat with brims, sunglasses, long-sleeve shirts, or using umbrella, sunscreen with sun protection factor (SPF) of 15 or higher, and minimizing sun exposure have been shown to lower the risk for skin cancer.

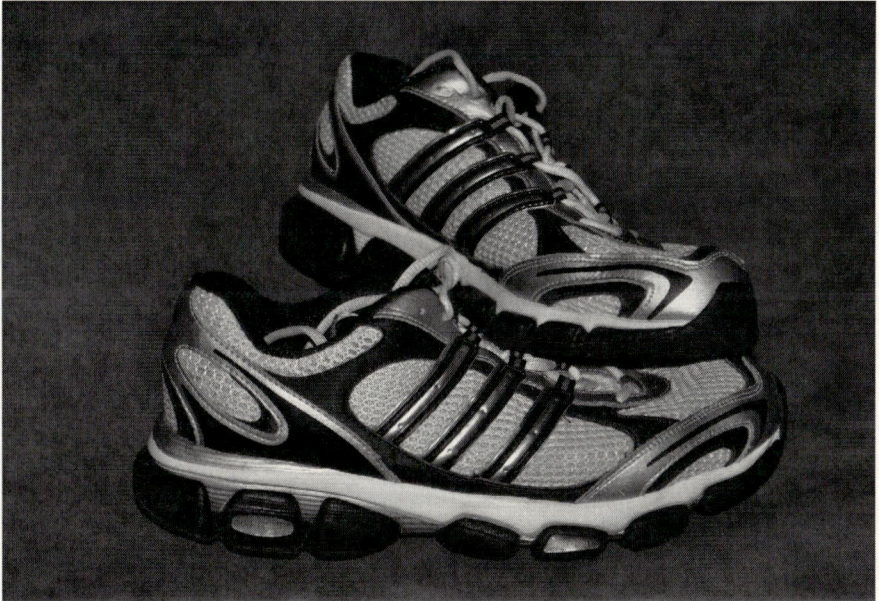

Physical exercise, as simple as walking, even leisurely for half an hour daily, can prevent a host of diseases, including cancer.

Cancer Cells in Our Body?

The Internet was recently flooded with a medical claim (allegedly from Johns Hopkins, which I doubt) that was scaring the public. Circulating in the e-mail around the world was the statement that said, "Normally, we all have dormant cancer cells in our body." Implied is the assertion that all healthy people are walking around with a time bomb within them, ready to explode.

This senseless, insensitive, and unkind fabrication is obviously the work of someone with an ignorant, or confused, if not twisted, mind.

The healthy person does not carry any cancer cell in their body, period. If every tissue in the body of a normal person is biopsied, or if a person who dies of any noncancerous disease, like heart attack or stroke, or trauma, is autopsied from head to foot, no cancer cells will be found. The only exception to this is if the person had an undiagnosed cancer, which is incidentally found on autopsy, a finding that excludes this person from being healthy in the first place.

If that ridiculous claim were true, then each person would be carrying around (from birth to death) "dormant" cancer cells in his/her brain, head and neck, breast, lungs, liver, pancreas, kidneys, intestines, prostate, and other organs in the body.

Our creator was more intelligent and more sensible not to make that mistake of intentionally designing the human body with such a grotesque built-in defect in it. Even humans don't do that when they design or build anything. God blessed us with a body that is a powerful generator, a great computer, with most efficient organs, a body amazingly functional and full of dexterity. The imperfections among us are caused by factors that are of our own (human) doings, even those congenital defects in some babies, etc., or illnesses we get are due to our own recklessness and unhealthy lifestyle.

Therefore, I am saying that all healthy individuals, from birth to adulthood to their death, do *not* normally carry, or have, any cancer cells in their body, unless they develop a malignancy. If they abuse themselves and subject their body to carcinogens, substances, or toxins that cause cancers, then the tissues of the organs involved (like the lungs among smokers, the esophagus or food pipe, and the liver, among alcoholics) could be so chronically irritated and damaged by the toxic agent for the cells of those tissues to change into cancer cells.

Normal Cells

The normal cells our body came with when we were born have a predetermined growth pattern and final adult size, from infancy to adulthood. As the cells, tissues, and organs attain their normal number and size, the cell growth ceases at the right time. That is why our organs, our body as a whole, have the average sizes and shapes, according to our genetic makeup. There is no runaway, uncontrolled growth in cases of normal cells. Muscle cells are greater in mass and stronger among those who exercise daily, especially among body builders. Fat cells increase in number and size when we overeat and become overweight. But even these "growths" are still within the expected "norm."

From time to time, as our activities and lifestyle "damage" our cells as a result of the wear and tear in our body, our older cells (including blood cells) die and are replaced by new cells efficiently and automatically. An example of this is our dead skin, which flakes off, to be replaced instantly by new skin. Worn out or dead cells in a normal body are constantly replaced with new ones almost every day. But all this happens in an organized, systematic, orderly, and "disciplined" process. Our body system's self-protective and auto-control mechanisms are always in control maintaining our health. If we do something that will adversely alter this natural internal balance and harmony, then disease sets in.

Cancer Cells Are Something Else

Cancer cells are different. They grow and divide with blatant disregard for the body's needs and limitations. They do not stop reproducing. There is random multiplication and replication that is out of bounds, without order and direction. These cells become very aggressive, attacking tissues and organs nearby, as in malignant tumors, where in many cases even spread to, and destroy, distant organs (like in cancer of the lungs with metastases to the brains, bones, adrenals, etc.).

Unless cancer cells are treated effectively to induce cure or remission when they first form, they are unstoppable in their growth and aggressiveness. This behavior and characteristic of cancer cells alone are a self-evident proof that normal healthy bodies do not have what is claimed as "dormant cancer cells." If any cancer cell forms in a person's body, it will continue to grow and multiply unceasingly and be clinically obvious in a matter of weeks or months in almost all cases.

Oncogenes

Normal (noncancerous) cells have a regulated, well-controlled cell division and growth, thanks to the genes that produce proteins that provide such auto-regulation and control. These are the proto-oncogenes and tumor-suppressor genes, which regulate the cell cycle and keep the cells in good control. Tumor-suppressor genes produce proteins that prevent the uncontrolled cell growth and abnormal cell division.

When the cells are constantly exposed to cancer-causing agents (either toxic substances, chemicals in food or drinks, excess sunlight, radiation, etc.), the body produces an abnormal proteins called oncogenes which cause the cells to lose their ability to control their regulation. The nonregulated cells then go wild and divide abnormally fast, uncontrolled, transforming the cells into cancer cells that lose their original characteristics and functions (like cancerous lungs tissues turning into a solid mass, losing their air cells and ability to oxygenate blood). The uncontrolled growth and replication of the cancer cells lead to large space-occupying masses in the body, crowding out other organs and pressing on vitals blood vessels and nerves. The most adverse outcome of this malignant process is the transformation of the cancerous organ into a useless hard mass of tissues and the loss of original function of the organ as in cancer of the lungs, liver, kidney, brain, breast, prostate, etc.

Conclusion

Normal, healthy, persons do not have cancer cells in their body. That includes the general population at large. Only individuals with a cancerous disease have cancers cells in them. And you can e-mail this medical fact to your friends.

Knowing how deadly cancers can be, it behooves all of us to live a healthy lifestyle and to be knowledgeable and keenly aware that cancer is best prevented. And if it still occurs, in spite of our diligence and discipline, it is best diagnosed early. A regular medical check-up is a prudent prophylactic health strategy in our fight against diseases, especially against cancer.

Cancer Is Self-Induced

On September 28, 2010, I was interviewed by Sky Cable. Besides the topics on heart attack and stroke and lifestyle in general as a preventive regimen in warding off diseases, the discussion also touched on cancer.

One of my statements alluded to the fact that most of the diseases known to man, including cancer, in my opinion, "are man-made, self-induced, brought on by us to ourselves thru unhealthy lifestyle, whether we realize it or not, inadvertently or otherwise."

Smoking (firsthand or secondhand), alcohol abuse, ingestion of processed and high-fat and high-cholesterol foods, absence or lack of vegetables, fruits, and high-fiber items like nuts and lentils in our diet, and exposure to environmental pollution (air and water), were among the culprits I cited.

I also stated that while genetics play a role in all this, our environment and our lifestyle appear to outweigh the hereditary factor.

Man's self-abuse and rape of his environment are almost certain to doom the world he lives in. The human factor in the causation of cancer includes all the pollution and damages we have done to our planet and the insults most of us do to our body every day.

How can we prove that cancer is self-induced?

To do this, we have to get facts, historical facts. We have to go not only a hundred years back, but millennia, in the history of man—as far back as the period of the dinosaurs.

Researchers from the University of Manchester, England, using massive data from ancient Greek and autopsy findings in hundreds of Egyptian mummies. Greek medical writings hardly mentioned cancer, and among these mummies (from the ptolemaeic period) only two (worldwide) were detected to have histological evidence of cancer. Obviously, cancer, in adults or children, was extremely rare during those times and not because their life expectancy was shorter compared to ours. The mummies studied were persons with arteriosclerosis, osteoporosis, Paget's disease, illnesses found in seniors who were old enough to develop cancer. Logic tells us that the carcinogens (cancer-causing agents) we inhale, eat, or expose ourselves to today were not present in the ancient times. The environment then was pristine, not polluted as it is now.

Then came the Industrial Revolution and the massive environmental pollution. This was followed by the explosion of the incidence of cancer, especially childhood cancer, not to mention other diseases now known to man: cardiovascular, metabolic, even infectious.

"So it has to be a man-made disease, down to pollution and changes to our diet and lifestyle," explained Professor Roselle David at Manchester University's Faculty of Life Sciences.

Professor Michael Zimmerman, a visiting professor at the KNH Centre, who made the first ever histological diagnosis of cancer in an Egyptian mummy, stated, "In an ancient society lacking surgical intervention, evidence of cancer should remain in all cases. The virtual absence of malignancies in mummies must be interpreted as indicating their rarity in antiquity, indicating that cancer causing factors are limited to societies affected by modern industrialization." It has also been pointed out that all the mummies at the museums in Cairo and Europe showed no evidence of cancer at all.

The research, which was published in NATURE, reported that, "Evidence of cancer and medical procedures, such as operations for cancers does not appear until the 17th century . . . Scientific literature depicting distinctive tumors have only been about for the last 200 years, when data started to be documented about chimney sweeps with scrotal cancer in 1775, nasal cancer in snuff users in 1761, and Hodgkin's disease in 1832."

It is lucidly clear from the data in this study, which included information from across the millennia, that cancer and most of the diseases afflicting mankind and the damages to our environment today are man-made and self-induced.

The vital question is: what do we do about this self-destructive, almost suicidal behavior of our species on planet Earth?

Vitamin D3 versus Cancer

The role of vitamin D3 as a cancer-preventing and fighting agent has been on the forefront of medical news these days. Medically known as calciferol, this vitamin was discovered in 1918 in cod liver oil and popularly called today as the sunshine vitamin.

New studies revealed that "vitamin D regulates cell proliferation and can hold in check the sort of wild cell growth that leads to cancer."

Several studies showed that among people taking high dose of vitamin D there was a decrease in the rate of at least 18 types of cancer and autoimmune diseases, including diabetes, rheumatoid arthritis, and 40% less risk for multiple sclerosis. Statistical analysis estimates that "thousands of caner deaths could be avoided in the United States each year if everyone gets enough vitamin D."

Vitamin D is the only vitamin humans can produce on their own when exposed to the ultraviolet B from the sun. In 15 minutes, a fair-skinned person, outside on a sunny day, can generate as much as 10,000 to 20,000 IU of vitamin D. This vitamin is recently in the limelight for being a "blockbuster" nutrient that confers even greater health benefits than previously recognized by the medical community. This rediscovery has put vitamin D in an altogether new perspective and importance.

Which vitamin D is preferred?

Vitamin D3 (choleciferol) is the recommended form since it is better absorbed and better utilized by the body compared to vitamin D2 (ergocalciferol).

What foods contain vitamin D?

Not many foods contain vitamin D. Milk is fortified with 125 IU of vitamin per glass. The following contain some vitamin D, but in themselves, do not provide the minimum daily requirement: organ meats, eggs, fish like tuna, mackerel, sardines, salmon, and herring. Having a balanced diet with enough calcium (1,000-1,500 mg) and vitamin D3 (400-1000 IU daily) will prevent osteoporosis (thinning of the bones, a common cause of fractures). Exposure to the sun for about 5-10 minutes, 2-3 times a week is enough help in the body's production of vitamin D.

How different is D from the other vitamins?

Besides being unique in the sense that it is the only vitamin our body can make on its own, vitamin D is also the only vitamin that influences the entire body as the findings have shown. Receptors that respond to vitamin D have been discovered in almost all the various kinds of human cells, from the brain to the bones.

What else is vitamin D good for?

Besides the old role vitamin D was popular for (boosting absorption of calcium which is essential for bone health), vitamin D has also been found over the past decades to have a broad range of added benefits. This includes the ability to help fight cancers and diabetes. Sixty-three independent studies showed that high normal level of vitamin D reduced the risk of developing colon, breast, and ovarian cancer by 50%. It is also a "pivotal feedstock" for a hormone that protects muscles and inhibits autoimmune diseases like multiple sclerosis, lupus, and inflammatory bowel illnesses. It also helps in easing some body aches and pain.

How does one prevent vitamin D deficiency?

Health education and awareness are essential. Human breast milk does not have enough vitamin D (40 IU/L), unlike fortified cow's milk (400 IU/L). Babies who are breastfed should have a physician's advice for possible oral supplement of vitamin D (300 IU per day) from birth to 6 months. Dr. Michael F. Hollick of the Boston University School of Medicine stated in their NIH-funded study, which involved 16,500 subjects, they have "found that lactating women need about 6,000 IU a day to transfer enough vitamin D into their milk to supply adequate amount to a nursing infant." In more urgent cases, like the studies done among adolescents in the Far East, one does of intramuscular injection of 2.5 mg (100,000 IU) of ergocalciferol given in the fall has increased the plasma level of vitamin D that lasted till spring the following year.

Experts now say that, together with normal sun exposure, 1,000 IU is the amount of vitamin D3 tablet we all should be getting daily. While researches have also shown the safety of the daily intake of up to 4,000 IU, studies are still underway to determine if the intake of 5,000 IU daily is better, is safe, and is devoid of the potential toxic side-effect (dangerous increase of blood level of calcium). Check with your physician first before starting yourself on this regimen.

Vitamin-cancer link?

The CBS health news telecast early in 2011 regarding the possible link between multivitamins and cancer has been confusing to many, taken out of context by some and exaggerated by others, creating doubt and fear among those who take them.

What WebMD reported was the preliminary data of a new research from the National Cancer Institute that basically stated "men who take many multivitamins may be increasing their risk of dying from prostate cancer."

What the study showed was taking vitamins "more than 7 days a week was linked to a 30% increased risk among those with advanced prostate cancer and a doubling of the risk of death from the disease."

Taking multivitamins, at the "regular recommended dose, one to six times a week, did not to increase the cancer risk, and excessive vitamin use was not associated with an increased risk among patients with early, or localized, prostate cancer."

The subjects referred to in this study were patients who already had prostate cancer to begin with, in varying stages of the disease, and the researchers were investigating what effects multivitamins had on their cancer. There were 8,765 men with localized prostate cancer and 1,476 with advanced prostate cancer diagnosed during this 5-year study, which included a total of 295,000 men enrolled in a diet and health research.

"More research is needed to confirm the association and understand how vitamin and other dietary supplements affect cancer risk," concluded NCI researcher Michael F. Leitzmann, MD, PhD.

Following our clarification of the medical subtleties in that CBS news, we are hoping that those taking multivitamins and minerals regularly can have the peace of mind, knowing that the study did not pertain to the general public.

Carbs: Good or Bad?

There is a confusing controversy, at least, in the public arena, whether carbohydrates are healthy or bad for us. This will, of course, depend on what type of carbohydrates we are talking about. There are carbs that are better for us than others. And then there is the quantity factor. How much is too much?

What are carbohydrates?

Carbohydrates are one of the 3 main classes of food and sources of energy. The other two are protein and fats. Carbs are organic compounds of carbon, hydrogen, and oxygen, which include the sugars and starches found in rice, bread, cookies, candies, ice cream, cakes, potatoes, popcorn, corn, milk, beans, cereals, fruits. All these are eventually broken down to simple sugars called glucose.

What types are there?

The old classification categorized them into simple and complex. This was modified into carbs with high glycemic index and those with low glycemic index. The latest measure is the so-called glycemic load, since glycemic index alone did not tell us how much carbs is contained in the food item. The glycemic load tells us both the amount of carbohydrates in the food, how fast they are absorbed, and its impact on the blood sugar levels. Low-glycemic-index foods, in general, are the healthier ones, because they are absorbed more slowly and increases the glucose level more steadily, not rapidly and abruptly like the high-glycemic foods are.

How do we calculate the glycemic load?

To get the glycemic load of the food item, multiply the glycemic index by the amount of carb calories the food contains. This may seem complicated, but the important caveat to remember is minimally processed whole-grain foods are healthier than highly processed grains, cereals and sugars. An example is brown rice, which is less processed, and therefore healthier, compared to white rice which has been thoroughly processed, from cleaning, husking, paddy separating, and milling (which strips off the bran layer, which is actually good for us), leaving only the starchy endosperm we call white rice. The more processed the food items are, the less healthier they are, even in processed, canned, or packaged meats, vegetables, and fruits, with preservatives.

Which are these food items?

Low-glycemic load (LGL) food items are high-fiber fruits and vegetables, bran cereals, and legumes, like chick peas, pinto beans, kidney beans, black beans. The medium glycemic load (MGL) ones include brown rice, oatmeal, bulgur, pearled barley, whole grain pasta, whole grain bread, and fruit juice without added sugar. The high-glycemic-load (HGL) foods include white rice, potatoes, French fries, potato chips, refined cereals, white flour. Nondiet pop drinks, candies, jelly beans, couscous, cranberry juice. Potatoes, for one, in any form, is both a high-glycemic-index and high-glycemic-load item.

Does our body need carbohydrates at all?

Yes, most definitely. To stay healthy, we need all the three types of food items: carbohydrates, proteins, and fats. But there are food items in each of these three classes which are healthier than others. The healthiest carbohydrates are the low-glycemic-load foods and some medium-glycemic-load items. The best source of proteins are fish, legumes, some seafoods, instead of red meats, especially not processed meat products. As for fats, we do not have to eat fat per se, since most of the other food items we eat as listed above already have fats in them. While our digestive system breaks down all other food items into glucose, the fiber foods cannot be broken down and pass through our GI tract undigested, helping us have more regular bowel movements and also in lowering the incidence of cancer of the colon.

Why are high-glycemic-index foods unhealthy?

In general, our body system is adversely affected by anything abrupt and drastic. It prefers more gradual and smoother fluctuations in the chemistry that is constantly occurring in our body. When we eat high-glycemic foods, especially nondiet soft drinks, candies, rice, potatoes, desserts, our glucose (blood sugar) level shoots up abruptly. This has been linked to an increased risk of diabetes and heart disease. Lower glycemic foods help control type 2 diabetes.

How much is too much?

The best gauge for our daily food (calories) intake is our body mass index, which, simply stated, is our expected weight according to our height. A person 5 feet four inches tall should normally weigh around 110 to 140. Weighing once a week (preferably the same day and time) will help guide us as to our daily calorie requirement. But as a rule, cutting down our carbohydrate consumption will help not only in maintaining a normal weight, but in preventing diseases such as metabolic syndrome, which includes diabetes, high blood pressure, and heart disease.

So what's the healthier choice?

Choosing healthier sources of proteins and carbohydrates as listed above and, of course, controlling the calories to achieve your normal weight, is the key. A two-decade prospective study of 82,802 women revealed that those "who ate low-carbohydrate diets that were high in vegetable sources of fat or protein had a 30 percent lower risk of heart disease, compared to women who ate high carbohydrate, low-fat diets . . . and women who ate low-carbohydrate diets that were high in animal fats or proteins did not have a reduced risk of heart disease." Eating a lot of green leafy vegetables, whole oats, legumes, yogurt, and fruits is healthier in general and will also protect us from a host of chronic illnesses, metabolic diseases, and cancer.

As always, what we sow is what we reap.

Carbs: Sweet killer

Like choosing your own poison when it comes to abusing any of the various alcoholic beverages around if you were a drinker, there are also different food types that are really hazardous to health when we consume them with abandon, without care.

While we have listed red meat as the most notorious on the list of what food to eat only sparingly, if at all, since it is not an essential food item, without which we can survive and even be healthier, carbohydrates (sugars) are the so-called "addictive white substance," the "sweet killer."

Unlike the white meat of chicken (minus the skin) when taken in moderation, red meat (pork, beef, etc.), even in moderation, increases our blood cholesterol and fats, which lead to clogging of our arteries, causing heart attack, stroke, blockage of leg arteries, and gangrene. High-fat and cholesterol also increase the risk for Alzheimer's, diabetes, arthritis, gout, and many forms of cancer. Processed red meats are unhealthy for all of us, especially for children.

Carbohydrates include table sugar, rice, bread, pies, cakes, ice cream, cookies, potatoes, all sweets, and anything made of flour, rice, or corn. A few vegetables have some carbohydrates in them also, but the health benefits from vegetables outweigh the little sugar in them. Fruits have a lot of sugar, called fructose, which is a better form of carbs. But those who are diabetics must include the calories from fruits they eat when they count their daily total calorie limits.

Why must we control our carbohydrate or sweet intake?

Carbs are more addictive than cocaine, believe it or not. Those who have sweet tooth who are not aware of the bad health effects of carbohydrates and become "hooked" often become overweight or even obese. This increases their risk to develop diabetes and metabolic diseases, heart attack and stroke, and Alzheimer's dementia. The consequent elevation of triglyceride in the blood further predisposes the person to even higher risk of all those diseases.

Once the craving for sweets is established, following frequent consumption of any of the carbs foods as listed above, which should include what I call "liquid candies" (cola or uncola soft drinks), reducing intake will lead to subtle withdrawal symptoms, just like among cigarette, alcohol, or drug addicts, albeit lot milder. Some develop intense desire to eat sweets or drink pop. Others may have headaches or sense of hunger, feeling down, irritable, or have mood changes.

Soft drinks, including the low—or zero-calorie ones, even one drink a day, are very unhealthy because they cause illnesses that creep in slowly, like heart disease, according to famous the Framingham Heart Study. There are 10 teaspoons (40 grams) of sugar in 12-ounce nondiet soft drinks, yielding 160 calories! While these "liquid candies" are unhealthy, even those no-cal soft drinks have been found to cause metabolic syndrome (high blood pressure, diabetes, heart attack/ stroke). Alcohol gives greater calories (7) per gram than carbohydrates (4 per gram).

To neutralize the sugar and the phosphoric acid in the liver, following consumption of just one can of soda, one needs to drink thirty-two 8-ounce (256 ounces) alkaline water. So why even ingest the "poison" in the first place, only to follow it with an "antidote" chaser?

What are the findings of the Harvard Research on soft drinks?

The study reveals that those who consumed one or more sodas a day have 31% greater risk of becoming obese and 44% increased risk of developing metabolic syndrome.

How much sugar do we consume?

The average individual in the United States eat about 142 pounds of sugar each year, which translates to about 48 teaspoon a day. Added to that amount is the sugar in the food and drinks we consume each day, which is about 4 pounds. That's a total of about 146 pounds a year. As a general rule for those who are not overweight,1/2 cup (4 heaping tablespoonful) of cooked rice per meal is sufficient. For those who are overweight or diabetic, lesser amount, or abandoning rice and sweets altogether, would be healthier. Remember, vegetables and fruits have carbohydrates as well. The main idea is calorie control.

What happens following sugar control?

Studies have shown that about two weeks of lowering your carbs intake or not eating rice, bread, etc., our body chemistry stabilizes, including the levels of serotonin and other neurotransmitters, and our metabolism and general well-being are enhanced. While sugar elevates the serotonin level, a feel-good hormone, the after-effect, when the blood sugar goes down (even to normal level for those "addicted" to and used to eating a lot of carbs) is the opposite. It is best for all our hormones to be on an even keel, in their natural normal levels most of the time, for normal physiology.

Vegetables, whole grains, nuts, and fresh fruits (not fruit juices loaded with sugar), with all their fibers, restore the body's pH (natural acid-alkaline) balance. This reduces sugar cravings and improves digestion. In general, berries and melons have lesser sugar contents than other fruits.

Do carbs affect our homeostasis?

Yes, excess carbs in our system, which is usually the case among most of us, disturbs our homeostasis, the proper internal balance of our body physiology and functions. High carb intake leads to disruption of hormonal production and release, including insulin, and compromises our immune system. Occasional indulgence in sweets is healthy, like pampering our body with special treat, a reward for discipline, if you will.

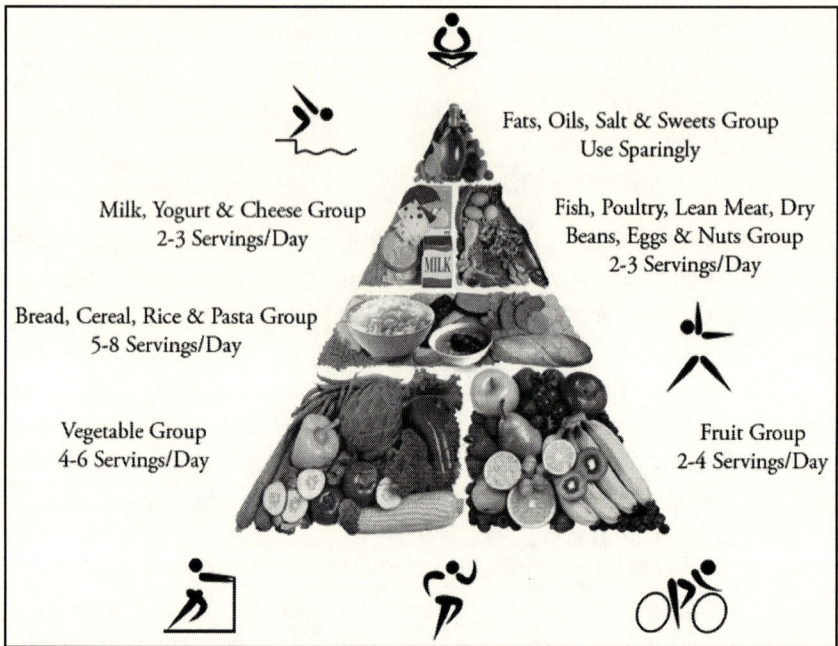

Fats, Oils, Salt & Sweets Group
Use Sparingly

Milk, Yogurt & Cheese Group
2-3 Servings/Day

Fish, Poultry, Lean Meat, Dry
Beans, Eggs & Nuts Group
2-3 Servings/Day

Bread, Cereal, Rice & Pasta Group
5-8 Servings/Day

Vegetable Group
4-6 Servings/Day

Fruit Group
2-4 Servings/Day

On October 10, 2008, I revised the original Food Pyramid issued by the US Department of Agriculture in 1992, and replaced its wide base of mostly carbohydrates with vegetables and fruits as shown in my version above, to comprise about 50% of the total daily diet. In "my" Food Pyramid, carbohydrates were reduced and moved up to the second tier. The new Food Plate (on page 37), which was introduced by the USDA and the First Lady June 2, 2011 to replace the 1992 Food Pyramid, emphasizes vegetables and fruits. The role of daily exercise is overwhelmingly essential, besides a wholesome diet, in the maintenance of good health and prevention of diseases. One regimen without the other severely reduces their combined potential health benefits.

Carcinogens in Our Home

Most cancers, in general, are caused by the body's repeated exposure to harmful chemicals in our environment. These include tobacco, alcohol, and all dangerous ingredients in common household cleansing agents, like laundry, kitchen, walls, windows, floor, and toilet detergents. Added to these are the variety of chemicals, solutions, or sprays we have in the garage, for cleaning cars and the floor underneath them. And the pollution of our rivers and lakes and oceans from industrial toxic wastes and air pollution from these same companies and from our car exhaust system destroy the protective ozone layer above us and are major sources of carcinogens. To boot, many of us regularly ingest with gusto two major cancer-producing substances: tobacco and alcohol, two culprit agents that account for most of the diseases, disabilities, and deaths in the world today. The diseases include cancer, lung illnesses, diabetes, hypertension, heart attack, and stroke. Many forms of cancer are literally "self-inflicted" and otherwise preventable.

Whether we realize it or not, our bad habits and our closets and shelves at home are the two of the most substantial sources of cancer-causing chemicals that we come in contact with, or inhale the fumes of, daily, which adversely impact our body, health, and longevity. The other carcinogens are from the environmental poisons forced upon us by irresponsible industrial corporations and pollutant-emitting vehicles.

Statistics show that most of the illnesses that affect, maim, and kill human beings today are brought on by these substances: alcohol and/ or tobacco (including secondhand smoke). These diseases include lung diseases (bronchitis, emphysema, lung cancer), cardiovascular diseases (high blood pressure, heart attack, cardiomyopathy, rhythm problems, and sudden death), metabolic diseases, like diabetes mellitus, and many forms of cancer. The other factors are likewise due to similar bad choices on our part: a high-cholesterol, high-fat, high-carbohydrate, high salt, low-fiber diet; and dangerously living a sedentary life (as a couch potato, doing only finger exercises with the TV remote and munching on all the junk foods around), simply getting fat. This scenario reminds us of the strategy to get the most weight on cattle and hogs before an early slaughter: keeping them in a tight "cage" where they practically cannot move and feeding them frequently to maximize their weight and fat. And it works. Much like our couches at home.

Living a healthy lifestyle will eliminate most of these diseases and provide us a healthier, happier, and more productive life. And this singular wonderful benefit in itself is worth all the sacrifices and hard work one needs to invest to achieve it.

On the household front, we agree that these chemical agents make it a lot easier for us to do our chores at home, but the potential side effects and complications from their use—possible diseases, disabilities and early deaths—are too high a price to pay. And for these dozen or more chemical agents we use at home daily, perhaps we can minimize the danger of toxicity by limiting their use. And maybe we can utilize more the old-fashioned nonchemical scrubbing and cleaning methods used by our great-grandparents and theirs for centuries. This will certainly appear to be one retrogressive step; but ultimately, I am sure, it will be evident that this is a great leap forward that will actually spell progress.

Cardiac Cath: "Supreme Court" of heart tests

What is a cardiac catheterization?

Cardiac catheterization is a medical test where radio-opaque dye is injected into the left (and as needed, also into the right) chamber of the heart and the coronary arteries of the heart to find out if there are any abnormalities of the inner walls of the heart, the heart valves, the strength of the cardiac contraction (pumping action), and any blockages in heart arteries.

Why is this test important?

Cardiac cath or coronary angio, as the procedure is popularly nicknamed, is what could be regarded as the "supreme court" of all heart tests. While EKG (electrocardiogram) and stress EKG (treadmill test), or even ECHO (echocardiogram) are studies used to detect the presence of coronary artery disease, these tests are noninvasive procedures utilized as preliminary or screening diagnostic methods. If they show normal results, then chances are there are no blockages in the coronary arteries. If the results are doubtful or positive, then cardiac cath is performed to make the final determination. Following cardiac cath, the physician can say with practically 100% certainty if the patient has coronary blockages or heart valve disease or not. Hence, it is considered the "supreme court" or "court of final resort" of cardiac diagnostic tests.

What are the possible complications of this test?

Allergy to the dye injected is one possible complication. An antihistaminic and steroid injection could be given by injection (before the procedure) for those with known allergy to the dye, or is used to counteract this allergy following the test. During the actual catheterization, there could be temporary heart irritation from the catheter in the aorta or in the heart, causing minor heartbeat irregularity or slowing of the heart rate. A tiny air bubble or tiny clot could travel to other organs or to the leg, but this is very rare and more of an exception. After the procedure and the catheter is removed from the puncture site at the groin, there could be bleeding. Usually, the oozing is very mild, and pressure applied to the area stops the bleeding. Cardiac cath is a widely used procedure every day all over the world and a very safe test.

Has there been any death reported from the procedure?

Just like many invasive medical tests, cardiac cath has possible risk, but the risk of dying from cardiac cath is much less compared to, say, accidental death from a car accident on a busy highway. The risk of *not* having the test at all and leaving the heart condition undiagnosed poses a greater risk than undergoing cardiac cath. In one study, it was shown that in 5,000 consecutive cardiac caths, there was no mortality at all. Indeed, cardiac cath is one of the safest tests and a most valuable and lifesaving one.

How vital is this test?

Prior to the introduction of cardiac cath in 1958, people developed coronary artery disease, undiagnosed, and died of heart attack without much hope. It was only after this test became popular that heart-lung machine, heart-bypass procedure came about, one rapidly following the other in historical development. And these three technologies prospered and exploded, hand in hand, to their present state-of-the-art popularity and service to humanity.

Should cardiac cath be done as preventive measure?

Not as a rule. If there are no symptoms and the patient is healthy and active, we do not recommend cardiac cath just to satisfy our or the patient's curiosity. Besides being expensive, the test has possible risk and complications (although mild and rare) as described earlier. One exception is for big corporation executive checkups and for airline pilots, where some companies require initial employment cardiac cath. The other exception, which is more of a medical indication, is for persons who have a strong family history of heart attack (a genetic predisposition), who are also hypertensive, diabetic, and a cigarette smoker.

What is a "widow-maker" lesion?

The possibility of the presence of the "widow-maker" blockage is also a medically accepted reason for doing coronary angiogram as a preventive measure, even if the patient looks healthy and has no symptoms whatsoever. When the stress test (EKG taken on a person walking on a treadmill of increasing speed and incline) shows findings suspicious of a left main coronary artery (LMCA) blockage (widow-maker lesion), which could have a 50% mortality within 6 months depending on its severity, coronary angiogram is a mandatory medical recommendation, even if the patient is totally asymptomatic. Indeed, this LMCA lesion has caused sudden deaths and all too many widows. I have seen many patients with this preventable catastrophes and deaths. So if in doubt, see your doctor, at least for a stress test, especially if you are 45 years and older.

A sage advice: "Take good care of your heart—it's the only one you've got."

Cardiac Pacemaker

What is a cardiac pacemaker?

Cardiac pacemaker is a self-contained battery-operated unit that sends electrical stimulation to the inner wall of the right ventricle of the heart to make it beat no lower than a certain pre-set rate. A heart pacemaker is implanted among patients, usually elderly, whose heart rate goes below 60 beats per minute, causing them to feel weak, lack pep, and even feel dizzy or actually faint and lose consciousness.

What is the normal heart rate?

Essentially, it is between 60 and 100 beats per minute. Anything below 60 is considered bradycardia (slow heart rate) and rate above 100 is called tachycardia (rapid heart rate). But what is normal is also relative. Well-conditioned athletes, for instance, could have heart rate lower than 60, maybe as low as 40, as their normal rate and feel very well. Almost all of us, in general, especially the elderly, would feel dizzy, weak, and even pass out if our heart rate dropped below 60.

Why does bradycardia cause this?

Slow heart rate obviously causes the heart to pump less blood to the brain and the rest of the body. The brain is very sensitive to diminished blood (oxygen and nutrition) supply. So when the "pump" slows down, the blood circulation and pressure going to the brain is also lower than what is normal for the individual. This fall in blood pressure and blood volume to the brain causes the weakness and fainting spells.

What causes bradycardia?

The usual cause of slow heart rate is called sick sinus syndrome (SSS), where the natural impulse generator (sinus node) of the heart is "ill" and not able to send enough electrical impulses to the heart to stimulate it to beat at the normal rate. The culprit is usually arteriosclerosis (hardening of the artery that supplies that "pulse generator of the heart"). For this reason, an artificial (electronic) pacemaker is used to function as the heart's stimulator.

If not treated, what happens?

Untreated persistent bradycardia leads to hypotension (lower blood pressure) and lesser blood supply to the brain, which could result in a stroke. Usually, the symptoms range from weakness, lack of pep or interest, sleepiness among the elderly, to chest pains and/or fainting spells or to actual syncope (passing out). Persons who develop bradycardia while climbing stairs could faint and fall and hurt themselves, and those who are driving could pass out and lose control of the vehicle.

How is the diagnosis made?

Simplistically, the diagnosis is made by history and physical examination. Listening to the heartbeat and checking the pulse to count the heart rate instantly reveal the diagnosis. An EKG tracing will confirm this on record. A more sophisticated method, like electrophysiologic studies (EPS), is now available. This test defines more precisely the nature of the rhythm problem.

Do all patients with bradycardia need a pacemaker?

No, not all. Only those bradycardeic patients with symptoms of weakness, dizziness, or fainting spells, and/or chest tightness need a cardiac pacemaker. If they feel well and are active, with none of any of those symptoms, they do not need an artificial cardiac pacemaker.

Do people with dizziness or fainting spells need a heart pacer?

If the heart rate is normal, the dizziness or fainting spells could be due to other medical causes, and therefore a cardiac pacemaker will not help and is obviously not needed. Having the correct diagnosis is very important in order to know the proper treatment regimen. Consultation with a physician is essential because some symptoms could be common among many diseases.

Can a person with a cardiac pacer live a normal life?

Yes, individuals with a cardiac pacemaker usually live a normal life, a lot safer and more comfortable life. The only exception would be those persons with an attendant illness that is debilitating. One famous political personality who had a cardiac pacemaker implanted and who is still very active in global political affairs is former US Secretary of State Henry Kissinger. Contrary to the myth, persons with heart pacer can safely use a microwave oven, as long as the door of the oven is intact and not leaking. Patients with a cardiac pacemaker are advised to prevent anything from hitting the left upper chest where the unit is, to prevent the pacer lead from getting fractured. Cardiac pacemakers have saved millions of lives and have made life more comfortable and more productive for millions more.

The Carnitine Craze

Like the snake-oil style scams claiming "the greatness, benefits, and safety" of dozens of so-called food supplements and herbals, which are very expensive, the addition of L-carnitine in drinks and other food items is nothing but false advertisement and public misinformation.

Carnitine is a normal substance in our diet. It is a hydrophilic amino acid derivative, produced in the liver and kidneys, from meat and dairy products we eat. Carnitine allows for the proper metabolism and conversion of fats into energy. We do not need any "extra" carnitine to stay healthy. Our body gets enough from the food we eat daily. To add another chemical substance to our food is totally unnecessary and may even be dangerous.

Primary carnitine deficiency, which is a rare inherited autosomal recessive pattern, affects 1 out of every 40,000 live births in Japan and 1 out of every 37,000 to 100,000 newborns in Australia. It is a congenital defect in babies and very young children but seen in adult very rarely. Primary carnitine in adults is almost unheard of.

In view of available medical facts, why are manufacturers adding L-carnitine to their food products for the general public? Besides, an infant or a child, or even the rare adult who has this uncommon disorder, would not be helped, much less cure the carnitine deficiency anyway, since the amount added to the food items is not in the therapeutic level.

The inference that the added L-carnitine to the food items in question is beneficial and safe for the consumers is another gimmick these greedy and unscrupulous vendors of ill will are using to earn a fast buck.

Manufacturers of unproven herbals and the umpteen numbers of "food supplements" on the market today continue to victimize the helpless ignorant consumers. And they obviously do so with impunity because they know they can get away with it.

The more important issue here is, therefore, why our government is not enforcing our laws governing truth in advertising and other pertinent regulations to protect the public?

Carpal Tunnel Syndrome

What is carpal tunnel syndrome?

Carpal tunnel syndrome (CTS) is a very common condition that causes persistent or frequent pains in the wrist and hand, especially after protracted use of the typewriter or computer keyboard and resulting from months or years of prolonged and repeated extension and flexion of the wrist or making the same hand/wrist movements over and over.

What is a carpal tunnel?

Carpal tunnel is an anatomical space within the wrist, much like a tunnel, comprised of a semicircle of wrist bones on one side and bounded on the other by transverse carpal ligament. Through this confined and unyielding channel pass nine tendons, the median nerve, and tenosynovial tissue. When these tissues swell (from chronic and repeated trauma of extension and flexion of the wrists), the median nerve is pinched, causing the syndrome. One or both hands/ wrists may be involved, frequently the one that is most often used.

What are the signs and symptoms of CTS?

Pain in the wrist, palm or forearm is common, which may also involve the shoulder, back and the neck in some cases. There may be numbness, tingling of hand or fingers, weakness of the hand, loss of grip, the hand my "fall asleep" on waking up in the morning, during the night, or while driving, or following any activity that requires elevation of the hands. The pains are usually more at night and may even wake the patient up. In women, more pains before menstrual period, in the third trimester of pregnancy, and the first few months after delivery (all these due to edema or fluid retention during these times).

Who are most prone to CTS?

CTS is most common among those whose work requires constant gripping, pinching, typing, with the wrist held in flexion (bent), like chronic computer users, typists, meat packers, violinists, mechanics, assembly-line workers, grocery checkers, carpenters, etc. Canoeing, playing golf, needlework can cause the CTS symptoms. Fracture of the wrist could also cause the syndrome. Women between the age of 40 to 60 are the most frequent target. CTS could also be due to diabetes, thyroid disease, or rheumatoid arthritis.

Is CTS serious?

No, usually CTS is not a serious condition. With prompt and proper treatment, the symptoms are alleviated and no permanent damage develops.

How is CTS diagnosed?

The patient usually describes the typical symptoms when seeking medical consultation. The physician will also ask the type of job the patient does and what illnesses he/she may have. Some of the tests include tapping the inside of the wrist to elicit pain or a sensation of an electric shock in the wrist or hand, bending the wrist for 60 seconds to see if symptoms of CTS develop, or ordering nerve conduction velocity test or an electromyography. Without all the above tests, the condition is often missed and not diagnosed accurately.

Does using a wrist support band help?

Elastic wrist support band may offer some help in minimizing the onset and the symptoms of CTS, unless the cause is one of the diseases mentioned above. Also, if the person does not reduce the hand and wrist repetitive movements, support band will not help. The anatomical size of the patient's carpal tunnel is obviously an important factor.

How can one prevent CTS?

Taking care of health and the way the hands and wrists are used allow one to prevent the development of carpal tunnel syndrome. Attendant medical diseases must be treated. Those who are overweight should lose weight. Stop smoking. Cut down on alcohol and caffeinated drinks. Be conscious not to bend, extend, or twist the hands (wrists) for a long time. Do not rest the wrists on hard surface for a long time. Switch hands. Hold objects instead of pinching them. Avoid or minimize using tools that vibrate a lot. Do not stand or sit in the same position the entire day; take a break from repeated hand/wrist movements to give them a rest. Prop up the arms with pillows when lying down. For computer or typing work, adjust the height of the chair so that the forearms are on the same level as the keyboard to allow you type without flexing the wrists.

What is the initial treatment for CTS?

If the carpal tunnel syndrome is caused by a disease, then the particular illness is treated first. If it is not, then the patient is advised to rest the wrist involved and to change the manner in which the hand and the wrist are used. A splint on the wrist may also be recommended to rest the wrist while use of the hand is allowed. The splint also eases the pain, especially at bedtime. Application of ice pack, massaging the wrist, and some stretching exercises may also help.

How about pain medications?

For control of pains, acetaminophen, aspirin, ibuprofen, naproxen, or ketoprofen may be used as directed by the physician. In some situations, local injection of corticosteroid may help in reducing the swelling and inflammation and ease the pains.

When is surgery needed?

Surgery is indicated if all those conservative measures fail and do not alleviate the symptoms.

What surgery is performed for CTS?

The basic principle of surgery for CTS is dividing the overlying ligament to release the constricting effect of the tunnel over the nerve and underlying structures in the tunnel. This can be done by open method where a cut is made on the wrist to expose the ligament, which is then divided. The close method is one where an endoscope is used (like a small telescope with a light), and the ligament is cut through tiny holes in the skin, which can later be closed without sutures.

What is the prognosis?

When diagnosed promptly and treated properly, the prognosis of CTS is very good. In majority of cases, with appropriate therapy, the cure is usually permanent and no residual damage occurs.

Hope for Cataract Patients

Our consultant for this topic is Emily C. Greenlee, MD, Assistant Clinical Professor in the Department of Ophthalmology and Visual Sciences of the University of Iowa Hospital and Clinics, 6th on the top ten list of Best Hospitals in America.

What are cataracts?

Cataracts are cloudiness or opacities of the lens of the eyes that impair visual acuity. Located behind the pupil of the eyes, the lenses help the eyes focus, much like that of a camera. If the photographic lens is "dirty" the picture taken will be out of focus or blurry. And if the lens is covered with very thick smudges, the camera may not be able to "see and focus" at all. The same thing is true with our eye lenses. Cataract is not a tumor or anything else but a cloudiness of the lens, causing change or decrease in the clarity of the lens.

What causes cataracts?

Practically everyone over the age of 65 has cataract in one or both eyes that causes visual impairment. Diabetes and medications, like steroids, hasten cataract formation. When the eyes are exposed to excessive X-rays (as among radiology technicians), penetrating trauma, chemical burns, intense sunlight, or exposure to excessive heat, this also contributes to cataract formation.

How about smoking?

Smoking has been shown to lead to a higher occurrence of cataracts compared to abstinence from tobacco.

How fast does cataract form?

Cataracts usually take years to develop, but some cases may worsen rapidly in a few months, because of the "dose" or intensity of the contributing factors at play. One or both eyes may be affected, usually both, simultaneously, and the severity in one could be worse than that in the other eye.

What are the symptoms?

The most common the person notices is hazy or blurred vision, poor night vision, or in very bright light, even glare from headlights of oncoming cars when driving at night. There could also be "ghost" images, a change in color vision, poor distant vision, and loss of contrast.

Do all cataract patients need surgery?

No. People with clear vision in spite of having cataracts do not need surgery. Only those with cataracts that impair vision and interfere with their ability to perform daily routine tasks (reading, driving, watching TV, etc.) and any other activities that require a good sight would require an operation to remove the opacified or cloudy lenses and restore clear vision.

Is cataract surgery common?

Cataract surgery is one of the commonest and most successful surgeries today. In the United States, more than 1.25 million such procedures are performed annually. The outcome of the procedure depends on the overall health of the patient, age, coexisting medical diseases (diabetes, hypertension, etc.), the severity of the cataract, and the presence of other abnormalities of the eyes.

How about non-surgical treatment?

Cataracts, when present in the lenses, never go away on their own or even with the use of medications. Only surgery can remove the cataracts. For temporary relief, until surgery is done, the use of eyedrops to widen the pupil of the eyes may help improve vision among some patients. The use of Polaroid sunglasses and visor to protect the eyes from sunlight to reduce the glare and the use of brighter light bulbs instead of fluorescent light may help the patient see better indoors. But these are all temporary measures. Only surgery can remove the cataracts.

What is the timing of the surgery?

There was a time in the past where ophthalmologists recommended a waiting period "to ripen" or to allow for "full growth" or "maturity" of the cataracts before doing surgery. Advances in eye surgery today recommend early elective removal to avoid complications and avoid making the surgery more difficult. The other factors in the decision-making are the patient's age, occupation, and lifestyle. Today's procedures are safer and more successful than ever.

How successful is the surgery?

Cataract surgery has a success rate of more than 95%. Most of these patients now have intraocular lens (IOL) implanted after removal of the cataracts. In those rare cases where IOL is not appropriate, the ophthalmologist may prescribe the use of contact lens and, in rarer cases, a thick and heavy eyeglasses may be an option. But in these cases the peripheral vision (side vision) is distorted. Since there are various operations available, it is prudent for the person to discuss in detail with the attending ophthalmologist as to which procedure is the best for him/her.

Are both cataracts removed at the same time?

No, there is an interval of 4 to 8 weeks or so between surgeries. And the operation on the second eye may not be necessary for visual acuity. The need is tailored to individual needs of the person. The trend in the procedure is using a small incision and ultrasound. Most sutures used on the eyes do not have to be removed, so the surgery is referred to as "stitchless cataract surgery."

What are the procedures performed?

There are two types: Phacoemulsification or "phaco" for short, also called "small incision cataract surgery," where a small incision is made on the side of the cornea and a probe is inserted that emits ultrasound waves that soften and break up the diseased lens so it could be removed by suction. The other procedure is the extracapsular surgery, where a longer incision is made and the entire cloudy lens is removed in one piece. Of the two, "phaco" is the most common procedure done today.

Are there risks involved?

As with any form of surgery, there are potential risks involved with cataract surgery. They are possible bleeding, infection, and retinal detachment, especially among those with myopia (nearsightedness). Patients must discuss with their eye surgeon the details of the reason for the recommended surgery, the type of procedure itself, and possible risks and complications. With rare exceptions, this surgery yields a most rewarding transformation—from a state of near blindness or total darkness to an instant and "miraculous" restoration of clear sight.

Cell Phone-Cancer Debate

The World Health Organization (WHO) announced on May 31, 2011 that "radiation from cell phones can possibly cause cancer." This is the boldest statement yet from this international body.

WHO's International Agency for Research on Cancer (IARC), stated that "radiofrequency electromagnetic fields have been classified as possibly carcinogenic to humans (group 2B) on the basis of an increased risk for glioma (brain tumor) that some studies have associated with the use of wireless phones."

Thirty one scientists from 14 countries conducted an extensive review of various studies on the safety of cell phones, specifically evaluating "the potential carcinogenic hazards from exposure to radiofrequency electromagnetic fields." Their findings were the basis for this recent WHO declaration.

What is the current theory?

It is suspected that the frequent and extended use of a cellular phone (where the phone is right at the user's cheek, the earpiece smack against the ear) might be associated with increased incidence of brain tumor.

How could the cellular phone "cause" harm?

The cellular phone antenna is the "probable culprit" in this medical concern. It is theorized that the antenna, which receives electromagnetic waves (EMW) or signals, transmits the same EMW to the brain of the person using the cellular phone (since the unit is in close proximity to the brain), and that these EMW might explain the suspected increase in the incidence of brain cancer among chronic users.

Is one cellular phone worse than the other?

The ones which are with dual band (1800 MHz) are said to be worse than the regular ones with only 900 MHz. Obviously, there are other factors, like length of exposure and proximity of the cellular phone to the brain, etc.

What other illness can cellular phone use cause?

The other condition often mentioned is leukemia. Again, we would like to emphasize that we do not have scientific data to support this suspicion at this time.

Are microwave ovens safe?

The normal use of microwave ovens is safe, provided the protective shield is not broken. However, we caution users not to bring their face near the oven door while the oven is on, because the microwaves can harm the eyes by causing premature cataracts. A leaking microwave oven can also affect (inhibit) cardiac pacemakers.

How about television sets?

Since television sets or computer monitors also emit some electromagnetic radiation, it is advisable not to go too close to the TV or monitor. The fact that medical science does not have any evidence that these EMW are harmful does not mean they are totally safe. It is best to be cautious and view the television at least 5 feet away from you.

Does cellular phone use cause infertility?

There is no factual basis for this concern. We do not have any reason to believe that infertility or impotence can be caused by the use of cellular phones or having one in a holster by the hip or in a purse.

In the advisory he sent to about 3,000 faculty and staff, he also suggested that "children should use cell phones only for emergencies because their brains are still developing."

How can we make cellular phone use safer?

First and foremost, use cellular phones only as briefly as possible. The lesser the exposure to the EMW, the better. The use of "hands-free" devices like earpieces with microphone and EMW ear shields will help lessen the exposure.

Any health risk in text messaging?

Text messaging, a very popular preoccupation among some people in these days of instant telecommunication, poses no known hazard to physical health, not even to the fingers used in the process. And since the cellular phone is held farther away from the body when text messaging, the exposure to the EMW is less.

Heart Chelation: A Scam

What is chelation therapy?

Chelation therapy is an accepted treatment for poisoning by many metals (like lead, cadnium, arsenic, zinc, etc.) and other toxic substances. These chelating agents "cleanse" the blood of these poisons. Some unscrupulous healthcare providers, however, are bilking the unsuspecting public of their hard-earned money by prescribing and giving chelation intravenous shots "to unclog heart arteries," a claim that is false and without medical basis.

Which drugs are used as chelating agents?

Calcium disodium edetate, dimercaprol, and penillamine are some of them.

Is this the "therapy" advertised to unclog arteries?

Yes, there are unscrupulous individuals in the United States, Europe, Asia, and other parts of the globe who dupe and victimize the innocent public with claims that intravenous injections of supposedly these drugs, which they call chelation therapy, can unclog arteries in the body to prevent a heart attack and stroke. These "practitioners," who advertise that chelation therapy can dissolve hardening of the arteries and therefore preclude the need for angioplasty or open heart surgery, charge exhorbitant fees for the "treatment." In the United States, charges range from 4 to 6 thousand US dollars for "the complete session."

How is chelation treatment given?

The patients are given a series of intravenous injections for so many days. What drug is actually injected or whether only plain saline or dextrose are administered instead of true chelating agents, no one knows. In the United States, this practice of using chelation therapy to dissolve hardening of the arteries is not approved by the Food and Drug Administration (FDA) and condemned by the medical community. There is no legitimate scientific proof or basis for the claim. Some physicians and doctors of osteopathy have lost their medical license for perpetrating this fraud.

How did this practice come about?

It is easy to surmise that since chelating agents are really effective in the treatment of poisoning with metals and other toxic substances, and "cleanse" the blood among these patients, some enterprising people conveniently "extended" the use of these agents to include unclogging blocked arteries. Since all adults develop hardening of the arteries, to one degree or another, sooner or later in life, and since heart attack and stroke are commonplace, financial greed and deception have overcome some of these "practitioners" (who may not even be licensed physicians) to go into this very lucrative business.

Why does the FDA not ban these chelating agents?

Chelating agents are legitimate and good drugs indicated for specific conditions: metal poisoning and toxicity from other substances. There is nothing wrong with these drugs. The issue here is that these chelating agents are being used for a condition for which they are not indicated or effective. They are useless as far as dissolving hardening of the arteries or unclogging arteries are concerned.

Is there any drug that can dissolve hardening of the arteries?

No. There is no known safe drug that can dissolve hardening of the arteries or unclog blocked arteries. The blockages in the arteries are so hard and usually calcified like teeth or bone that to date, medical science has not discovered any medication that can dissolve hardening of the arteries. In the recent meeting of the American College of Cardiology, another study confirmed that chelation therapy for coronary artery disease is baseless, useless, and ineffective.

How about the enzymes injected to treat acute heart attack?

These enzymes (streptokinase, urokinase, TPA, etc.), which cardiologists administer intravenously in the emergency room or ICU when the patient is diagnosed to have an acute heart attack that is 4 to 6 hours old, are substances that dissolve the solid but still soft blood clot that blocks the coronary artery causing the heart attack. These enzymes cannot dissolve arteriosclerotic plaque or hardening of the arteries.

How are patients adversely affected by this scam?

Not only do unsuspecting patients lose their hard-earned money for a treatment that has been proven by medical science as ineffective, but they are also deceived and given false hopes, which can delay the proper diagnosis and treatment of their heart illness. Needless to say, this unwarranted delay could lead to worsening of the disease and a higher morbidity and mortality rate.

Chlamydia Sex Infection

Today's more liberated and permissive society has seen an increase in sexually transmitted diseases (Stds). The most common is genital chlamydia infection (GCI) in men and women. It is not as infamous as gonorrhea or syphilis, but it could nonetheless cause serious complications.

What is chlamydia infection?

This STD results from infection with bacterium *C. trachomatis* (serotypes D-K), which is transmitted primarily through sexual intercourse, but cases have been seen in the newborn (from maternal infection), by direct and indirect occulogenital (eye-genital) contact during delivery.

How prevalent is this STD?

In developed countries, genital chlamydia infection is the most common sexually transmitted disease. Over the past decade, there has been a 20% increase in incidence of genital chlamydia infection, most commonly among women between ages 16 and 19. There are about 1,300 new cases per 100,000 population in the UK each year; 1,900 cases per 100,000 in Sweden; and about 2,536 per 100,000 in the United States. Among men, the peak age is between 20 and 24, with about 965 per 100,000 new infections per year in the UK and USA and about 1,200 per 100,000 in Sweden.

What are the signs and symptoms of GCI?

About 80% of GCI do not have symptoms and the victims may not even know they are infected. This is a situation which promotes the transmission of infection to the sexual partner(s) and geometrically spreads uncontrollably. Among women, the sign could be vaginal discharge and bleeding between menstrual periods. In men, it could also be asymptomatic or manifest as dysuria (painful urination) from urethritis (inflammation of the urine channel within the penis) and penile pus discharge.

What is complicated GCI?

When the GCI infection becomes worse and goes beyond those symptoms and signs described above, it is termed complicated GCI. In women, the infection could spread "upwards" to the inside of the lower abdomen leading to pelvic inflammatory disease (PID) in 30-40% of cases; and in men, it could lead to epididymoorchitis (inflammation of the sperm tubules and testicle). Both can also cause eye infection and infertility.

Do sore-free genitals mean absence of infection?

No. This is a very common myth. Without exception, all STD infections can be present without any obvious external sign. Only laboratory examination (culture techniques or nucleic acid amplification test) can diagnostically confirm the presence or absence of the infection. As we have reported in a previous column, oral sex increases the risk of throat cancer from human papillomavirus infection.

Can chlamydia cause blindness?

Yes. Trachoma, also caused by chlamydia trachomatis bacterium, is the world's leading cause of preventable blindness, second to cataract. Trachoma victimizes about 150 million persons globally, mostly children; and as a result, 5.5 million of them become blind.

Does chlamydial infection lead to AIDS?

No, GCI does not lead to AIDS, which is caused by HIV, which is also sexually transmitted. But having chlamydial infection, which may coexist with other STDs, may facilitate and enhance the risk of getting HIV infection.

What is the prognosis of GCI?

Untreated chlamydial infection leads to pelvic inflammatory disease in 30-40% of women. After just one episode of GCI, 11% of women will develop infertility, and the chance of ectopic pregnancy (outside of the womb) increases 6 to 7 times, compared to healthy uninfected women. Maternal-to-newborn transmission leads to opthalmia neonatorum (eye infection) and pneumonia in 30-40% of the newborn whose mother carries the infection.

How can this STD be prevented?

Like all diseases in general and sexually transmitted diseases in particular, chlamydia infection can be prevented by practicing healthy personal behavior, discipline, and discretion. Although not a guarantee, the choice of intimate partner helps minimize the risk of exposure. The proper use of condoms (2-3% of which are defective) also reduces the chance of infection. Having multiple relationships exponentially increases the risk.

What is the treatment for GCI?

Like with most diseases or infections, prevention is key. Early diagnosis where the infection has set and prompt treatment are crucial in the prevention of complications. The drugs used for the treatment of GCI are antibacterial pills like levaquin, azithromycin, deoxycycline, erythromycin, amoxicillin are prescribed for specific medical situations of the chlamydial infection. For complicated cases, appropriate management is customized to individual cases.

Is self-medication safe?

Except for managing common cold, influenza, and other relatively nonserious medical conditions, self-medication can be most dangerous, especially when dealing with major or potentially life-threatening diseases (high blood pressure, heart disease, diabetes, etc.), including STDs like chlamydial infections. When in doubt as to whether infection is present or not or whether treatment is necessary, it is best to "err" on the safe side. The preservation and maintenance of health are worth the inconvenience and expense associated with trips to your physician's clinic.

Chocolate: Cardio-Good?

In a previous column a few years back, we reported that one person in the United States died of heart attack about every 60 seconds. The stat has almost doubled. Recent studies show that in America, one succumbs every 33 seconds to this number 1 killer in America and in many well-developed countries around the world. Hypertension is common among heart patients and a most frequent cause of stroke. About 80%-85% of all primary hypertension are mild enough to be effectively controlled by modification in lifestyle alone, sans drugs.

Scary statistics

To put those frightening statistics in their proper perspectives and truly understand the gravity and impact of cardiovascular diseases on all of us, one person in America has already died of CVD the past 33 seconds (2500 will die today from cardiovascular diseases.)

Chocolate to the rescue?

Scientists now say that chocolate, especially the dark variety, is good for our cardiovascular system. Health experts claim that this mouthwatering and practically "addictive and decadent" food item improves the circulation and lowers the blood pressure. For centuries, cocoa has been used for medicinal purposes in Europe and the Americas.

The 2006 study of a team of researchers from the University of California-Davis and the university of Dusseldorf in Germany confirmed that "the compound epicatechin found in cocoa is directly linked to vasodilation and improved circulation and other hallmarks of cardiovascular function." The flavanol-rich compound causes relaxation of constricted blood vessels (especially the arteries) "mediated by nitric oxide (NO), a key signal released by the inner lining of the arteries," same action as Viagra, Cialis, or Levitra in their ability to vasodilate (open up) and fill with blood the veins of the penis, to effect engorgement, as a treatment for erectile dysfunction. The relaxed blood vessels are less prone to clotting and blockage. This effect also leads to reduction in the blood pressure among hypertensives (persons with high blood pressure).

A separate study in Tufts University and the University of California, San Francisco, confirms the U of C and Dusseldorf findings on vasodilation and added the information that consumption (in moderation) of chocolates did not increase the lipid (cholesterol) level. Review of other studies reveals that "flavanoids from chocolates have an anti-inflammatory effect by controlling the activation of several pro-inflammatory agents in the body." A University of Buenos Aires scientist, Cesar G. Fraga, found that there was a rise in the procyanidins in the blood following ingestion of cocoa-based foods, which protected the circulating lipids from the bad oxidation process.

Chocolates also have a cardio-protective effect via its effects on prostacyclins, which work like low-dose aspirins, with their mild anticoagulation (blood thinner) action, preventing blood clots by reducing platelet clumping, a process that induces blood clot formation.

Procyanidin and flavanol in cocoa have significant antioxidant (free radical fighting) properties, which protects the heart and the vascular system, by protecting the cell membranes and minimizing the oxidation of the LDL (bad) cholesterol, thus slowing down hardening of the arteries. Oxidation in our body is a major cause of aging among human beings and other animals. (This process is akin to the oxidation that transforms a brand-new car paint into an old-looking, faded, shine-less, aged appearance, and the metal parts corroded, lusterless, and damaged.) This is why fruits and vegetables, which are loaded with antioxidants, are strongly recommended for us to eat at least 3 times a day. Red meats, egg yolks, smoking, lack of exercise (sedentary lifestyle) have the opposite effects, besides their bad-fat-/cholesterol-elevating properties.

Dark chocolate, which contains the highest level of cocoa (at least 60%), is the one that confers (almost exclusively) the best cardio-protective benefits. The flavanoids are found in cocoa beans but not in the milk, cream, sugar, and other additives that make chocolates lighter or whiter. Preferred are the chocolates processed without "dutching" or alkalinization, because these methods destroy a significant amount of antioxidants in cocoa. Heat also destroys these flavanoids, so chocolates that are cold-pressed are better than those "pressed with heat."

Together with a healthy lifestyle and in moderation, one may "sinfully" savor dark chocolate a couple of times a day without guilt . . . and enjoy a happy heart.

New Stunning Reports on Cholesterol

A recent study revealed that getting cholesterol to super low levels can stop the progression of arteriosclerotic heart disease, the culprit responsible for blockages in our coronary arteries which supply blood to our heart muscles. This was reported by Steven E. Nissen, the cardiologist who headed the investigation at the Cleveland Clinic, where the cholesterol-lowering drugs, Lipitor and Pravachol, were used in more than 500 patients. The study shows that taking 40 mg of Pravachol did not offer the same slowing effect on heart disease, even though some patients were able to achieve the same superlow LDL levels. Heart disease in the Pravachol-treated patients was about 3% worse after 18 months of treatment. Lipitor seems to be superior in this regard.

Nissen also observed that Lipitor stopped progression of plaque in a variety of patient groups including younger and older patients as well as people with diabetes and high blood pressure. But for Pravachol it was a different story: "We were unable to stop progression in any of the subgroups in the Pravachol group," he says. Nissen based his findings based on ultrasound images inside the arteries in beating hearts. This technique is still in its infancy and needs to be correlated and confirmed with clinical results. However, evidence-based medicine has shown that these statin drugs, like Lipitor and Pravachol, among others, reduce deaths and complications from coronary heart disease.

Nissen added that "in addition to bigger drops in LDL cholesterol with Lipitor, patients taking Lipitor also had much greater reductions in C-reactive protein: 36% vs. 5%." C-reactive protein, CRP, is an inflammatory marker found in the blood. High levels of CRP have recently been identified as a heart disease risk factor. "The potent anti-inflammatory effect seen with Lipitor might be a factor in the observed differences between the two treatments," according to Nissen.

Is there a skin test for cholesterol?

Skin test for cholesterol is still being developed. In the mean time, cholesterol level or Lipid Profile are still performed thru blood (serum) test. Screening should start at age 20 because 33% of young adults have been found to have a cholesterol level above 200. Among young children whose parents have a cholesterol level of 240 and higher should likewise have cholesterol screening.

What are the markers of heart disease?

The markers of coronary heart disease among those with blockages in their heart arteries are: high white blood count, high fibrinogen (blood clotting factor), high c-reactive protein (suggesting inflammation), and Lipoprotein-associated phospholipase A2. These findings suggest the presence of coronary heart disease, which could be (and, if the patient is symptomatic, needs to be) confirmed by coronary arteriogram.

How does one lower his/her cholesterol level?

The initial step, which is quite successful in majority of people, is by not eating red meats or meat products made of pork or beef, nonskim dairy products, eggs (the yolk of which is in itself very high in cholesterol). The diet should consist of fish, vegetables, white chicken meat (no skin) and fruits. Indulging a bit in red meats during the holidays is acceptable, except among those whose cholesterol and LDL are very high and the HDL is very low. If this recommended diet regimen is followed religiously, chances are the cholesterol and triglyceride levels will come down to the desired levels. Medications to lower the cholesterol and triglyceride levels are reserved for those where months of strict fish, vegetable, and fruit diet has failed to bring the cholesterol and triglyceride level down to normal. Some of these are people have a genetic predisposition (two out of 100 people) to having high cholesterol level, and therefore would need the help of cholesterol/lipid lowering drugs. However, many of us have been on unhealthy diet for years and will definitely benefit from these medications. Your physician will be your best partner in planning an effective strategy for you.

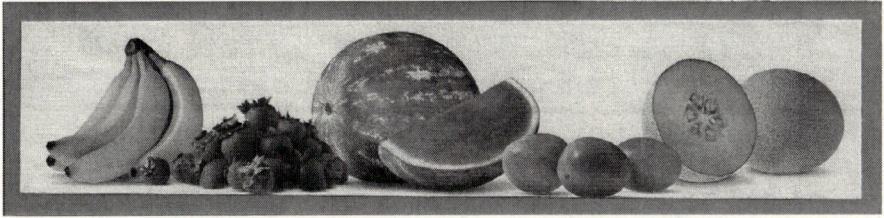

Fruits are loaded with potent natural antioxidant ingredients and fiber, and fortify our ability to fight illnesses, including cancer. When eating fruits, individuals with diabetes should calculate the added calories in their computation.

Christmas Ailments

Is there an illness called Christmas disease?

Yes, there is, but it has nothing to do with the Christmas season. Christmas disease is a blood disease, also known as hemophilia B or factor IX hemophilia. It is a hereditary bleeding disorder due to deficiency in coagulation factor IX. This condition is X-linked recessive inheritance, affecting only males, and occurs in 1 in 100,000 male births. This illness causes spontaneous bleeding in the joints.

What is Christmas blues?

Christmas Blues is a form of mild depression (known as SAD: seasonal affective disorder) that happens to some of us, normal and healthy people, during the Christmas season and other seasonal festive events. Empty nest syndrome, where the grown up or married children have left home, creating an empty and lonely feeling in the parents, especially the mothers, is one such type of emotion that is magnified by family occasions like Christmas, New Year, birthdays, etc. Frequent visits from the children or family reunions during the holidays minimize these "blues" and provide a sense of parental security and happiness, especially among the elderly parents. The other common cause of this extreme sadness is poor financial situation in life, where self-pity, panic, a sense of hopelessness, and helplessness prevail especially on a holiday like Christmas.

Is guilt more common at Christmastime?

Yes, somehow this season of the birth of Christ, according to psychologists, brings out in most of us our good and better qualities, such as a more youthful exuberance, honesty, sincerity, compassion, and humanity. During this season, many of us become more critical of ourselves and our past actions (sins of omission or commission against our parents, siblings, or friends, or our less privileged fellowmen) and hence the feeling of guilt is more common on this holiday and also a contributing factor to Christmas Blues.

Are accidents and injuries more common during Christmas season?

Yes, and the reason is obvious. There are more activities going on everywhere, at home, on the streets, in stores, etc.; so there are more people, more traffic. And this lends to a higher prevalence of accidents and injuries. Alcoholic consumption is increased, people light firecrackers, people climb to install Christmas lights, children play with these lights or with lit candles, more cooking takes place in the kitchen, and all these are potential sources of accidents and injuries. Most hospital emergency rooms in America are more than 75% busier during the Christmas season and the New Year's Eve celebration. Compared to all holidays, New Year's Day has the greatest increase in traffic fatalities (64%), about 40% of these involving drunk drivers.

Is diarrhea more prevalent during the Christmas season?

Yes, just as diarrhea is also more common during holiday celebrations. Ingestion of either contaminated food or food that is spoiled (especially those left exposed to the warm weather or room temperature and not refrigerated right away after meals) are the usual causes of diarrhea. Common food contaminants are *Staphylococcus aureus, E. coli,* and amoeba; and water contaminants are (nontyphoidal) salmonella and shigella. Staphylococcal food poisoning is due to the enterotoxins produced by the staph bacteria. The diarrhea—sometimes accompanied by stomach cramps, vomiting, headache, and fever—starts about 2 to 8 hours after eating contaminated food. The potential outbreak is high when the food handlers with skin (staphylococcus aureus) infection touch and contaminate foods left at room temperature. Proper food handling, dishwashing, and hand washing are hygienic practices that will significantly minimize, if not prevent, these bacterial and parasitic contaminations. When the diarrhea persists for more than two days, consult your physician.

How long could food be left safely at room temperature?

Different types of food have different "spoilage time." Fish, processed meat, cream-filled pastries, custards, fruits salads, noodles, food cooked with tomatoes provide good media for bacterial growth after more than 6 hours of exposure to room temperature, depending on how warm the ambient temperature is. Some dishes could last for even a week in room temperature without spoiling, unless contaminated by handlers. The prudent thing to do is to refrigerate the leftovers as soon as the meal is completed.

Do alcoholic beverages protect people from diarrhea?

To some extent, yes, but the dose of the enteroxins determines the potential seriousness of the condition. Imbibing alcoholic drinks during a (contaminated) meal does not confer guaranteed immunity from these bacterial or parasitic diarrheas. The low alcohol content of all these drinks is not enough to "sterilize" our gastrointestinal tract.

Are more people taking antacids during the holidays?

More people take antacids (Tums, Rolaid, Alka Seltzer, Tagamet, Pepcid, etc.) during or after the holidays because of overindulgence in alcohol or food, leading to heartburns and /or indigestion. These medications (alkali) counteract the high acid contents of the stomach following these binges during holidays.

What is holiday heart syndrome?

Prevalent during holidays, this symptom complex is mainly characterized by cardiac arrhythmias (heart rhythm irregularity), mostly due to alcoholic binges. The excitement brought on by the festivities and ingestion of a lot of caffeine (coffee, chocolate, cola drinks) during the holidays could also play a role in this syndrome.

Clots in the lungs

How do clots get to the lungs?

The commonest sources of blood clots in the lungs are the veins in the pelvis and in the legs, where the clots form and travel to the lungs. This condition is called pulmonary embolus, or PE for short, where clots are "filtered" and caught in the pulmonary artery (the main artery of the lungs), causing obstruction of blood flow into the lungs, resulting in hypoxia (diminished oxygen blood level). Pulmonary embolus is a serious condition which could be fatal, if not detected and treated promptly.

How prevalent is it?

In the United States, more than 650,000 cases of PE are diagnosed each year, making it the third most common causes of death. It also ranks as the first or second most common causes of unexpected death in most age groups. Sixty percent of hospitals deaths among patients admitted and treated for other illnesses were found to have PE on autopsy. The diagnosis of PE is usually missed in 70% of cases because of the subtle and treacherous nature of the condition.

Which patients in the hospital are prone to have PE?

The likely target of PE are as follows: those medical patients placed on bed rest for at least a week (10-13% of them are prone to develop PE), patients in medical ICU (29-33%), patients with lung disease on bed rest for 3 or more days (20-26%), post-heart-attack patients in coronary care Unit (27-33%), and, those patients with no symptoms, recovering in the hospital after coronary bypass surgery (48%). Because of this fact, early ambulation is encouraged among these patients; and most, if not all, are placed on blood thinner of one form or the other to prevent blood clots and PE.

Is the condition dangerous?

Very risky, in severe cases. It could even be life-threatening. What happens is the pulmonary artery becomes filled with blood clots and eventually blocked off. This will prevent much of the blood from going to the lungs to be oxygenated. As a result, the person's blood oxygen level drops dramatically (hypoxia), a condition that could lead to severe shortness of breath, massive chest pains, shock, and cardiac arrest.

Are there mild forms of PE?

Yes, when the blood clots lodged in the pulmonary artery are small ones and not significantly blocking the blood flow to the lungs. Mild subclinical PE, those without symptoms where persons are not even aware they have blood clots in the lungs, occurs much more commonly than we realize. Many times, the discovery of PE is made during autopsy. Normally, the lungs automatically lyse (dissolve) blood clots; but if the clots are very large and overwhelming, the enzymes will not be able to dissolve the clots, and the dangerous situation described earlier will come into play.

Why do clots form in the legs and pelvis?

The most common reason is the presence of varicose veins in the legs and in the pelvic veins, where blood pools and stagnate. This slowed circulation and stagnation promotes thrombosis (clot formation). If the clots are not firmly attached to the walls of the veins, normal body movement could send these clots flowing with the stream of blood, all the way to the pulmonary artery and to the lungs.

What promotes blood clots?

The major factors that encourage clot formation includes dehydration (poor fluid intake), smoking, inactivity, birth control (estrogen) pills, standing for a long period of time on one spot, and varicose veins (both of which cause blood pooling in the leg veins). All these factors have a common denominator: they make the blood thicker and more prone to clot.

What is the prognosis for PE?

Those with markedly compromised cardiopulmonary function (preexisting bad heart and lung diseases) have a greater than 25% chance of dying from a severe pulmonary embolism. Those who are otherwise healthy would succumb to PE only *if* the obstruction in the pulmonary artery is greater than 50%. If the PE is so severe that death is inevitable, it usually happens within one to two hours. About 10% of patients diagnosed with acute PE die within the first hour. About thirty-three percent of those undiagnosed will die. In the USA, about 100,000 patients die because of undiagnosed PE. Those with massive PE, 80% will die within the first two hours from onset of the condition. A scientific study on PE called the USET trial showed that thrombolytic (clot-dissolving therapy) did not improve or reduce the mortality rate. For massive PE, prompt emergency surgery with the aid of the heart-lung machine is performed as a last resort. Although massive PE is often fatal, early diagnosis and treatment can reduce the mortality rate dramatically.

How can one prevent PE?

To prevent or minimize pulmonary embolism, one has to avoid all those factors that promote blood clot formation. Doing daily exercises; low-fat, low-cholesterol diet; abstinence from smoking; strict moderation in alcohol intake; drinking at least 8 glasses of water a day, elevating the legs and wearing support stockings for varicose veins; avoidance of prolonged sitting, moving around and exercising the legs often (as on a long flights)—all these tend to prevent blood from thickening and, thus, from clotting. Medical consultation is paramount, especially among those with varicose veins or those who have had frequent thrombophlebitis (painful inflammation of the leg veins, with clots). Where indicated, blood thinners may be prescribed by the physician.

Coconut Oil and Health

The controversy about the health effects of coconut oil has been going on for decades. The question still remains: is coconut oil ingestion beneficial or harmful to our body?

Those who are promoting the sale of coconut and coconut oil hail the products as a healthy food ingredient across the board. However, those in the scientific community carefully make a clear distinction between regular hydrogenated coconut oil and virgin (nonhydrogenated) coconut oil.

Coconut oil and juice extracted from coconut are high in fats (92% saturated fats), commonly used for baking, cooking, and in cosmetics. In cosmetics, coconut oil is undisputed for being excellent, especially for the hair. No question or debate there. But for cooking, baking, regular coconut oil is unhealthy because of the saturated fats and trans fats it predominantly contains. On the other hand, virgin coconut oil, which has not undergone hydrogenation (or any processing that uses chemicals), is free of trans fats.

Saturated fats (pork, beef and other red meats, eggs, coconuts) have been proven to cause hardening of the artery, and the resultant cholesterol deposits on the walls of the artery block the blood supply to organs (like the heart, brain, major blood vessels, leading to heart attack, stroke, etc.). Saturated fats have also been linked to obesity and cancer.

What are the false claims?

In view of this, the common coconut oil has gained the bad reputation of being unhealthy for regular or frequent consumption. The marketing and commercials on coconut oil, however, have misrepresented the facts. They apparently advertise coconut/coconut oil as healthy food items that lower cholesterol, increase metabolism, aid in weight control, and have some antiviral, antibacterial, and antifungal action.

And what is the truth?

Some scientific studies suggest that the virgin (nonhydrogenated) coconut oil (with its polyphenol) possibly (?) has these good effects and that the common regular hydrogenated, chemically processed coconut oil and coconut meat, which are the most commonly used form for cooking and baking, are definitely unhealthy, except for cosmetic use and perhaps, hopefully, as bio-diesel engine fuel in the future. Actually, coconut oil has more saturated fat than butter, beef tallow, and even lard. Coconut oil raises LDL (bad) cholesterol as much—or higher—and is worse than animal fats.

Coffee Reduces Diabetes Risk

Does coffee drinking reduce the risk for diabetes?

A new study published in the Annals of Internal Medicine January 6, 2004, suggested that regular coffee drinking "reduces the risk" for the development of type 2 (adult onset) diabetes mellitus.

Which type of coffee?

The research, which was conducted by the Harvard School of Public Health and Brigham and Women's Hospital, showed that caffeinated or decaffeinated coffee are both beneficial in lowering the risk for the adult onset diabetes; but the decaffeinated brew is somewhat weaker.

Wasn't coffee supposed to increase the risk?

Yes, older studies have reported that caffeine might, in fact, increase the risk of developing diabetes. However, the new theory is that other beneficial chemicals in coffee are able to offset the damage caused by caffeine.

How about tea?

In a separate report and not a part of this Harvard study, tea has been found to improve insulin activity up to 15 times. This includes green, black, or oolong teas, but not herbal tea (which does not have this beneficial effect). Since the active ingredients do not last long in the body, one should drink a cup every few hours to benefit from it. Also, no milk (not even soy milk) must be added, because this renders the "good chemicals" useless to the body.

How was the study done?

The Harvard research studied about 42,000 healthy men and more than 84,000 healthy women from 1980s through 1998, sending them questionnaires every 2-4 years for 18 years, to assess their intake of both regular and decaffeinated coffee and the development of diabetes. Compared to those who did not drink coffee, men who had more than 6 cups of caffeinated coffee a day lowered the risk of developing type 2 diabetes by 50%. Among women, there was a 30% reduction in the risk. "This is good news for coffee drinkers; however, it doesn't mean everyone should run out for a latte," Frank Hu, an associate professor at the Harvard School of Public Health, stated in a release. "We still don't know exactly why coffee is beneficial for diabetes, and more research is clearly needed."

How does coffee do it?

The exact mechanism is still unclear. In another research (Nurses Health Study), it shows that the 2,000 women coffee drinkers in its survey had significantly lower (13%-14%) levels of C-peptide hormone, a component of insulin in our body, compared to noncoffee drinkers. Higher level of C-peptide, which indicates the body is unable to use insulin (called insulin resistance) are linked to the increased risk of developing adult-onset diabetes. The good effect was more apparent among obese and overweight women, 22% and 18%, respectively. So if coffee reduces C-peptide, then the risk is reduced.

Is this hormone working alone?

This is still not fully understood. Both regular and decaffeinated coffees have a lot of antioxidants in them, like chlorogenic acid (the ingredient that gives the "addicting" coffee flavor), phytoestrogens, and magnesium. These chemicals improve sensitivity to insulin and may play a vital role in lowering adult onset diabetes. Caffeine itself is also known to affect insulin secretion.

How much coffee is needed?

The Harvard study stated 6 or more cups per day. The research on the same subject in Finland (which has the highest per capita coffee consumption in the world), involving 15,000 healthy men and women (ages 35-64), as reported in *The Journal of American Medical Association*, showed that women who consumed 10 or more cups a day had 79% lower risk, and men, about 55%.

How many cups of coffee are safe?

Since the long-term effects of coffee (especially caffeinated) on diabetes, cardiovascular diseases, and other illnesses are not totally clear, the so-called "safe level" is an individual issue. One cup of regular coffee may be too much for one person, who might develop heartbeat irregularity, like palpitation, or insomnia, when taken before bedtime. Three cups a day may not be enough to satisfy another. There is more leeway for consumption of decaffeinated coffee if you plan to follow this study, but even this should be tailored to your tolerance. The final word on this issue is not settled, but the preliminary results as presented above are most encouraging. More long-term studies are definitely needed before this becomes a medical dogma.

Colonoscopy: Lifesaver

The devastating statistics about deaths from colon cancer have put the spotlight on a dreaded disease which today could be detected early with a relatively simple diagnostic regimen, which includes colonoscopy.

A recent German study involving more than 3,600 patients shows that the overall risk of developing malignancy (cancer) among those who underwent colonoscopies is reduced by 77%. The study also shows that the procedure has no "blind spot" and detects malignancies both on the left and right side of the colon. This confirms once again that colonoscopy as a tool against cancer is a lifesaver.

What is colonoscopy?

Colonoscopy is a procedure where a flexible endoscope (malleable tube with a telescope), equipped with fiberoptic lighting and (video CCD) camera, is passed through the anus, to view and examine the inner walls of the colon (large bowels) and distal part of the small bowels for any abnormality, like bleeding, ulcers, or the presence of benign poly(s), or cancer. Thru the colonoscope, excision of polyps or biopsies may also be performed for a definitive microscopic tissue diagnosis. A sigmoidoscope is another scope that examines the final two feet of the colon, while the colonoscope examines the rest of the entire colon which is about four to five feet long. Many times it is done in conjunction with colonoscopy.

Are meat eaters more prone to colorectal cancer?

It appears to be so, because colorectal cancer is found more prevalent in populations whose diet is low in fiber and high in animal proteins, fats, and refined carbohydrates. The incidence of colorectal cancer is indeed high among those who eat red meat (pork, beef, etc.) compared to those who eat high fiber diets (vegetables, fruits, wheat, bran, etc.) and fish. The other predisposing factors include chronic ulcerative colitis, ganulomatous colitis, and familial polyposis. The older the person is, the higher the risk. Smoking, in general, severely increases the risk for cancer formation of the lungs and various organs in the body, not to mention pulmonary diseases, heart attack and stroke.

What are the signs and symptoms of colorectal cancer?

The person may not have symptoms at all. It could be so subtle, like fatigue and anemia. Blood in the stool (black or bloody red stools) is one common sign. The others include change in the bowel habits, diarrhea or constipation, stools more slender or flatter than usual, stomach discomfort, bloating, fullness, abdominal cramps, frequent gas pains, unexplained weight loss, a sensation that the rectum does not empty completely. Not all these symptoms and signs need to be present, or necessary, to suspect possible presence colorectal cancer. Any one of these, if persistent, should alert one to seek medical help.

When should colonoscopy be done?

Everyone 50 years old and older should have an annual fecal occult blood test (FOBT), a rectal digital exam, and a prophylactic colonoscopy every 3 to 5 years. Since blood in the feces is one of the earliest signs of colorectal cancer, testing for blood in the stools yearly among those 50 and older is essential, and could be lifesaving. And so with prophylactic rectal digital examination and colonoscopy.

How do we prevent colorectal cancer?

As alluded to above, a high-fiber (vegetables, bran, oat, wheat, fruits) and fish diet will tremendously reduce the risk of colorectal cancer. Therefore, staying away from animal protein, like red meat (pork, beef and anything made of these) is a big factor in preventing the development of colorectal cancer, besides heart attack and stroke. Daily exercises make our body healthier and more resistant to illnesses. Abstinence from tobacco is a must. Checking your stools for blood every time you defecate and reporting any warning signs listed above to your physician will help. Recta Exam and colonoscopy are strongly recommended as stipulated above.

What is the treatment for colorectal cancer?

Depending on the stage and location of the colorectal cancer, the primary strategy is wide surgical resection of the cancer and regional lymphatic drainage. Cure is possible in 75% of surgical patients. For cancer limited to the mucosa (surface lining of the wall of the colon), 5-year survival is about 90%; those cancer going deeper into the muscularis propia (muscle-layer of colon), 80%; those with positive lymph nodes, meaning cancer already spreading to the lymph nodes, 30%. Other modalities of treatment includes pre-operative radiotherapy, adjuvant radiotherapy, chemotherapy. When surgery and/or any of these other modalities are indicated will depend on the location, extent, and stage of the colorectal cancer.

What is the outlook for colorectal cancer patients?

There is no question that the outlook for colorectal cancer and most other cancers in general is much better today, depending on their stages when first diagnosed. This is why we cannot overemphasize the common-sense wisdom that prevention is the best "treatment," especially when dealing with any potentially deadly disease like cancer, heart attack, stroke, AIDS, etc. New hopes for cancer victims are in the pipeline of dozens of research/clinical laboratories in the United States and other countries around the world. Before the advent of the oral medications for pulmonary tuberculosis, this disease acted like cancer, spreading from the lungs to the brain, bones, liver, kidneys, spleen, lymph nodes, etc. We predict that someday, hopefully in the not-too-distant future, many forms of cancers, if not all, will be cured by simply taking anticancer pills. In the meantime, it behooves each one of us to play an active role in protecting ourselves from becoming cancer victims by living a healthy lifestyle and by being ever-vigilant about our health and that of our loved ones.

Computer Health Hazards

Is using a computer safe?

Yes, computing, just like other human activities, is safe unless abused. Computers are indispensable. In this age of technology revolution, everybody, if possible, should learn how to use computers in order to keep up with these exciting times of the shrinking world, to be competitive. Anyone with a computer and Internet access can obtain practically any information desired, from movie trivia, to travel guides, health matters, shopping, banking, investing online, to history and sociocultural information, etc., to name a few. The computers have really leveled the playing field for all of us in this fantastic informational age.

Does computing lead to blindness?

No, that is a myth. The same was also once "suspected" and linked to the use of microwave ovens and even to having frequent sex. These are all not true. There are no medical evidences to substantiate any of these. So get on with it. Computing, I mean.

What injuries are associated with computing?

A condition called carpal tunnel syndrome (CTS) has been linked to extensive computer (or typing) job. Any prolonged, repetitive flexion and extension of the wrists (typing on keyboards) could result in compression of the median nerve as it passes through the carpal tunnel in the wrist, hence the name. This is especially true when the typist rests his/her wrist against the edge of the computer or typewriter. It is best to type with the rest "floating in the air" rather than resting (pressing) on a hard surface. Even cushioned wrist "pads" do not help much. Simply allowing your wrists to "float" while you type on the keyboard while minimizing extreme flexion and extension of the wrist will help prevent CTS. Give your wrists (and your whole body) rest and relaxation regularly at frequent intervals to minimize computer-related stresses.

Is computing addictive?

Addictive is not the right word. It is more habituative or habit-forming, where an individual, who is extremely interested in computer games or Internet surfing, emailing, chatting, etc., has developed a strong and regular compulsion and a habit of "bonding" with the computer. This is especially the case among those who are "loners" or "alone." And the condition could be so severe as to be abnormal and unhealthy. There was a student who was reported missing from his classes for days, only to be found "holed up" in one room in an uninterrupted marathon of computing.

Are computer games good for children?

It depends as to what the nature and goal of the games are. If they are about "violence and killing people," even if they are the designated "enemies," the threshold for restraint to kill among these children (chronic) viewers is lowered. Studies have shown that some children (and even adults) exposed to much violence on the television, movies, or computer games have higher tendencies to violence and senseless killing themselves. The games involving role models like James Bond, Batman and Robin, and Superman, Spiderman, etc., are healthier for children.

Does computing lead to truancy and absenteeism in school?

There is no doubt that this is happening because of unguided, unsupervised use of computers among undisciplined young children and teenagers. Hardcore sex on the Internet is also a major problem we now face. That is why laws should be passed in the country (or in each city and town) to restrict the proximity to schools and churches of Internet cafes and legislations on how to deal with pornography on the Internet. But the best guide and "law enforcers" are the parents or guardians, who must be precise and firm in their "house or family rules" for the children. Compassion, understanding, and discipline are the keys to good parenting in general. And they apply to the proper use of computers are home, in school, or at Internet cafes as well.

Does computing lead to bad posture?

Spine alignment or posture could be caused by how one habitually sits, especially for a prolonged period of time. Whether it is computing, typing, or simply writing, a good posture is important. Children must be reminded of this constantly.

Does chronic exposure to computers lead to cancer?

No evidence supports this. The radiation is minimal and safe as far as present legal guidelines are concerned. Nonetheless, breaks and rests should punctuate computer use, simply to relax, if for nothing at all, because computer related stress is real. Too-loud audio in computer games and looking at a bright computer monitor screen for prolonged period day in and day out can lead to hearing and visual impairment, respectively.

How about the effect on the psyche?

This computer age has tremendous advantages not only for businesses but for everybody, especially for the children. They learn more and faster. They become more self-reliant, resourceful, independent, confident, and more positive in their outlook of their future. The feel empowered by having available to them limitless information, facilities for domestic and international communication (voice mail, e-mail, chat, surf), and games and recreation, etc. This empowerment has created thousands of young multimillionaires and billionaires, led by Bill Gates. Our youngsters of today feel more confident than ever before that they too someday could reach their star.

COPD

What is COPD?

COPD is chronic obstructive pulmonary disease, a lung disease that severely limits normal airflow in and out of the lungs, making the patient short of breath. The airflow obstruction is progressive and associated with an abnormal response of the lungs to noxious particles and gases in the environment, either actively or passively inhaled (like cigarette smoke, etc.).

How prevalent is COPD?

In the USA alone, 12.1 million adults 25 and older had COPD diagnosed in 2001, about 8% greater in 2006, where the death rate was 46.4% for men and 34.2% for women, per 100,000. Twenty four million smokers have impaired lung functions. More than 120,000 die of COPD and complications each year. COPD is the 4th leading cause of death and projected to be the 3rd by year 2020. This disease cost the government $32.1 billion in 2002 alone. Since women have started smoking and surpassed men, COPD victimizes more females than males.

What are the symptoms of COPD?

Deep, wet, crackling cough with sputum production, even before airflow limitation ensues. Dyspnea (shortness of breath) on exertion is progressive. These are most noticeably common among smokers. The severity of COPD is gauged by stages, from stage 0 where there is chronic cough and sputum production but the lung function is still normal, to stage 4, where there is severe airflow limitation and severe shortness of breath, where quality of life is poor, and exacerbations become life-threatening.

What causes COPD?

The single most essential risk factor is cigarette smoking. Cigar, pipe, tobacco chewing, and other types of tobacco smoking in many countries are likewise risk factors for COPD. The other risks and causes of COPD are long-term exposure to occupational dusts and chemical vapors, indoor pollution from biomase fuels utilized for heating or cooking in poorly ventilated factories or homes, outdoor air pollution.

How about passive smoking?

Most definitely, passive smoking (inhaling smokes from a smoker nearby or in a room filled with cigarette smoke) also contributes to the risk and development of COPD. Passive smoking also causes children to develop reduced lung function and respiratory ailments as they grow, making them more prone to COPD as adults.

What are the tests for COPD?

Tests to diagnose COPD, besides the classical history of smoking and the clinical symptoms, include spirometry (test of patient's breathing capability), bronchodilator reversibility test, chest X-ray, arterial blood gasses, and alpha-1 antitrypsin deficiency screening.

How can one prevent COPD?

The first and foremost is abstinence from cigarette (tobacco) smoking. "Quit before you start!" is the best prophylactic strategy. Not starting the habit at all is the best way to prevent this debilitating disease that makes patients gasp for breath and cripple them with suffocation, every minute, day in and day out, making life miserable. Some even "drown" in their own sputum, because even their ability to spit it out is severely impaired. Those who smoke should quit because it is never too late. Quitting helps minimize progression and worsening. For those who work in factories exposed to chemical vapors or dust, the use of the approved industrial mask is recommended. Homes must be well ventilated; and smokers should step out of the house to smoke, instead of forcing their spouse and children to passive smoke, which is more dangerous than active smoking.

Obviously, the other essential lifestyle practices are equally important, like low-cholesterol, low-fat, low-carbohydrate, low-salt, high-fiber-and-grain diet (basically fish, vegetables, nuts, fruits); and daily physical exercises. All these make the body and its immune system fit and strong to fight, not only lung disease but metabolic diseases (diabetes, etc), cardiovascular illness (high blood pressure, stroke, heart attack), and cancer in general.

What is the treatment for COPD?

COPD is not curable. Once the lungs are "burned" by tobacco smoke or other pollutants, the lung tissues are irreversibly damaged. Part of the management includes patient education, drugs to lessen the symptoms, bronchodilators to help ease the shortness of breath, steroids to reduce some inflammation, antibiotics for secondary infection, mucolytic agents to help thin out thick mucus for easier elimination, antitussives for cough, rehabilitation, and oxygen therapy. Flu vaccines reduces the risk and death rate by 50% Among patients with COPD.

How about surgery?

Surgery is limited because destroyed lung tissues are useless. If there are lung "bubbles or balloons" (emphysematous bullae), these could be resected to provide the lungs more room and allow the remaining lungs to expand. For stage 4 patients who are relatively young and otherwise healthy, lung transplantation may be an option on a selected-case basis. But the cost and the risk are high. And results are not guaranteed.

The million-dollar question is: why even smoke and allow all these miseries to happen to your body and cut your life short?

Coronary Angioplasty

What is Coronary Angioplasty?

Commonly called angioplasty, the procedure is technically known as percutaneous transluminal coronary angioplasty (PTCA). *Percutaneous* refers to "the needle puncture thru the skin," transluminal means "the inside channel of the artery," *coronary* is the name of the "arteries to of the heart," and *angioplasty* is "repair/dilatation" of the blocked artery using an inflatable balloon.

How is angioplasty done?

Once a significant blockage (more than 50% obstruction of the arterial channel) is detected by the coronary angiogram in a patient with chest pains, the cardiologist doing the procedure gets a special catheter that has an inflatable balloon toward the tip. The angiogram catheter is pulled out and the special balloon catheter is inserted to the femoral artery thru the same sheath. The balloon is still deflated at this time as the catheter is directed into the blocked artery under continuous X-ray guidance. Once the balloon is inside the segment of the artery that is tightly blocked, the balloon is inflated to push open the obstructed artery. This dilates the narrowed segment. A stainless steel stent (a tiny spiral coil spring) is then inserted within that dilated segment to prevent the walls from collapsing (reblocking) the lumen of the artery.

Can PTCA be done on an outpatient basis?

Yes, this procedure is being done in some centers in the United States as an outpatient procedure, where it is done in the morning, and the patient is discharged the same evening. Some cases are kept overnight for observation. The decision is based on the patient's condition, the nature of the blockages, the response to the angioplasty, and the presence or absence of any complication.

Is the patient put to sleep for the angioplasty?

No, it will be more risky to give general anesthesia for this procedure. Nobody does that. The accepted standard of practice for this procedure all over the world uses moderate sedation for the patients, keeping them comfortable and less anxious, plus local anesthetic injection to numb the area in the groin where the sheathed needle is to be inserted. This is the safe technique which has been proven in hundreds of thousands of cases and well accepted by patients around the globe.

What are the possible complications?

More common possible complications of coronary angiogram include allergy to the dye, bleeding in the puncture site in the groin, hematoma (blood clots) under the skin in the groin, blood clot within the artery (thrombus-embolus) that cuts off the leg circulation, and irregularity of the heartbeat. For angioplasty, all the above possible risk plus tear in the artery being ballooned, causing bleeding or even dissection, where part of the hardened wall of the artery cracks during balloon dilatation and blocks the entire artery, cutting off circulation to the heart muscles, leading to a heart attack in some cases. But in experienced hands, these complications are rare, and the procedure is medically safe.

Is angioplasty a substitute for Bypass?

No. While angioplasty is a lot less invasive a procedure compared to heart bypass surgery, it is not beneficial and not indicated for all cases of coronary arterial blockages. There are arteries that are so severely blocked and hardened that the balloon cannot dilate or open them. When multiple coronary arteries are severely blocked and the anatomy is not amenable to angioplasty, coronary bypass surgery is the safer and prudent choice. When the blocked vessel is the left main coronary artery, which is a life-sustaining artery, then bypass surgery is the accepted and the uncontested standard of treatment. Cases are individualized based on many complex, some subtle, medical factors, and in some situations, also on the patient's preference, so long as it is medically reasonable.

What is sirolimus-coated stent?

A stent, coated with sirolimus (rapamycin), was reported on June 6, 2002, in the *New England Journal of Medicine* as being much superior to the currently used stents. The sirolimus stent has been found in independent studies (in Europe, Brazil and in the USA) to lower the current restenosis (reblockage) rate of 35% to 50% within six months after the angioplasty, to almost 0% in 6 months. In other words, practically all patients studied on whom the sirolimus stent was used had patent (opened) arteries after six months. More recent studies have shown that the restensosis rate was higher than originally suspected, but still much lower than with the use of the old "noncoated" stents. Extensive clinical studies and trials are being done all over the world. We look forward to the progress of this investigation with eager anticipation.

Coronary Bypass

Do you really stop the heart during coronary bypass?

Yes, we stop the heart during coronary bypass surgery, but circulation and oxygenation of the blood continue since the patient is connected to a heart-lung machine that temporarily acts as the patient's heart and lungs. This is a standard and routine technique used by cardiac surgeons all over the world.

Why stop the heart during the procedure?

In doing the bypass, we (suture) hook up the graft (the vein or artery to be used as the new channel) to the area beyond the blockage to supply blood through this new channel to the muscles of the heart that was deprived of blood because of the obstruction. The connection (anastomosis) is similar to the sleeve of the shirt "hooked up" to the side of the shirt. Because the coronary arteries are very small (about the size of a round toothpick or the lead in a pencil) the heart is stopped to facilitate the "hookup" of these two vessels. In some selected cases, OPCAB (off-pump coronary artery bypass) may be done, using a special instrument, where bypass is done on a beating heart and without the use of a heart-lung machine.

How is the heart stopped?

The body temperature is cooled down to 28 degrees Centigrade and we inject ice-cold (about 4 degrees Centigrade) potassium chloride solution. This stops the heart in a relaxed state (diastole). This step is done to protect the heart by transforming it into a "hibernating" state. This is one of the advances in cardiac surgery that makes it a lot safer procedure compared to, say, 40 years ago.

How is the heart restarted?

When all the anastomoses ("hookups") of the grafts to the coronary arteries are completed, the patient is rewarmed to normal temperature, and the heart is perfused (supplied with rewarmed blood) through the new grafts. This invariably restarts the heart. Occasionally, the heart needs to be "shocked" to restart its beating. This electrical defibrillation is not harmful to the heart or the patient.

How many bypass grafts could be done?

Depending on the number of coronary arteries that are blocked, there could be four, five, or even more grafts implanted.

Where do the grafts come from?

One of them is the internal mammary artery that is behind the breastbone. This is used as a graft and so with veins from the leg. These leg veins are the ones stripped, removed, and thrown away, when they are varicosed (engorged and ugly-looking leg veins). These same leg veins, when NOT varicosed, are routinely used as vein grafts. Since there are lots of veins in the leg, removing the superficial vein and using it as a graft does not cause harm to the leg.

After bypass surgery, can the patient live a normal life?

Yes. More than 98% of patients do lead a normal life. This is in fact the goal of coronary bypass surgery. However, modification of life style is part of the treatment in coronary artery disease, like having low-cholesterol diet (fish, vegetables, whole grain, nuts, fruits), daily physical exercise regimen, stress management, quitting cigarettes, regular medical checkups. As a matter fact, this modification of lifestyle leads to a healthier and more normal lifestyle. This is good for everybody, not only for heart patients.

How soon can patients have sex after coronary bypass surgery?

Depending on the speed of recovery and general condition of the patient, bypass patients may have safe sex even as early as a month after discharge from the hospital. The advice is for the patient to be the passive partner in the act for at least six months. Since each person is different in his/her capacity, patients should consult their cardiologist/ family physician before indulging in any exertional activities.

Can heart patients use ED pills?

Yes, so long as the patient is not taking any nitrates, is under a physician's supervision, and the heart is strong enough. This is why medical supervision is a must. Taken properly as prescribed by the attending physician, Viagra, Cialis, Levitra are safe and effective drugs in the treatment of male erectile dysfunction (ED). It can work wonders.

Could a person have coronary artery disease without symptoms?

Yes, many of them do not have symptoms. In some individuals, the first symptom could be sudden death or a massive heart attack. This is the reason why we recommend yearly medical checkup and a stress test among persons who are 40 years and older. For those with high blood pressure and/or a strong family of heart disease, we recommend stress test even at a younger age. The standard EKG alone does not reveal the accurate picture of our heart condition, especially if it turns out to be so-called "normal." The best first step is to see your physician regularly, have your blood test and cholesterol and triglyceride levels checked, and have a yearly stress test.

CPR must be a required course

Each day, more than 820 active persons, or 300,000 a year, develop unexpected cardiac arrest in the United States. Of these victims, less than 10% of them survive if it happens outside the hospital and less than 20% when the event happens in a hospital setting.

Clinical studies have likewise shown that for every minute delay in instituting cardiopulmonary resuscitation after the arrest, the survival rate goes down by 10% to 15%. The rule of thumb is for CPR to be performed within 3 to 4 minutes of the event. The sooner, the better. Bystander's prompt initiation of CPR doubles, or even triples, the chances of success in reviving persons with cardiac arrest.

As a cardiac surgeon, I am hoping that our legislators and educators in the country would make the "art and science" of CPR a part of our educational system, our community, and our nation.

What is CPR?

CPR stands for cardiopulmonary resuscitation, the strategy and technique of reviving a person who stopped breathing or whose heart stopped beating due to a heart attack or other causes of cardiac arrest.

Why learn CPR?

Learning how to perform CPR is vital, because one who knows how to do it effectively could save the life of a loved one or someone else. This knowledge could spell the difference between life and death for the victim. Indeed, knowing how to perform CPR properly is very important.

When should be CPR be done?

When confronted with a person who has collapsed, one should determine within 5 to 10 seconds (not minutes!) if the patient is breathing or not, if the pulse at the wrist by the base of the thumb is present or not (it is good to learn how to check the pulse beat before emergencies occur). Putting your ear right on top of the upper mid chest (between the left nipple and the breast bone where the heart is) is another way of checking if the heart is beating or not. This is a most crucial period, and time must not be wasted here. This determination of breathing and heartbeat must not be more than 10 seconds. If in doubt, it is safer to presume cardiac arrest has taken place and CPR started without delay. At the same time, paramedics must be summoned immediately by another person present.

What is the crucial period?

The crucial period is the first 3 to 4 minutes after cardiac arrest or pulmonary (breathing) arrest. That is all the time the victim has to maximize survival. Beyond that time, the chances of success becomes less and less as minutes go by, and the brain sustains irreversible damage from hypoxia (inadequate oxygen). So it is obvious that an efficient and super prompt CPR is needed to be successful in saving lives of arrest victims.

What is new in CPR?

With the old technique of performing CPR, one person was performing chest compression while another was sequentially doing mouth-to-mouth breathing for the victim, or one person doing both at proper intervals. The new method is specially designed for nonmedical people or for untrained individuals. The "revised" technique, as popularized by the Mayo Clinic, entails continuous chest compression of about 2 inches "deep" at about 100 times a minute, without the mouth-to-mouth component. The chest movement from the compression allows air-exchange in the lungs, enough to provide the brain and the coronary arteries sufficient (though not optimal) oxygen to sustain the victim under the situation. This has been found to be as effective and successful as the old method, and a lot simpler to do, especially for the untrained person. Even children can be taught how to do it. No official certification is needed to perform this new method of CPR.

The CPR-trained personnel may do alternate 30 chest compressions and two rescue breaths (mouth-to-mouth or with a resuscitation bag), achieving 100 compressions a minute. Either method may be used by those trained in CPR.

How long should CPR be done?

CPR should be continued until the paramedic or medical help arrives or at least for an hour if no expert help is available or expected to come. There have been medical reports of victims of drowning in a body of water that is cold (like in a lake during winter) who were successfully revived after three (3) hours of continuous CPR. This is true especially among children. The ice cold water protects the brain and the other vital organs in the body from deteriorating due to lack of circulation and oxygen, since cold body temperature slows down the body metabolism and requires practically no oxygen during that temporary "hibernation."

What happens if CPR is not done?

If CPR is not done to a person with cardiac or pulmonary arrest, as when the victim is alone at the time, or no one knows how to do it, the sequence of events starts with the heart quivering (not beating, not pumping), resulting in a heart that balloons out and unable to beat. The more dilated the heart is, the less chance it will have to respond to CPR. With no effective heartbeat, the circulation to the brain ceases, and brain-cell damage ensues within 5 to 10 minutes in the usual environment. The other vital organs are similarly affected, but the brain is much more sensitive to lack of blood supply (oxygen) and deteriorates the fastest.

Can CPR be done to oneself?

Yes, but not in the same manner described above. When one feels his/her heart rate is slowing down (which can cause dizziness and fainting), or the heartbeat is irregular causing some chest discomfort, one can do preventive "self-CPR" by taking a big deep breath, holding the breath (not exhaling) and straining (like trying to move your bowels), and coughing forcefully hard for about 15 seconds or so. This should be repeated as long as the symptom persists, until you reach the emergency room. This technique is called Valsalva maneuver, where the expanding lungs on both sides squeeze and "jolt" the heart. This technique could also be done if the heart is beating too fast. Discuss this idea with your physician the next time you visit him.

Where can one view the technique of CPR?

The Internet is a most helpful site. *YouTube* has a video on the new method of performing CPR. For more information, you may Google "CPR" or cardiopulmonary resuscitation. One can also find out from the Red Cross and hospitals when and where CPR courses are being offered in your area.

Ideally, CPR should be a required subject in our school curriculum, from mid-elementary and up.

Learn how to perform CPR. The life you save may be that of a loved one. Or even your own.

Why Not CT Scan Everyone?

This is indeed an interesting and a logical question, even from the scientific point of view, if we are to consider the fact that the earlier the condition or disease is diagnosed, the sooner the physicians can treat the illness (or even prevent diseases in some cases) and minimize, if not preclude, the malady from getting worse or causing complications. A good example here is cancer. Majority of cancers can be treated with a great deal of success, or even cured, if detected at their very early stage.

Tests, like CBC (complete blood count), lipid (cholesterol) profile, blood sugar for detecting diabetes, and urinalysis to check for infection or other conditions are done routinely. The so-called "executive panel" (which includes 26 blood and urine tests), for example, is regularly performed to detect abnormalities early, even among those without symptoms. So why don't physicians order total-body CT scan or MRI as routinely on all patients? Wouldn't these imaging tests not detect diseases in their very early stage and therefore allow prompt treatment and help physicians achieve better medical and surgical outcomes for their patients?

Again, all these questions from our readers appear logical, and the replies to them seem straightforward and obvious. But realistically, the answers to these questions are very complex and intricately woven into our system, a standard of medical practice that precludes this overly simplistic approach to making the diagnosis.

The reasons are many. The most compelling one today is economics. Insurance companies in the United States or in any other countries will not cover the cost of routine total-body X-rays, much less scans or MRI, unless the patient has symptoms of a probable disease (where the specific test is justified per criteria of the health insurers) and that initial simpler (lesser expensive) diagnostic procedures had been done and found not diagnostic. For the affluent who are able and willing to pay for the test on their own can certainly have access to full-body CT scan or MRI, even without having any symptoms.

But the medical community, in general, with its current standard of care, will frown upon this shotgun diagnostic strategy—and for a reason: total-body CT scan or MRI for everybody in our general population who seeks medical care will have a very low diagnostic yield (finding a disease), "too insignificant" statistically (per our current healthcare system) to justify the massive cost of this random imaging on everyone. Then there is the question of possible risk, no matter how negligible it might be with today's advanced X-ray and scanning technology. And more significantly, behind all this are the third-party payors (HMO being the worst per decades of experience in the USA), who will go to all lengths to save a buck, while their CEOs (as reported by the *Wall Street Journal* a couple of years ago) received millions of dollars a year in bonuses.

In a perfect world, where all these imaging tests, among others, could be done for free for everyone, total-body imaging may not be a bad idea, especially for those 35 years and older with a strong family history of cancer. And even if the test, when done on everyone at random, has a low diagnostic yield, one life saved, even in a thousand, is one life spared. In our imperfect world of today, however, even this particular "preemptive strike" against cancer is considered "not justified for coverage and reimbursement" by insurance carriers.

A few particular situations in my practice of cardiovascular and thoracic surgery in the United States the past 3 decades reinforce my own personal belief that some relaxation of the current regulations against prophylactic (preventive) diagnostic imaging (like full-body CT Scan) may be a valid consideration, one that could save lives and even lower the cost of medical care for these insurance companies themselves, in the long run, thru early diagnosis and prompt treatment.

A recent case in point involves a close friend and medical colleague of mine. This physician was healthy and symptom-free and had been going to the Mayo Clinic yearly for routine medical checkup. During his last visit his blood tests, which included liver profile, all came back normal. But because of a mild elevation of his diaphragm seen on the routine chest X-ray, the attending physician ordered a CT scan to find out what was pushing the diaphragm up. The result of this imaging test showed a huge (12 cm) cancer of the liver, which had already spread.

Retrospectively, everybody is wondering: "Since the tumor has grown that large, it has obviously started several months before that visit, and therefore could have been diagnosed earlier when it was small and before it had spread (and still operable) if a CT Scan had been performed 3 or 6 months earlier, in spite of the absence of symptoms and normal blood tests." What my friend went through was the accepted state-of-the-art "standard of medical care" practiced today by competent physicians at the Mayo Clinic and in other medical centers around the world.

Although the yield of random total-body scanning would be "very low and too insignificant for reimbursement" as far as insurance carriers are concerned, the unfortunate reality is that there will always be individuals, like my friend, who will inevitably fall through the crack of this current system and suffer from a cancer discovered too late that will totally devastate, not only his life, which will be cut short, but also the lives of his loved ones.

Dr. Google and Cyberchondriacs

The advent of the computer and cyberspace technology has led to the explosion of, and instant access to, seemingly endless volumes of information in the various fields of human endeavor, including in medicine, via the Internet.

This modern "virtual library" on the Web, accessible to practically anyone, any place in the world where the Internet exists, has leveled the playing field for people around the globe. Practically any information is instantly available in different languages, to any individual within a second or two on the World Wide Web, with a simple click of the mouse. I dare say, the world today is, metaphorically speaking, fundamentally flat as far as the access to data about science, medicine, art, technology, and other human enterprises are concerned.

However, as can be expected, progress and advances in our civilization also inherently bring with them some possible "negative side-effects," or potentially "unfavorable consequences," for some of people.

An example of this includes the birth of "Internet addicts," not only among young children and teenagers, to the dismay of some parents, but even among those in their sixties and older, to the dismay of some spouses. Indeed, computer works, surfing the net, exploring the Web, navigating the cyberspace, are addicting. I can personally relate to this, because I myself am hooked and have been a certified Internet addict for years. My personal computer is my constant companion, and I am most dependent on it. The first thing I do when I wake up each morning is to turn on my notebook, even before turning on the coffeemaker. I never leave home without my laptop. I feel "naked" and insecure without my notebook. It is my security blanket, my ectopic brain, my library, and my connection to the world out there. As a cardiac surgeon and a health columnist, I find the Internet a most valuable tool for me.

Cyber-navigation has also created a group of individuals who are known as "cyberchondriacs." Like the hypochondriacs many of us know or have heard or read about, "cyberchondriacs" are the Internet-driven version of these "self-diagnosticians." They are people who imagine and actually believe to have whatever illness, or medical complications, they read about on the net. Indeed, as the old adage says, "A little knowledge is a dangerous thing." More so among those with insecurity and fertile imagination. The obsession for self-diagnosis on the Internet has led to the rise of "cyberchondriacs," who are often misled by some inaccurate online information or by their erroneous interpretation of medical data on the Web. Consulting a physician can certainly help these individuals sort out facts from fiction, truth from falsehood, and reality from perception.

*   *   *

Touring some major cities in Ireland and Scotland in 2008, on my way for an induction ceremony into the Bohemian Paradise in Prague, I saw the large headline on the November 10 issue of *METRO*, a newspaper in Edinburgh, which said "Doctors urged to Google for cures."

Ever since search engines came into our midst, many physicians have been surfing the net and taking advantage of the power of the Web in keeping themselves abreast with the state-of-the-art medical information about diseases, their epidemiology, diagnosis, complications, and treatments, from renowned medical institutions in the United States and around the world.

After long years of medical schooling, internship, residency training, and optional fellowship, which training could range between 12 and 16 years, the physician should be medically competent. With the rapidly evolving advances in medical science and technology, the Internet is playing a major supplementary role in providing continuing medical education for the physician in his/her quest for the latest and the best in patient care.

While the implication of that headline might inadvertently suggest incompetence on the part of the physician as the driving force to Google for diagnosis or for cure, the truth is obviously far from it. As a matter of fact, it is the exact opposite. The competent medical practitioner is the one who knows his/her limitations in this era of rapidly exploding advances and progress in medical science. The good physician is the one who tends to be more of a "perfectionist," more exacting, more concerned, more meticulous, and more curious, one who wants to learn to the max, in order to provide excellence in the diagnosis, treatment, and total care of the patient. This is the quality physician we all want for ourselves. The more our physician knows, the better it is for his patients, regardless of his method of choice for acquiring the most current and relevant cutting-edge medical information needed for their care.

"Honeymoon Cystitis"

What is cystitis?

Cystitis is inflammation of the urinary bladder. This affects women much more than men. About 80% of women have suffered from cystitis at some time in their lives.

Why is cystitis more common in women?

Women have a very short (about one inch) urethra (the opening anterior to the vaginal orifice through which urine comes out); and hence bacteria from the anus, vagina, or from the contaminated skin in the area can easily enter the urinary bladder. Men have much longer urethra (about 5-6 inches, inside the entire length of the penis), and bacterial access into the bladder is obviously much harder.

Why the name "honeymoon cystitis"?

Cystitis is very common among those on their honeymoon, especially among women on their first sexual experience. Since lovemaking involves physical activities that could lead to some trauma to the genital and the urethral orifice and bacterial contamination from the fingers or mouth of the either partner, cystitis is highly prevalent among honeymooners, especially among females.

What bacteria is the usual culprit?

The most common bacteria that cause cystitis are called *E. coli* (*Escherichia coli*), which normally live in the bowel. In the colon, these bacteria do not cause any harm to the bowels, and may even be useful; but in the urinary bladder or other organs, *E. coli* causes infection and harm. *E. coli* thrives in an acidic milieu; and because urine is acidic, these bacteria multiply rapidly in the urethra and in the urinary bladder, causing inflammation (cystitis). If not treated, *E. coli* can spread upward to the ureters (the two tubes that bring urine from the left and right kidneys down to the bladder in the pelvis) and cause infection of the ureters and, in the neglected cases, the kidneys (pyelitis). If not managed early and properly, the damage to the kidneys can be serious and irreparable.

What are the other causes of cystitis?

An ill-fitted diaphragm, contraceptive foam or jellies, herpes and trichomona infection (sexually transmitted diseases), nonbacterial infection (like thrush) from contraceptive pills, kidney stones or cysts, etc., can all cause cystitis. Some women seem to be more prone than others to acquire cystitis, many of them having the infection 3 to 4 times a year.

Do children get cystitis?

Yes, children, even babies, can develop cystitis. This is also more common among girls than in boys. Most of the time, babies with cystitis come down with a fever, become fretful, and may even vomit. In younger girls, they may have the classic pain and urges to urinate often.

What cause cystitis in children?

Not drinking enough fluid can cause the urine to be concentrated and therefore irritating to the urethra, leading to inflammation. Congenital abnormality in the kidney or bladder, which are rare, can cause cystitis also; but the most common cause is contamination with feces. The proper technique of wiping (or even washing) after defecation is from the front to the back, since the urethra and the vaginal orifices are anatomically located in front and the anus behind. This will prevent the fecal dirt and bacteria in the anus from contaminating the "front" where the vagina and the urethral orifices are. All females, young and old, (and even males) should use this technique habitually for better personal hygiene.

What are the symptoms of cystitis?

The urinary bladder is a muscular bag that holds urine until it is voided. When the bladder is inflamed, the symptoms include frequency of urination and urges to urinate even if the bladder is empty, pain on urination, and sometimes blood in the urine (making it appear as dark as tea or cola drink, instead of light yellow). Among women, the first sign could be that of pricking pain, burning and scalding sensation during urination. This then develops into a sharp pain in the lower abdomen.

Can dry sex in women cause cystitis?

Cystitis invariably results if the vagina is not moist and well-lubricated during sex. The bruising and irritation to the vaginal and urethral orifice due to the dryness make women prone to this infection. Also a source of infection are bacteria under the foreskin of the penis among uncircumcised men.

Can cystitis be due to hormonal imbalance?

Yes, changes in the female hormonal cycle predispose women to suffer cystitis. The attack can occur shortly after the onset of menstrual cycle, during pregnancy, after delivery, during menopause, or after a hysterectomy. Stress or depression can disrupt the hormonal cycle. Hormonal changes affect the acidity or alkalinity of urine and the level of moisture in the vagina.

How can one prevent cystitis?

Some of the causes of cystitis mentioned above should be avoided. Drink enough water (6 to 8 glasses daily) and cranberry juice (it destroys E.coli bacteria); urinate whenever you feel the urge to avoid urine retention; use proper wiping/washing technique (from front to back); take a shower (wash genitals and hands well) before and after sex; avoid using perfumed soap, talcum powder, or antiseptics on the genitals; do not use bubble bath or bath oils in the bath; use vaginal lubricant during sex if needed; avoid tights and tight jeans and nylons (cotton pants are better when afflicted with cystitis); and avoid spicy foods, coffee, and especially alcohol.

When does one see a physician?

When the first symptoms of cystitis occurs, drink a pint of bland liquid (cranberry juice is best) right away, and half a pint every hour for 8 hours. Sodium bicarbonate (Alka-Seltzer or Bromo-Seltzer, etc.) helps make the urine more alkaline (less acidic) and discourages bacterial growth. However, if the symptoms persist for than 24 hours, medical consultation is recommended. Children with cystitis should be seen by a physician sooner.

Date-Rape Drugs

What are date-rape drugs?

Date-rape drugs, sometimes referred to as party drugs or simply ecstasy, are medications that can be slipped into drinks and make a person unconscious for 15 minutes or so. There have been reports of dozens of women in the United States who were under the influence of a date-drug known as GHB (gamma hydroxybutyrate), a clear and flavorless liquid, when they were raped.

What is this drug legitimately used for?

GHB, manufactured by Orphan Medical, a drug firm in Minnesota, was developed for the treatment of narcolepsy. In smaller doses, this drug induces euphoria (a sense of well-being). As a date-rape drug, GHB causes the victim to fall into a deep sleep, oblivious of the sexual assault until they wake up. Some do not even remember what had transpired.

What is narcolepsy?

Narcolepsy is a rare sleep disorder which causes the persons to nod off without notice. They just suddenly and rapidly fall asleep. There are about 100,000 people in the United States with this ailment. Orphan Medical states that GHB can help the patients who have the form of narcolepsy that is accompanied by temporary muscle paralysis.

How safe is GHB?

Used as a prescription drug for narcolepsy and taken as directed by the physician, GHB is safe. Its abuse as a date-rape drug has led to countless comas and several hundreds of deaths from overdose.

Is GHB legal?

Twenty states in the United States, including Illinois and Michigan, have banned GHB, allowing police arrest those who manufacture or sell this drug. Eight states have listed GHB as a controlled substance with varying degrees of criminal penalties, making it available only as a prescription drug.

What other drugs have been used?

Ketamine and rohypnol are both controlled substances which have been used as date-rape drugs. Other perpetrators have tried ordinary sleeping pills, which do not act fast enough and do not induce a deep enough level of unconsciousness, thus foiling the rape attempt.

Are some sold as dietary supplements?

Yes, the Food and Drug Administration of the United States warns the public against "more than half a dozen sleeps aids and party drugs in the guise of dietary supplements sold in health food stores and on the Internet," which are substances that are unregulated and can maim and kill. Parents and children alike must be aware and vigilant about this, if date-rape, or even death from this drug, is to be prevented.

Under what other names are they sold?

The FDA cautions the consumers not to use products containing GHB, GBL (gamma butylrolactone), or BD (1,4 butanediol). Some such drugs are sold under the name Revitalize Plus, Weight Belt Clenaer, GHRE, Serenity, Thunder Nectar, SomatoPro, Enliven, Tetramethylene glycol or 23H)-Furanone di-hydro, and NRG3. These drugs can cause severe nausea, vomiting, dangerously slow breathing or cessation of breathing, unconsciousness, seizures, and death.

Are there date-rape drinks?

Yes, three of them are Cherry fX Bombs, Orange fX Rush, and Thunder Nectar. The claim that these drinks are from Kava plant and are safe is not true. These and other date-rape beverages have BD (1,4 butanediol, an industrial solvent) in them.

How is the date-rape drug used?

The usual modus operandi of the perpetrator is to invite the woman to go out on a date with him. Most of these men are friends or acquaintances of the women. Some target victims are casual pickups in lounges and bars. The drug is discreetly poured into the drink, and moments later the victim is taken from the bar to a vehicle or to a secluded area or motel room, or raped right in her own home or wherever the party was.

Do victims have memory of the assault?

Some date-rape drug victims do not remember what had happened to them until they physically felt that they were assaulted. The drug blurs the memory somewhat for the most recent event. Some people are so sensitive to the drug that they overdose on it easily even on moderate amount.

Is there an antidote a woman can take?

No, the only "antidote" a woman can use to avoid date-rape drugs or date-rape is discipline, common sense, will power, and vigilance. There is no medication one can take to ward off the bad effect of date-rape drugs.

How can women avoid these drugs?

The question may sound trite and the answer obvious, but nonetheless it is a most fundamental one, especially for the young and uninitiated ladies. The following set of advice may sound an over simplification but could be life-saving: (1) Never go out with a "stranger." Having a liaison with a man you just met is risky and dangerous. (2) Also remember that many of the apprehended perpetrators were friends of the victims. (3) When on a date, at a restaurant or at home (his or even yours) watch your drink and your food with vigilance and care. (4) If you suspect "something," stop drinking your cocktail and eating your food, and excuse yourself and leave, or call a trusted friend to join you ASAP. (5) If you do not feel well at this point, get the assistance of the bartender, the waitress, or any woman. (6) Do not go with your date to the car. (7) If your suspicion is really strong, or if you actually witnessed your date slipping a drug into your drink or food, ask the waitress to "bag" the food for you to take home and have it tested for drugs at the toxicology lab of a hospital. (8) If this tested positive, hand over the evidence to the police as you file a criminal complaint.

A Billion Deaths

Worldwide, a billion people will die from smoking this century, according to the World Health Organization.

Smoking kills. It is that plain and simple. There is no more doubt today that tobacco (cigarette smoking) is the predominant cause of lung cancer, besides other malignancies and cardiovascular diseases that maim, kill men and women, and hurt our society, especially our children. In the United States alone, almost half a million die each year from smoking-related illnesses. These are preventable deaths! Demographic studies have shown that smokers are about 10 times more prone to die premature deaths than nonsmokers. This unnecessary loss of lives is at an immense direct cost for nonsmokers in terms of increased health risks from passive smoking, in higher health insurance premiums and taxes, not to mention personal and family tragedies in all shapes and forms.

As we have alluded to in a previous column, secondhand smoke is even more dangerous. Innocent bystanders are forced to inhale cigarette smoke at their workplaces or in public places, thus increasing their health risk. In one stick of cigarette, there are about 4,000 chemicals and 200 of them cancerous. The Environmental Protection Agency engineers have shown that even the best available ventilation and air-moving equipment were unable to reduce carcinogenic (cancer-causing) air contamination to a safe level for a nonsmoker sharing work space with a habitual smoker. Physical isolation of the tobacco addict is most essential as shown by these scientific studies.

Tobacco use leads to four times as many excess deaths annually compared to all other drugs and alcohol abuse combined, ten times more than all automobile fatalities per year, twelve times more than deaths from AIDS, and much more than all the American military casualties (in all wars) in this century put together. That's how dangerous and damaging tobacco is to the human body and to society as a whole.

At the beginning of the past century, lung cancer was almost an insignificant health problem for the world. It became a minor problem in the 1930s (death rate of 5 per 10,000). Today, it has become the main killer among men and women. Since women started "really" smoking in the 1950s, "because it was glamorized in ads by actresses and models as a sophisticated and fashionable habit," lung cancer in females has increased at least six-fold, an alarming rate, with death rate comparable to that in males. Women also have added risks: osteoporosis, thrombophlebitis (vein inflammation and blood clot formation), arthritis, infertility, cervical cancer, and menstrual irregularities. Pregnant smokers face miscarriages, stillbirths, low-birth weight, and SIDS (sudden infant death syndrome) babies. Almost 30,000 female lives are snuffed out every year as a result of smoking. Of the 4 billion cigarette-related deaths in the world each year, about half a billion are women. It is now the top killer among women. Today, one woman dies from cigarette-related illness every three minutes!

Dengue

What is dengue fever?

Dengue fever is a severe, potentially fatal hemorrhagic febrile disease caused by dengue viruses, which are carried and transmitted by the female day-biting *Aedes aegytpti* mosquito, the same mosquito responsible for yellow fever. Dengue was first reported in Australia in 1897. Most of the victims are children.

What is the global picture?

Today, about 2.5 billion (2/5 of the world population) are at risk from dengue, and 50 million are infected worldwide annually, with a mortality rate ranging from 1% to 2.5% for those who receive treatment, according to WHO statistics. For those without treatment, the death rate could be 20% (one in 5) or higher.

How does one catch this disease?

One catches dengue through the bite of a female *Aedes aegypti* mosquito. It is not transmitted directly from person to person. The vector (carrier) mosquitoes inhabit and rapidly breed in stagnant pools of water or in tanks of drinking or bathwater in the backyard of homes, which makes the situation more dangerous. They do not thrive in dirty contaminated water as some may think. The disease is more widespread during the rainy season. In 1999, there were 57,000 cases. This year, 2010, the dengue cases could go up to 70,000, if the trend continues.

What are the symptoms of dengue fever?

In areas where dengue is found, any abrupt onset of fever (38-40 degrees) 2 to 7 days duration must be suspected as dengue till proven otherwise. More specifically, there will be (but do *not* wait for these before seeing a physician) skin rash, malaise, pain behind the eyes, headache, joint and bone pains, anorexia, vomiting, nose and/or gum bleeding, easy bruising, coffee-ground loose stools, and cough. This may be followed, after 2 to 5 days, by rapid deterioration in the patient's condition and collapse.

What can be done to prevent dengue fever?

Personal protection (mosquito nets, protective clothing) helps. However, the best measure is to eliminate the breeding sites to get rid of the mosquitoes. No mosquitoes, no virus. No virus, no dengue. Pure and simple. So the most prudent strategy is to eliminate all possible breeding places of mosquitoes around us, like pools of stagnant water (in tanks for drinking or bathing, pools of water in the ground, in discarded auto tires, bottle, coconut husks, plastic container, etc.) Tanks of drinking or bathwater must be covered. DEET (N, N-diethylmetatoluamide) mosquito repellent is helpful. In addition to DEET, US health authorities are recommending two more safe repellents: picaridin and oil of lemon eucalyptus. Permethin-coated curtains are also effective in repelling mosquitoes. The chemicals used for fumigation (fogging) have potential health hazards and do not kill the infective larvae. Vaccines for the prevention of the different types of dengue fever are not available.

Depression

What is depression?

Depression is a state of emotion where the individual has some or all of the following senses, feelings, or moods: downhearted, unhappy, anxious, irritable, unable to concentrate, socially withdrawn, empty inside, has inordinate fatigue and reduced interest in activities which used to be fun, hopelessness, indecision, impaired sleep, misery, helplessness, confusion, monosyllabic speech, or abnormally quiet.

What is morbid mood?

The morbid mood in depression may be so severe that the patient is unable to cry (tears dry up) or to feel the usual emotions like pleasure, grief, or joy. The whole world appears lifeless and colorless to the patient, who could be preoccupied with a sense of guilt and self-denigrating and destructive ideas.

What is melancholia?

It used to be called endogenous depression. Its features include marked slowness in thinking and activity, agitation, worthlessness, weight loss, restlessness, wringing of the hands, inability to experience pleasure or well-being, difficulty falling asleep and has insomnia, following arousal from sleep, with diminished or loss of sexual desire. The patient usually has the feeling of guilt that he/she has committed a grave crime, with hallucinations (voices of people accusing the patient of bad deeds or condemning him/her to death. Others believe that they have incurable diseases like cancer or AIDS). Very rarely, the patient with this psychotic depression kill family members ("to save them from future misfortunes in life") and kills himself/herself.

How rampant is depression?

In the United States, depression affects about 17 million Americans. More than 2/3 or 75% of them do not benefit from proper therapy because of patient's inability to seek counseling, misunderstanding of the condition, or misdiagnosis. Most people do not seek professional help because the condition is very common and many of them mild or subclinical (with no obvious symptoms). Sometimes, even physicians miss making the correct diagnosis in earnest, thinking the patient's complaints could be due to some medication interaction.

Are there screening tests for depression?

Yes, there are. Mental health specialists can administer preliminary tests such as the BDI (Beck Depression Inventory), or the HRS (Hamilton Rating Scale), which is composed of 20 questions to screen the patient. Today, computerized phone interviews are gaining effectivity as a screening tool. These tests are only a small part of the evaluation process, because the specialists have the symptoms of the patient and other criteria to aid them make the correct diagnosis.

Don't we all get depressed sometimes?

To some degree, when the situations demand it, normal people develop a mild form of depression, which is transient, self-terminating, and not a disease. As long as the resultant symptoms are trivial and temporary and do not debilitate the person, the condition does not need any medical treatment.

What foods relieve depression?

Foods that are high in tryptophan, an amino acid involve in serotonin production, provide relief to some people with depression. Niacin (vitamin B3), which is essential in the production of tryptophan, can be found in dried peas, beans, whole grains, dried fortified cereals, and especially in oily fishes like salmon and mackerel. It is reported that omega-3 polyunsaturated fatty acids in fish oil may actually reduce depression. PMS Escape, a high-carbohydrate drink, is claimed to increase tryptophan level and may control the depression related to premenopausal syndrome for about 3 hours. However, there are impurities in the L-tryptophan diet supplements that are associated with EMS (eosinophilia-myalgia syndrome), which increases the white blood cells and causes muscle pains. In 1989, there was an epidemic of EMS.

Does calcium help alleviate depression?

Calcium supplements and vitamin B12 have been reported to reduce premenstrual depression. Also, some studies showed that among depressed people who drink caffeinated beverages have a lower incidence of suicide, which seems to suggest that coffee or tea reduces depression.

How about exercises?

Believe it or not, physical exercises may be as effective as psychotherapy in the management of mild to moderate depression. Prolonged aerobic workouts lead to higher levels of serotonin, adrenalin, endorphins, and dopamine in the brain (producing the popular term "runner's high"). Physical exercises, brisk walking, ballroom dancing, yoga, tae-bo, etc., lead to better emotional health. As an extra bonus from physical exercises, weight loss and improved muscle tone lead to the sense of well-being and higher self-esteem.

What about the spiritual venue?

This is one great aid in the management of depression, especially the mild and moderate ones. Those individuals with strong spiritual faiths have a relatively lower predisposition to depression. These people might benefit from meditation, yoga, and other techniques for obtaining spiritual security, inner peace, and happiness.

What are the therapy guidelines?

Among adults who suffer from major or chronic depression, a trial of antidepressant drugs is used together with psychotherapy that is designed for the particular patient. For those who do not improve with this strategy, ECT (electroconvulsive therapy) has been found to be effective and safe. If this fails, psychosurgery might be indicated.

How about for children?

Children and adolescents with major depression have been found in clinical studies to respond as well to placebos (sugar pills) as to tricyclic antidepressants, especially the newer ones, the SSRIs (selective serotonin reuptake inhibitors). For these group of young patients, a trial of psychotherapy (cognitive-behavioral or supportive therapy) is preferred before they are placed on antidepressant drugs.

Do you have depression?

If you do, it is most prudent to seek medical help, not necessarily psychotherapy. The first thing to do it to consult your family physician, who can help guide you. With early proper medication and/or advice, depression in most cases can be managed effectively and eliminated faster than one can imagine. Physicians today have invaluable tools in their armamentarium for the diagnosis and treatment of depression. Many individuals with depression, who have sought medical care, are so "cured" with simple oral medications that they look, behave, function, and live as normally and happily as anybody else.

Warning on DHEA

If you are one of those who have succumbed to the commercial claims on DHEA and are now taking this so called "food supplement" to make you feel younger, you better think again. You may not be in only for what you bargained for. There may be some disastrous surprises ahead of you.

What is DHEA?

Called by marketers as "superhormone, mother of all hormones, fountain of youth," DHEA is a steroid hormone (dehydroepianderosterone), a chemical cousin of testosterone and estrogen. This is produced by the adrenals, small glands that sit on top of the two kidneys. Very little DHEA is produced the first five years of life, more around six or seven. It peaks at mid-20s and steadily declines after age 30. A 75-year-old will have only about 20%. The males have higher DHEA levels than females in their lifetime.

What are the claims?

DHEA has been tagged by the medical community as the snake oil of the '90s. Too much hype has been accorded this over-the-counter drug, which manufacturers and dealers claim to increase longevity, make one feel younger, aid in weight control, prevent cancer, stroke, heart disease, Alzheimer's, and cures AIDS and many infections. Public ignorance and gullibility have contributed to the popularity of this potentially dangerous substance. The extensive marketing claims have fooled people, including some in the medical fields themselves, into taking DHEA.

Aren't these claims familiar?

Indeed they are, from the commercial ads of so many food supplements flooding the market today, victimizing the unsuspecting and gullible public who are eagerly seeking for an easy way, the "quick fix," to better health and longevity, sans dieting and exercise. If these claims were true, the ones who introduced these "miracle" food supplements should be awarded the Nobel Prize in Medicine for coming up with one single pill or juice that could cure all illnesses on earth from athlete's foot, to high blood pressure, infections, heart disease, liver ailments, kidney and prostrate illnesses, to diabetes and other metabolic conditions, Alzheimer's, AIDS, and even cancer. Obviously, these claims are unsubstantiated and false. The only thing these food supplements can do is to make their manufacturers and distributors grow richer and richer.

What do experts say?

"The one thing you should tell your readers is that we know very little about DHEA. The hype is out of control, and I can't stress enough that it should be used with caution, IF AT ALL, until we know more," says Samuel Yen, MD, professor of reproductive medicine at the University of California, San Diego.

"No one should take DHEA except under the supervision of a physician, who should routinely check steroid and cholesterol levels, glucose tolerance, and prostate health in men," says John Nestle, MD, professor of endocrinology and metabolism at Virginia Commonwealth University, who studies DHEA's effects on diabetes and blood clotting.

"It makes me very nervous that people are using a drug we don't know anything about. I won't recommend it," says Elizabeth Barrett-Connor, MD, professor and chair, Department of Family and Preventive Medicine at the University of California, San Diego.

"Selling potent steroid hormones in health food stores or by mail could be a disaster in the making. DHEA should be classified as an investigational drug and used only in clinical research until we figure out what it does and its side effects," says Peter Hornsby, PhD, associate professor of cell biology at Baylor College of Medicine. His team has just identified the body's DHEA-making cells.

Why such harsh statements about DHEA?

Simple: to date we know very little about DHEA. There is no valid scientific proof that the DHEA "supplement" being marketed is effective at all for anything, and there is no evidence to show taking it is benign and that after taking it for months or years, a person will not come up with brain, kidney, liver problems, or even cancer, etc. "Unfortunately, we don't see the problems associated with hormone use until years later," says Peter Casson, MD, assistant professor of obstetrics and gynecology at Baylor College of Medicine. He cited as an example the higher incidence of breast cancer in women who took diethylstilbestrol (DES) to prevent a miscarriage, which was discovered only after years of use.

Arthur Feinberg, MD, in his article in the *New England Journal of Medicine* says: "The potential for irreversible side effects is real. So given that there's no convincing evidence for any benefit of DHEA, I feel strongly that people should not take it." Indeed, there could be serious risks and complications down the road.

Diabesity: A Massive Epidemic

A relatively new descriptive term combining two closely related disease entities, diabetes and obesity, is spreading like wildfire in the clinical setting, posing great challenges, not only to the patient and the physician but also to society and human race as a whole. Diabesity is now a major epidemic, the most massive man has ever faced.

As Professor Paul Zimmet, director of the International Diabetes Institute in Melbourne, Australia, recently stated on a WebMD telecast, "What HIV/AIDS was in the last 20 years of the 20th century, diabetes and obesity and their consequences will almost certainly be in the first 2 decades of the 21st century."

Worldwide, in the last few decades, victims of diabetes have increased more than twice and expected to grow from its current 285 million to 439 million in 19 years, by 2030. Among this, 25.8 million are children. Each year, 3 million people die from diabetes and its complications.

In a previous writing, I commented that the rapid growth in the incidence of diabetes mellitus was a metabolic time bomb that was waiting to explode, brought on by, among others, "super-sizing" of America, where 90% of Type 2 diabetics were (are) overweight. The causal relationship between obesity (being overweight, even only to a moderate degree) and the higher risk of developing diabetes is a medically proven fact.

Actually, 2 out of 3 (66.6%) adult Americans and 15% of the children are overweight. Before insulin was discovered in the early 1920s, type 1 diabetes had 100% mortality. In the past 10 years, there has been a 33% increased in the number of diabetic patients. It is indeed scary.

The other grim statistics that confirm the radpidly developing epidemic of diabetes include the following:

1. An infant born in the USA in year 2000 has 1 in 3 chances (33%) to get the disease.

2. Shortening the life span by 10-15 years, diabetes is now the 6th leading cause of death, killing 210,000 people a year in the United States alone.

3. Diabetes is also the major cause of heart and kidney diseases, leg amputation and blindness.

4. The incidence of clinical depression is 3 times more among diabetics.

5. In the United States (population: about 312 million), there are about 18.2 million diabetics (9.3 million are women), about 1.3 million new cases a year ago, and 5.2 million undiagnosed or unaware. Five to 10% have type 1 (juvenile), and the rest, type 2 (adult onset) diabetes. An additional 16 million Americans are in a "pre diabetic" stage.

6. By year 2050, about 29 million Americans will be diagnosed with diabetes.

7. The United States is spending $218 billion a year in direct healthcare cost and in loss of productivity due to diabetes.

8. In a small country, like the Philippines, with a population of 91 million, there are more than 300,000 Filipinos who suffer from diabetes mellitus.

9. Worldwide, with its population of almost 7 billion people, there are about 285 million type 2 diabetics and more than 18 million type 1.

During our parents' time, diabetes was a disease of old people. Today, physicians are seeing patients as young as 4 with diabetes. Overeating and obesity are blamed for this and for the rising number of cases of adult-onset diabetes in general, worldwide. It is clear today that our diet should not only be calorie-controlled, low-fat, and low-cholesterol but also low in carbohydrates (like rice, bread, nondiet soft drinks, fruit juices and milk shakes, sugar-loaded morning cereals, cakes, cookies, ice cream, and sweets in general).

A diet of fish or chicken (white meat minus the skin), vegetables, and high-fiber whole grains and nuts has been shown to be healthier and better for longevity. Eating red meat has been associated with an elevated risk of developing any of the various types of cancers, like of the breast, colon, prostate, pancreas, etc. Smoking also increases the risk for diabetes, not to mention cancer of the lungs and other forms of cancers.

Antidiabetic Diet

A study published in the *British Medical Journal* May 30, 2008, suggested that individuals "who eat a Mediterranean-style diet are less likely to develop new-onset diabetes," reported WebMD. The findings also showed that the benefit was especially more among those persons who were at a higher risk of getting diabetes (the overweight, those who had high blood pressure and strong family history, etc.) Earlier studies have established a link between Mediterranean diet and the lowered risk of metabolic syndrome, of which diabetes is a component, but this recent study is the major one which showed this specific diet to reduce development of diabetes. Other studies have also suggested that this diet may reduce the risk for myocardial infarction (heart attack) and mortality from heart attack.

"Our prospective cohort study suggests that substantial protection against diabetes can be obtained with the traditional Mediterranean diet, rich in olive oil, vegetables, fruits, nuts, cereals, legumes, and fish but relatively low in meat and dairy products," stated Dr. Miguel A. Martínez-Gonzalez (University of Navarra, Pamplona, Spain) and colleagues, who did the research.

Minimizing red meat is key in this diet regimen, and moderate intake of wine is also a feature of the typical Mediterranean diet. While physical exercise was not a part of the study, various scientific researches have found beyond any doubt that exercise is an essential preventive factor in overall health, which can significantly ward off the development and reduce the risk of cardiovascular diseases and cancer.

It is very clear that we can minimize death from heart disease and other causes, including metabolic ailments, and even cancer, by following a diet that is low in saturated fats and sugar and high in fish, fruits, legumes, vegetables, and whole grains, in combination with proper weight maintenance and daily physical exercises.

According to the Heidemann Study published in the July 15, 2008, issue of *Circulation,* people who faithfully adhered to the Mediterranean diet "had a 17 percent lower long-term risk of premature death from all causes, and a 28 percent lower risk of death from cardiovascular disease, compared to women with a low adherence to this pattern."

Other studies have shown that early detection of the prediabetes stage (before obvious and full blown diabetes develops) significantly prevents the onset of type 2 (the commonest kind of) diabetes. Prediabetes can be treated and cured for good, with religious compliance with the proper diet and exercises alone, without medications. Done faithfully, this regimen will bring down the blood sugar level to normal. And if adopted as a lifestyle, this discipline can ward of the development of diabetes, cardiovascular and metabolic illnesses, and cancers. Minimizing these last three diseases alone, especially the Big C, are great bonuses in themselves.

Type 2 diabetes is, to a great extent, preventable. The question is, are we willing to discipline ourselves, do some sacrifices, control our appetite and weight through healthy lifestyle changes to escape this much-dreaded, severely debilitating, and costly global epidemic?

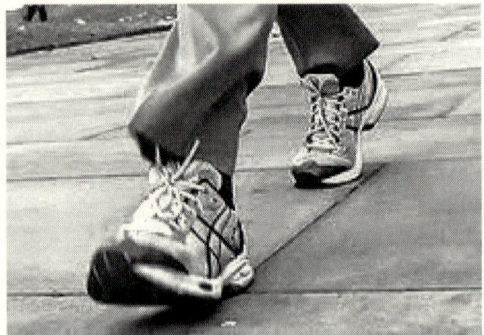

Indeed, diabesity is one of the greatest public health challenges the world is facing in the 21st century. It is a battle the human race cannot afford to lose.

Simple walking exercise, at least 5 times a week, boosts the immune system, oils the joints, tones muscles, and strengthens the cardiovascular system.

Artificial Pancreas

The pancreas is a thumb-shaped glandular organ, about 6 inches long, located right under and behind the stomach, attached to the C-curvature of the first part of the small intestine called the duodenum. The pancreas produces enzymes that aid in the digestion of food and contains alpha and beta cells, which manufactures glucagon and insulin, respectively. These two hormones control the blood sugar metabolism to maintain a normal glucose level.

The APS Advantage

For insulin-dependent diabetic patients, the implantable insulin pump has been in use but incidences of hypoglycemia (dangerously low blood sugar level) among these patients have caused some concerns among clinicians. An artificial pancreas appears to be a logical goal for the maintenance of a more constant and smoother level of blood sugar.

At Massachusetts General and Boston University, researchers have done the first clinical trials of an artificial pancreas system (APS) utilizing two hormones, insulin and glucagon. This APS "closely mimics the body's blood sugar control mechanism and was able to maintain near-normal glucose levels without causing hypoglycemia in a small group of patients."

The study, which appeared in *Science Translational Medicine*, reported that the system, "combining a blood glucose monitor and insulin pump technology with software that directs administration of insulin and the blood-sugar-raising hormone glucagon was designed at Boston University (BU)."

The FDA approved first clinical trial conducted at Massachusetts General Hospital (MGH) confirmed the feasibility of an approach utilizing doses of both hormones, according to Steven Russell, MD, PhD, of the MGH Diabetes Unit, who co-led the research team with Edward Damiano, PhD, of the BU Department of Biomedical Engineering.

A More Natural Balance

To preclude the risk of hypoglycemia, the BU researchers "developed a system that both accounts for the rate of insulin absorption and also incorporates glucagon, a hormone naturally released by the pancreas to raise blood sugar levels."

"Our system is designed to counteract moderate drops in blood sugar with minute doses of glucagon spread out throughout the day, just as the body does in people without diabetes," reported Dr. Damiano.

Once confirmed to be safe and effective in larger clinical trials, the artificial pancreas system will revolutionize the management for insulin-dependent diabetes mellitus. It will eliminate the need for patients to constantly stick their fingers to monitor their blood sugar and make treatment decisions several times a day. The APS will do the job for them and with more precision. While this would not be a cure, a perfected artificial pancreas system would certainly make life much better and more comfortable for hundreds of millions of insulin-dependent diabetics around the world.

Diabetes and Sex

Is sex affected by diabetes?

Yes. In men, diabetes mellitus can cause a varying degree of erectile dysfunction (inability to attain or sustain erection satisfactory for intercourse) as the diabetes progresses. Most of the time, however, the exaggerated and unfair condemnation of diabetes as causing severe erectile dysfunction leads to a psychological deterrent and a self-fulfilling prophecy in most men. Many well-adjusted and well-treated diabetics enjoy sex without problems. In women, loss of vaginal lubrication is a major sexual effect of diabetes.

How common is erectile dysfunction?

It is very common. While impotence affects very few men, erectile dysfunction affects an estimated 10 to 20 million men aged 19 and older in the United States. The prevalence is 52% in men aged 40 to 70 and increases with age. However, today, men and women can enjoy sexual activity throughout life, with proper care and strategy. Erectile dysfunction is not inevitable with aging, even into the 70s and 80s. With proper medical counseling and aids like Viagra, Cialis, or Levitra, most males and females can enjoy sex at any age.

What are the other complications of diabetes?

Diabetes has a lot of potential complications. Among them are the effects on the small arteries and big arteries in the body, causing blockages in the circulation, leading to damages (poor supply of blood, oxygen, and nutrition) to the various organs of the body: the eyes (retinopathy that results in blindness), kidneys (nephropathy resulting in kidney failure), legs (resulting in leg an feet ulcers, gangrene and amputation), nerves (neuropathy that causes numbness and pains in the feet), and cellular immunity (weakens the immune system leading to infections). This is the reason why all diabetic patients must be under the care of a physician and why the blood sugar must be well-controlled at all times.

What are the causes of erectile dysfunction?

Erectile dysfunction is rare in diabetic men until their mid-30s. Erectile dysfunction is very common in the general male population, especially in these modern times. Contributing to cause this condition are psychologic factors (severe anxiety, fear of intimacy, fear of unwanted pregnancy, sexual guilt, depression), drugs (most medications for high blood pressure and coronary heart disease, psychotropic drugs, CNS depressants-tranquilizers, etc., do affect erection), arteriosclerosis/vascular (blocking arteries that supply blood to the male organ), and, rarely, biogenic (associated with low testosterone levels and reflecting disorders of the hyphothalamic-pituitary-gonadal axis).

Does alcohol affect erection?

Alcohol definitely affects erection, either in diabetics or nondiabetics. While the first shot of alcohol may cause a little euphoria and a sense of well-being in most persons and, therefore, perhaps helps in improving the sexual climate, the second and subsequent drinks will impair erection in most men, depending on their tolerance to alcohol. As Shakespeare wrote, "Alcohol increases the desire but diminishes the performance."

Does diabetes cause gangrene of the male organ?

This is a myth that has been used to scare men to seek medical treatment for diabetes in the olden times. While there was wisdom in the intent, the medical truth is that the small arterioles in the penis have not been found to be affected by arteriosclerosis (hardening of the arteries) compared to arteries of the heart, brain, kidneys, abdomen, and legs. If there is any report in the medical literature about diabetes causing gangrene of the penis, it must be so rare physicians have not encountered it. On the other hand, trauma and other conditions, like priapism (abnormally prolonged, painful and persistent erection), have been well-known to cause gangrene, when intractable and not amenable to treatment.

What is the treatment for these side effects of diabetes on sex?

Making the correct diagnosis is very important, since the treatment depends on the cause. Once the diagnosis of erectile dysfunction is confirmed, ED drugs (Viagra, Ciaslis, Levitra) are the current drug of choice. Persons on nitroglycerine (medications for coronary heart disease) are strictly warned against taking ED drugs, because the combination could cause irreversible shock and death. It is essential that the diabetes is well-controlled at all times. Quitting smoking, exercising at least 4 times a week, and a conducive environment will tremendously help in improving sexual performance.

If ED drugs do not help, what next?

Erectyle dysfunction drugs help alleviate poor erection in about 90% of diabetics and more in nondiabetics. Other assistance may come from sex therapy. Other medications (penile erection suppository, yohimbine, which is still controversial, prostaglandin E1); vacuum constricting devices; male hormone testosterone, which is rarely needed and which increases the chances of cancer of the prostate; and surgery (aorto-iliac procedures for blocked arteries in the pelvis that partly supply the male organ) and implantation of penile shaft prosthesis are the other aids. With the advent of ED drugs, most of these "other aids" have been relegated to the background and used only as a last resort.

How about in diabetic women?

Among diabetic women, the major sexual side-effect is loss of the natural vaginal lubrication, which makes sexual encounters most uncomfortable and even painful. Master and Johnson, pioneering sex researchers in the 1960s, stressed the importance of vaginal lubrication during the initial sexual arousal in women and throughout the sex act. The wet cavity allows the male organ to slide in and out more easily, increasing both partners sense of ecstasy. The lubrication also increases the sensitivity of the vaginal lip and clitoris to touch, increasing the responsiveness and pleasure to digital caress. With proper vaginal lubrication, proper "ambiance," and well-controlled blood sugar (and other medical conditions, if any), diabetic women can enjoy pleasurable sex at any age.

What are the other causes of loss of vagina lubrication?

Other causes of loss in vaginal lubrication are stress or psychological factors, undesired partner, drugs (tricyclic antidepressants, like Elavil, Anafranil, Tofranil, Sinequan, birth control pills, antihistamines, cold formulas, etc.), alcohol, cigarettes, and marijuana. Other conditions include jet lag from travel across time zones, excessively prolonged foreplay or lovemaking, and pregnancy and childbirth.

Is there a remedy for loss of vaginal lubrication?

There is an easy remedy to this problem. There is practically no excuse why women should not enjoy sex as men do. Loss of vaginal lubrication happens to majority of women past 40 years old, some even as young as in their 20s and 30s. The cause among menopausal women is hormonal, but stress, as stated above, could play a great role also, especially in the younger women. There are now a lot of commercially available sex lubricants.

The Diabetes Epidemic

What is diabetes?

Diabetes mellitus is a hereditary condition characterized by hyperglycemia (high blood sugar), glycosuria (sweet urine), and is caused by an impairment in insulin secretion/and or insulin action. Insulin is a hormone produced by the beta cells of the Islet of Langerhans in the pancreas and is responsible for glucose metabolism. Insulin transforms glucose to energy. When these beta cells are destroyed (by an autoimmune process or by virus), the insulin production is diminished or halted, leading to the body's inability to metabolize glucose, thereby causing hyperglycemia (high blood sugar), the condition we call diabetes mellitus.

How prevalent is diabetes?

In the United States, there are about 18.2 million diabetics and about 1800 new cases are diagnosed each year. Type 1 Diabetes, used to be called Juvenile Diabetes, is insulin-dependent (the person's pancreas does not produce insulin), meaning insulin injection is needed to treat the condition. It is medically known as IDDM (Insulin Dependent Diabetes Mellitus) found most commonly among persons younger than 30 years old and associated obesity is not common. It accounts for 5 to 10% of all diabetics. Type 2 (Adult-Onset) Diabetes is NIDDM (Non-Insulin Dependent Diabetes Melllitus), which can be treated by pills (sulfonyl ureas, antihyperglycemic drugs) rather than insulin, is most commonly found among those who are older than 30, and associated obesity is frequent. It accounts for majority (90 to 95%) of diabetics. It has tripled the past 3 decades due to the obesity epidemic. The third type is Gestational Diabetes, seen among pregnant women. In the USA alone, the estimated cost of the treatment of diabetes is about $174 billion dollar a year.

Are there environmental factors that cause Diabetes?

Yes. Viruses (german measles, mumps, coxsackie B) may incite the development of autoimmune destruction of the beta cells in the pancreas. Exposure to cow's milk rather than maternal milk during infancy (where the albumin from cow's milk may cross-react with islet protein) have been postulated to be a factor in the causation of diabetes too. Geographic location appears to play a role as the incidence of type 1 diabetes is alarmingly high in Sardinia and Finland, compared to the rest of the world.

Is type 2 diabetes also genetic in origin?

Genetics also play a role in the etiology of type 2 diabetes, but lifestyle is a bigger factor. This type of diabetes tends to run in families, and genetics can increase the tendency. However, type 2 diabetes is largely a disease of overeating, obesity and lack of exercise. In spite of the genetic predisposition, type 2 diabetes can be prevented by an effective diet, weight loss, and exercise program under a physician's supervision.

Can pregnancy cause diabetes?

Yes, but fortunately not every pregnancy leads to diabetes mellitus. When it occurs, it is called gestational diabetes and develops more than halfway through pregnancy. At about the 24th week, the placenta starts to produce hormones that increase insulin resistance for the duration of the pregnancy. If the insulin resistance becomes severe enough, the woman develop gestational diabetes. As in type 2 diabetes, obesity and age over 30 are key factors for Gestational Diabetes.

When should pregnant women be tested for diabetes?

Prenatal care is very essential. All women, starting from the 24th week of pregnancy, should be tested for insulin resistance and gestational diabetes. Those who are at a higher risk of this condition should be tested earlier, even at 16 weeks, and, if negative, should be retested in 24 to 28 weeks. In the United States, Diabetes complicates about 4% of pregnancies, with gestational diabetes accounting for 88%, or an estimated 135,000 pregnancies a year. Diet is the cornerstone in the treatment of gestational diabetes. An estimated 75 to 90 percent can be managed successfully with diet and exercise. If untreated or not properly treated, this could lead to birth defects. This is the reason why it is prudent for all pregnant women to have a regular prenatal checkup, which will include the above mentioned tests.

What are the signs and symptoms of diabetes?

Persons with diabetes usually have excessive thirst and hunger. There is also frequent and excessive urination and weight loss. The blood sugar is elevated and abnormal amount of sugar is found in the urine.

What is the treatment for diabetes?

For type 2 diabetics, who are still able to produce some insulin, although not enough, oral medications are usually effective in controlling blood sugar level. Today, there are many superior oral drugs to manage diabetes compared to a decade ago. Your physician will prescribe the best one suitable to you. Sometimes, the addition of, or switching to, insulin may be needed to control your blood sugar level. This is the reason why management of this condition requires constant medical supervision.

What is an insulin pump?

The state-of-the-art method of administering insulin to insulin-dependent diabetic patients is by the use of an implantable insulin pump. The small device is implanted under the skin, and the catheter connected to it is inserted into a vein. The computerized pump contains insulin in its chamber and delivers a precise dose of insulin at a preset time schedule. The insulin chamber is refillable. This pump replaces the needle injection as a method of giving insulin.

How about cell transplant?

Experimental works on embryonic stem cell transplant to help type 1 diabetes are showing great promise, but progress here is being hampered by the controversy over stem cell research.

What about gila monsters' saliva?

The exendin-4 hormone has been isolated from the saliva of the poisonous gila monster (lizard), which eats only a few times a year and basically turning off its pancreas the rest of the time. When the rare mealtime comes, exendin-4 wakes up the hibernating pancreas to start secreting insulin, which controls its blood sugar during the binge. This hormone, now manufactured synthetically by Amylin Pharmaceutical and Eli Lilly and Company, under the name *exanatide,* which is for type 2 diabetes, has shown encouraging results on clinical trials.

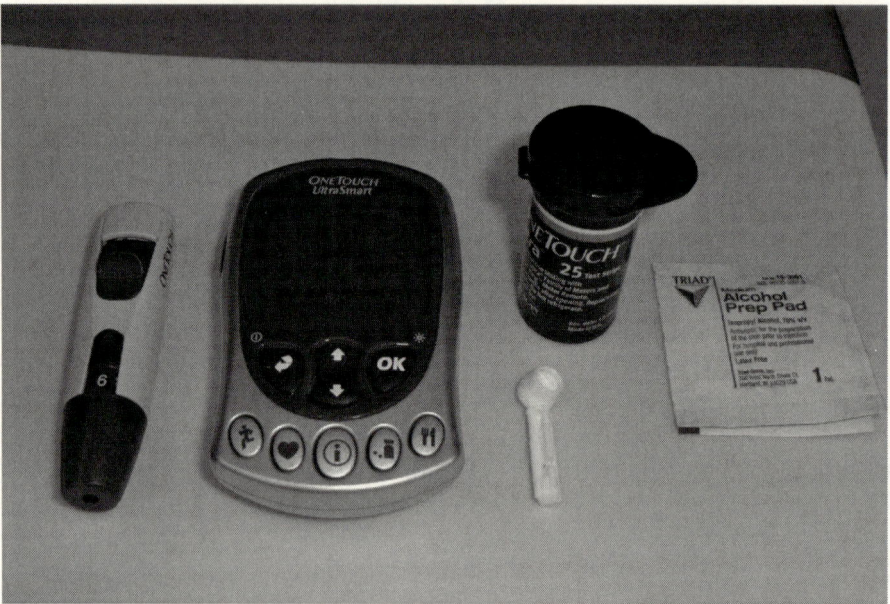

For diabetics, monitoring blood glucose with the use of a glucometer as directed by the physician can help manage the condition more safely.

Diet and Health Myths

Myth: Its all in the genes. There's no need to diet.

Fact: While heredity plays a vital role in our body's metabolism, the environmental factors are equally, and in some cases, more important than our genetic makeup. So it is not totally hopeless for those who are overweight. Done properly under a well-established and scientific regimen, dieting could do wonders.

Myth: I can eat all I want. My young body can take care of it.

Fact: Hardening of the artery, a major cause of hypertension (high blood pressure), heart attack, and stroke starts to develop in young children as early as 5 years of age, or even earlier. Eating a lot of foods high in fats and cholesterol (like eggs, dairy products, red meats (pork, beef, etc.) and foods made of these will lead to hypercholesterolemia and/or hypertriglyceridemia that thicken blood and cause plaques (calcium deposits) on the inner walls of the arteries all over our body. This will reduce the caliber (inner diameter) of the artery and eventually clogs up and deprive tissues and organs (heart, brain, kidneys, etc.) of the much-needed blood, oxygen, and nutrition.

Myth: Heart attack and stroke happen only to old people.

Fact: Statistics show that heart attack and stroke, and even sudden cardiac death, could happen to men and women younger than 30. The youngest patient I did heart bypass on was a 28-year-old female, who had high blood pressure, diabetes, and high blood cholesterol and triglycerides.

Myth: High cholesterol/triglycerides levels are due to hereditary traits.

Fact: Actually, only one and 500 people who have familial hypercholesterolemia are familial or hereditary (inherited from their parents). While that particular individual has the "excuse" to have high levels of cholesterol, the 499 of us do not. And since many of us have hypercholesterolemia, it only means we are abusing our body and our health. This is from the high-fat, high-cholesterol food we shove down our foodpipe.

Myth: Heart attack and stroke are part of our fate, our destiny.

Fact: This is untrue and a misguided way of thinking. This hopeless acceptance is unhealthy in itself and contrary to the mountains of scientific data and proofs we have today, to show that heart attack and stroke, and even high blood pressure and diabetes, are preventable illnesses.

Myth: Not eating carbohydrate is a healthy way to control weight.

Fact: While totally eliminating carbohydrates (rice, bread, pop beverages, cakes, candies, ice cream, desserts, etc.) will lead to weight loss, it is not the healthy way of controlling weight. Our body needs some carbohydrates, about 100 grams a day. It is when we eat this in excess that is bad, not only for our weight but for our heart, etc. The right way is to minimize or avoid refined carbohydrates that are nothing but sugar (like the list of food items listed above). Instead, it is best to eat carbs like whole grains, nuts, fruits, and vegetables. And brown (red) rice and wheat bread are healthier to eat than white rice and flour bread. These last six items can also minimize the risk of colon cancer, besides heart attack and stroke.

Myth: Diet foods on the market are safe for weight control.

Fact: Most diet foods being marketed are not really necessary for weight control. Some of them may even be downright dangerous, with side effects, etc. Not to mention the fact that they are as much as 200% more costly than regular food items. Many of them have trans fat and sugar that are not healthy. The best, safest, and cheapest a way to control your weight is by controlling the amount of food (calories) and quality of food you eat. Weigh daily, and adjust the amount of food intake until your desired weight is achieved. Daily exercises will help a lot, not only for weight control, but for maintaining a healthy body and mind.

Myth: All fats are the same

Fact: Like not all carbohydrates are the same as pointed out above, not all fats are the same. Healthy fats are monosaturated fats (found in olive oil, nuts, avocados) and polyunsaturated fats (in safflower-canola-oils, soybean, vegetables). They help ward off cardiovascular diseases, besides weight control, when used in conjunction with other healthy lifestyle practices (proper diet, no smoking, daily exercises, minimizing alcohol, managing stress and relaxation). Saturated fats (red meats, eggs, etc.) and trans fat (as shown on the labels of many food products), on the other hand, are bad for us, and have been linked to heart attack, stroke, and even cancer. Simply replacing as little as 30 calories of carbs a day with the same amount of trans fats practically doubled the risk of heart disease. On the other hand, replacing the same ratio of carbohydrates with polyunsaturated or monounsaturated fats reduced the risk of heart disease by as much as 30% to 40%.

Persistent Diet Myths

In today's health-oriented world, the four major players—diet, exercise, smoking, and alcohol abuse—are in the spotlight. Diet weighs heavily in this equation and has also been a subject of a lot of pervasive myths and misinformation. Today, we shall review some of the most popular misconception about diet.

Fasting is the best way to start

Fasting is the wrong way to start, or even punctuate, your dieting schedule. Fasting has no place at all in controlling weight or quality of nutrition for our body. The temporary weight loss resulting from fasting is thru water loss (dehydration). The best way to maintain your weight is to burn the calories your take in daily (example: if you take in 2,000 calories, you should exercise off 2,000 calories that day). It is a matter of intake and output, an obvious common-sense approach. If one is overweight and wants to lose weight, then the calories burned should be higher than the calories ingested, until the goal is reached. And at that point, the maintenance intake and output formula should prevail. Those who want to gain weight to reach the ideal weight, obviously, should have more intake than output of calories.

Low-carb, high-protein diet is best

Not true. Those on low-carbohydrate diet alone, but on high protein (meats, eggs, etc.) had good initial weight loss, but regained the weight after six to 12 months, as shown by some studies. They fared better than those on low-fat diet, which is actually more healthy as far as cardiovascular diseases, metabolic illnesses, and cancers are concerned. However, low-carb diet combined with low-fat diet and exercise has been found to be the best regimen. This means the diet mainly consists of fish and bean curd, beans, grains, and nuts (as the main source of protein and oil) and a lot of green leafy and other vegetables and fruits. Among diabetics, fruits should be included in the calculation of the total daily restricted calorie intake.

Eating late at night leads to more weight gain and fats

This is no more true than the myth that Elvis Presley is alive. Of course, it is best not to have a full stomach close to bedtime. Going to bed 3 to 4 hours after a meal is fine. The calories taken at night have the same effect as those taken during the daytime. While you burn less calories while sleeping, you lose these when you get up in the morning and start your daily routine, especially if you exercise every day.

Slimming tea works

This is a myth. Slimming tea or other drinks that are advertised as effective for weight reduction, are per se, useless and a waste of money. Any beverage, so long as they are zero-calorie drinks, can help in weight reduction, if taken in lieu of a ton of calories. And I repeat, in lieu of. Not together with thousands of calories. If you drink them and still eat more calories than you burn, then you will gain weight, regardless of what fluid you drink. There is absolutely *no* beverage on the market that will lead to weight reduction, per se. There is no easy solution to being overweight; it takes education, discipline, determination, and hard work. But the dividends are worth the sacrifices.

Drinking a lot of water leads to weight gain

Only if you heart or kidney is not healthy. Heart or kidney failure patients tend to retain water, so water restriction is part of the treatment among many of them. However, for someone who is otherwise healthy except for excess body weight, drinking two glasses of water before each meal is a great strategy in appetite and calorie control (it fools the brain into thinking the stomach is already full), which reduces the food intake, and, subsequently, the weight. The recommended fluid intake is at least 8 glasses of water a day. However, if the beverage ingested is loaded with a lot of calories (like regular cola drinks, fruit drinks, smoothies, etc.), then rapid weight gain results. Fruit juices (fresh fruits are better than the juice) should be limited to 4 oz a day since it has a high concentration of added sugar. Sugar-loaded pop beverages are among the top culprits in the calorie explosion of today and should be avoided. Purified water is the healthier and cheaper universal beverage for all seasons.

Eating grapefruit will help burn body fats

A caveat to remember: there is no food known to man today that can burn or "melt" body fats or that can reduce weight without proper dieting. Eating grapefruit is good, if done (again) in lieu of eating tons of calories. Grapefruits, like many fruits and vegetables, are loaded with good antioxidants that protect our body from the ravages caused by free radicals. So eating them daily is healthy for us, but for fat and weight reduction, the only guaranteed formula is our basic common sense principle: output must be equal to intake (calories taken in = calories burned) in order to maintain a certain weight. And you can extrapolate from there to suit your personal goal.

DNA: Who Is the Daddy?

What does DNA stand for?

DNA stands for deoxyribonucleic acid, the "substance" that is analyzed in the state-of-the-art test to determine paternity and, in other cases, maternity. The genetic information or "genetic code" of a person is carried in the DNA of the chromosomes and mitochondria. An individual's genetic composition is called genome and is established at conception. We have 100,000 genes encoded by 3 billion chemical pairs in our DNA. Each person is, indeed, an individual, with a unique genome.

How accurate is DNA testing?

Like fingerprints, DNA is very accurate. If nine ministrands of DNA coding match the suspect's, odds are billion to 1 that the suspect is "the one." The test is useful not only in determining paternity but in murder, rape, and other cases. In the news all over the world in 1998 was the semen stain on Monica Lewinsky's dress, which matched the DNA from a blood sample taken from President Clinton, which discovery ultimately forced him to admit his famous "inappropriate relations" with Monica.

When was DNA fingerprinting developed?

DNA was discovered in 1953. In 1984, Alec Jeffreys of the University of Leicester in Britain invented "genetic fingerprinting" to identify individuals, using unique sequences of DNA. It was a year later when this test was first used in a criminal investigation. The National Center for Human Genome Research of the United States was created to oversee the 3-billion-dollar project to map and sequence all human DNA by year 2005. In 1990, the formal launching of the International

Human Genome Project was done. Two years later, the US Army started collecting blood and tissue samples from all new recruits as a part of a "genetic dog tag" program to better identify soldiers killed in combat.

How far along is the technology?

In the fall of 1998, the power of DNA technology catapulted exponentially when the US Federal Bureau of Investigation activated its new Combined DNA Index System, a database that contained gene prints of 250,000 convicted felons and 4,600 DNA samples left at the crime scene of unresolved cases. In England, where genetic databases were in operation since 1995, suspects are routinely screened in this manner, and they have more than 360,000 gene prints online. Police remove the profile from the record when the suspect is cleared. Each week in Britain 500 matches are made between specimen taken at crime scenes and the database entries, and police claims a 70% success rate in cracking crimes. In the United States, more than 200 outstanding cases have been solved by DNA typing.

How does DNA benefit the convicted person?

DNA testing does not help only the people investigating crimes, but also the "innocent" but convicted persons. At least 75-death row inmates in the United States have been saved from execution when their convictions were overturned. Ten of these reversals came on the basis of new DNA evidence. DNA typing was partly responsible for the increase in the number of fathers acknowledging paternity to triple from 512,000 in 1992 to 1.5 million in 1998. In about a third of welfare cases and another 10% of other cases, it was conclusively proven that the man named by the mother (who was asking for financial support) turned out not to be the biological father.

What is store for DNA testing?

The use of DNA fingerprinting is limited only by the imagination. It is now predicted that within a decade, investigators may be able to use DNA information to draw a sort of genetic police sketch of a suspect's appearance, including race, facial shape, build, etc., and expedite the conviction of criminals.

How long does the DNA specimen last?

Accurate DNA testing has been done on mummies in ancient Egyptian tombs. Last year, DNA testing proved that U. S. president Thomas Jefferson had a child with one of his slaves, Sally Hemings, settling an age-old historical dispute. Obviously, the specimen lasts "forever."

How is the specimen collected for DNA testing?

Taking blood samples used to be the only method of collecting specimen for DNA typing. Today, obtaining the specimen (smear) from a buccal (inner cheek, mouth) swab has been found to be as accurate as blood. Public commercial DNA-typing laboratories all over the world use this simple buccal swab method, although blood is still being used in some centers.

How much does each test cost?

Commercial Laboratories in the United States charge about $450 to $600 per DNA typing, and the result is ready in 2-3 weeks. For an added fee, the result could be obtained within 72 hours. In the past 10 years, DNA-based paternity testing has more than tripled to about 247,000 cases.

In what other situations has DNA typing helped?

In resolving inheritance disputes, babies switched in maternity wards, determining recent or historical claims on ancestry or lineage, identification of human remains, resolving criminal cases, etc.

After a negative DNA paternity test, then what?

Heartbreaking stories associated with DNA testing are common. One such account was that of a recently divorced man, who, after 15 years, found out through DNA typing that the teenage son he thought was his was actually not fathered by him. He broke down and cried. Later, after he regained his composure, he told his lawyer, "I cannot throw this boy out of my life on account of a laboratory test result. I have loved and cared for him for 14 years as a father, and DNA typing cannot and will not change all that." Indeed, parenthood is more than just a biological linkage of sperm fertilizing an ovum or a womb carrying the fetus. It is the selfless love and unceasing moments of caring over time that makes a man a father and a woman a mother. The great advances in science and medical technology, as always, should be tempered with good ethics and moral values, justice, compassion, and above all, love and wisdom.

Dog Diagnostician?

Highly skilled explosive—or drug-sniffing dogs are fairly common and in great demand these days, thanks to Osama bin Ladin. But what's equally, or perhaps, more interesting is the dog's ability to learn how to detect diseases, like cancer of the lungs or breasts, simply by using its nose. Even more amazing is the degree of accuracy of "their diagnosis," which ranges up to 99 for lung cancer, 88 for breast cancer.

Trained dogs can also detect skin cancer called melanoma, prostate cancer, termites, fertile cows, and dead bodies buried really deep. In 1999, a UK scientific study was published, reporting the ability of dogs to detect seizures among their owners 15 to 45 minutes before the convulsion occurred.

Physicians undergo at least 18 years of schooling and often use diagnostic tools to make a definitive medical diagnosis, but all the dog need is its nose and, perhaps, a commendation pat on the head. No stethoscope. No X-ray. No CT scan. Just a supersensor nose. (Incidentally, in Africa, trained rats are used to detect tuberculosis.)

The olfactory lobe (sense of smell center in the brain) in dogs is about 4 times greater than in humans, where it is rudimentary. They also have 20 to 40 times more receptors ("detectors") in their nasal (nose) cavity than humans, so a dog's sense of smell is that much more powerful and acute. Dogs can detect differences in the concentration of individual odors, with their highly attuned sense of smell. They are like the ultrasensitive "breath analyzer" gadgets commonly used by police to detect the level of alcohol in the body of drivers suspected of DUI (driving under the influence).

Actually, medical students and residents are trained to use all their senses, including the sense of smell in working up patients and making diagnosis. The older physicians of the past centuries were more astute in the art. In the 1988 Academy Award Best Picture, *The Last Emperor*, for instance, the "nurse" caretaker smelled every bowel movement of the 3-year-old Emperor Aisin-Gioro "Henry" Pu Yi to detect any abnormality or illness. More commonly recognized smell or odor indicating an ailment is that of "ammoniacal breath" (uremic fetor) among those with severe kidney disease, in end-stage liver disease, and even in helicobacter pylori gastric ulcer; or there is the typical strong smell of decaying flesh of a gangrenous leg among diabetics or those with blocked leg arteries, which anyone can smell several meters away. But these are the strong and obvious ones our nose can identify.

What the trained dogs can detect effortlessly and almost instantly with a sniff is the "specific scent" of individual illnesses, explosives, drugs we humans cannot even smell at all, much less differentiate them. Dogs are also excruciatingly sensitive at detecting air, particles, and vapor.

All these observations suggest the possible presence of a distinctive biological marker or a subtle chemical scent or vapor in each disease condition. And if that were so, perhaps science can find out how dogs senses or detect the "odor." And from there, we can certainly utilize our modern technology to invent a supersensitive artificial bio-sensor ("sniffer-machine") for these various scents and biological markers for a more expedient detection and diagnosis of diseases.

For more than 12,000 years, dogs have been known to sniff out prey for the hunter. Today, seeing-eye dogs are helping millions "see" and cross the streets. As pets, they also soothe the emotion of menopausal women, sick children, and old people in hospitals and at home. Besides being bomb detectors, drug sensors, escaped-prisoner finders in the K-9 patrol team, dogs are also fast becoming celebrities as medical diagnosticians of late. (Watch out, Doc!)

With these great findings on our best friend's probable additional fabulous acumen, will the doctor's offices, clinics, and hospitals soon be "equipped" with a four-legged "medical assistant"? No, not yet.

The studies are very limited and the reports are preliminary at best. As you read this, hundreds of scientific studies are already ongoing on this particular fascinating subject. This doggy inspiration could lead to great advances in medical science and technology in the future, which will be a great boon to better patient care.

In the meantime, our most loyal canine pet will continue to remain as our best friend, house guard, and protector. And, of course, still the happiest and most eager greeter who celebrates our homecoming each day.

Warning: Drug Resistant TB

One of the easiest to catch infectious diseases is pulmonary tuberculosis. And most often than not, people get infected without even knowing they have it and who and where they got it from. The so-called open lesion and infectious tuberculosis could be spread in public places, especially crowded areas, movies, sports arenas, schools, congested stores, practically from any place at all. Doorknobs, stair or escalator handrails, any top surface of furniture or counters touched by a person with infectious TB could be a mode to transmission, besides inhaling thru his breath or by kissing, sharing food utensils, or even any object touched and contaminated by someone who is in the infectious stage.

Pulmonary tuberculosis, popularly known as TB, which used to kill millions and millions of people around the world before treatment was discovered, acting like a form of cancer that spreads from the lungs to the bones, brain, kidneys, liver, spleen, and other organs in the body has now "returned" with a more deadly form: the multiple drug resistant tuberculosis, or MDR.

Cases are almost at an epidemic proportion in the former Soviet Union ("the MDR capital of the world"), and obviously, it poses a potential global problem since it is very contagious and could easily be spread by world travel. Untreated, it is a death sentence; and even if treated, MDR could still be a formidable killer.

A recent WHO report on the regular form of tuberculosis states that this infectious airborne illness affects about 9 million people annually and kills 2 million of them. It is estimated that about 300,000 new MDR cases are diagnosed each year. A prompt and concerted global multilevel (government and the public) response to this imminent catastrophe is needed to prevent a pandemic of MDR because no country is exempt and every country is vulnerable.

What is tuberculosis?

Tuberculosis is a chronic, recurrent, infection caused by *Mycobacterium tuberculosis, M. Bovis,* or *M. Africanum.* In the United States, where tuberculosis was practically under control, there has been a resurgence attributed to immigrant carriers. Many of these cases were also found to be resistant to the conventional multiple drug therapy against TB, hence named MDR. Even the regular TB is still a major global public health problem today.

How is Pulmonary TB transmitted?

Tuberculosis of the lungs is transmitted by inhalation of the M. tuberculosis organism dispersed as droplet nuclei from a person with pulmonary TB whose sputum is positive. The bacteria may float in the air for several hours. Other modes of transmission is by direct hand or mouth (kissing) contact with infected saliva.

The preventive measures are obvious. If one is near a person known to have active TB, one should cover his/her nose and avoid handling items previously touched by the patient, including eating utensils. Doorknobs, stair or escalator handrails, any top surface of furniture or counters touched by a person with infectious TB could be a mode to transmission, or even any object touched and contaminated by someone who is in the infectious stage.

Washing hands following an unavoidable contact is a good practice. If one suspects the possibility of having TB, it is most prudent to consult a physician without delay.

What are the signs and symptoms of PTB?

Some people with pulmonary TB may not have any symptom whatsoever. The first sign could be a bloody sputum, or a chest X-ray finding of TB, or a conversion to "positive" of a previously "negative" tuberculin skin test, or recurrent cough and/or loss of weight. The symptoms could even be so subtle to escape attention.

How much PTB goes unrecognized?

As much as 90% to 95% of primary TB infection go unrecognized. Besides the primary or initial infection, the other stages of PTB are latent or dormant and recrudescent or adult-type TB. The disease may become active after 1 to 2 years after initial infection, but may be delayed for years, even a decade, and activate after the onset of diabetes mellitus, during the period of stress, after steroid treatment, or when the immune system is impaired, like in AIDS.

What are the drugs used for the treatment of PTB?

About 80% of MDR are caused by "super strains" of the bacilli that are resistant to 3 or 4 of the main drugs that are effective for the treatment of the regular strain of tuberculosis. The commonest drugs are: Isoniazid, Rifampin, Streptomycin, Pyrazinamide, Ethambutol, and Capreomycin. These medications have potential side effects that can be serious and therefore should be taken only under the advice and supervision of a physician.

Dying to Look Good

To take the risk of possible death from surgery that is necessary to save life or to maintain or restore health makes intelligent sense. But to die from an elective cosmetic procedure performed for vanity, or for whatever reason, is obviously reckless and foolhardy.

In medicine, one death out of 100,000-300,000 surgeries or, at most, a one-to-two-percent mortality rate from, say, major heart surgery procedures, is considered acceptable and normal range. There are some less major procedures where practically zero death rate is the norm. The death rate from liposuction, which is done primarily for beauty's sake, is about 19 out of 100,000, which is even higher than the mortality rate from car accidents. A recent survey of plastic surgeons in the United States revealed that "compared to other kinds of operations, more people die during liposuction." The death rate for liposuction is indeed alarmingly high and unacceptable.

In 2003, there were 1.8 million patients who underwent major cosmetic surgeries, including face-lifts, nose job, removal of eye bags, breast augmentation, liposuction, tummy tuck, etc. In Florida and a few other states, liposuction and tummy tuck have recently been banned as office procedures (pending results of investigations) in view of the overly high death rates.

However, some people appear to be willing to risk their life to get rid of some extra fat! Dying to look good seems to be a preoccupation among some individuals, not only among those in the show biz. Besides paying a hefty surgical fee for this risky procedure, whose benefit is not lasting or permanent anyway, the risk to life is too high and can never be justified by the sought-after gain, which is transient at best.

In a report published in the *Journal of Plastic and Reconstructive Surgery,* Dr. Frederick Grazer of Penn State University and Dr. Rudolph de Jong of the Thomas Jefferson Medical College "suggest that outpatient elective lipoplasty may not be safe," which is actually putting the issue quite mildly.

Any procedure for cosmetic purposes should have a near-zero mortality. The risk/benefit ratio should be overwhelmingly proportionate, tipping the scale toward the benefit. In other words, it is only logical to expect that the safety and benefit of any procedure should be much greater than the risk. With liposuction, this is not the case. The risk is too high for the potential temporary benefit to be gained. To lose life in the pursuit of losing a few pounds of body fat is senseless. Besides, chances are the fat will "recur," unless one goes on a strict diet and do daily exercises, which healthy regimen alone (if it was done religiously for years before) could have prevented the fat problem in the first place.

What causes the deaths in liposuction?

During the liposuction (which is like vacuuming the fats out), the fat cells are disrupted; and because the fats have veins that normally bring blood back to the pulmonary (lung) circulation, some of the fat cells could embolize (travel) to the lung circulation. Since fats are solid substances, they tend to block the circulation that brings blood to the lungs. A small fat embolus becomes a nidus that grows larger and larger, totally obstructing the blood flow to the lungs. This causes severe lack of oxygen in the blood (akin to choking, where a person could not breathe and unable to get enough oxygen to sustain life), resulting in cardiac arrest. There are also reports of other complications like anesthetic deaths and infection with "flesh-eating" bacteria, causing deaths.

Is fat embolization preventable?

Realistically, there is no absolute way to prevent fat emboli to the lungs in liposuction. This is a natural risk of the procedure, even in the best of hands. Doing the procedure in a hospital setting might be safer than in a doctor's clinic, not in lowering the chances of fat emboli, but in the ability of the surgical team to manage the complication of fat embolism better when it happens, with the more sophisticated facilities available in the hospital (like the presence of cardiac surgery team and heart lung machine, when needed).

How about "tummy tuck?"

Abdominoplasty or "tummy tuck" is another major plastic surgery procedure that is very popular and which has a significant mortality rate. The death rate is one for every 617 procedures (0.16 percent), about the same compared to deaths from hang gliding, 1:600. The risk is higher when combined with liposuction. About 10% of patients undergoing a tummy tuck would need blood transfusion, a hospital stay of about 12.4 days, and a complication rate of between 24% and 65%. The data reported in *Journal of Plastic and Reconstructive Surgery* showed that on the average, only about 55% of patients got good or excellent result and about forty-five percent did not achieve positive results.

Is mortality higher in combined procedures?

In 2002, there were 83,000 abdominoplasty and 373,000 lipoplasty done in the United States. The mortality rate was recorded as 1:47,415 for lipoplasty and 1:2324 for tummy tuck alone. When the two procedures were combined the death rate was 1:3281. The increased in deaths in the combined procedures is definitely significant. The other common cosmetic procedures being performed appear to have low acceptable risks compared to these two.

Is abdominoplasty benefit permanent?

Unfortunately, like in liposuction, the cosmetic benefit from tummy tuck is not permanent, unless the person changes his/her lifestyle as far as dieting and daily exercises are concerned. For those morbidly obese, who have religiously tried dieting and daily exercises and have failed, these two plastic procedures may have a justified medical role. If the patient, following these surgical procedures, continues to eat wantonly and not have adequate daily exercises, the weight gain will obviously continue, together with more fat accumulation in the body. The aesthetic benefit would be gone all too soon, almost as fast as the huge amount of money paid to the surgeon.

Dying to look good, are we?

As our culture and social pressure dictate, we must look our best, especially in public. I admire men and women who are well-groomed. Many girls, with proper and stylish attires, are gorgeous even in their natural self, sans makeup. Appropriate makeup, when applied in good taste, adds to the beauty of any woman. Today, we do have almost everything (nonsurgical) to make us look better. I strongly feel that major risky plastic surgery procedures are indicated only for those who, unfortunately, were born with birth defects that are disfiguring. But I won't be adverse to some cosmetic surgeries, if to be performed at all, that are simple and do not pose a significant risk to health or life. For more complicated cosmetic procedures the consequences could sometimes be costly and devastating.

We Are What We Eat

"We are what we eat" is an old expression and lay wisdom almost as old as civilization. With the sophistication of modern science and technology and our highly educated society, this "primitive" and previously unsubstantiated theory is now a conventional scientific fact. The voluminous medical research and clinical data in our advanced world of the 21st century have proven beyond any doubt that, indeed, we are what we eat.

Obviously, we are talking about how the foods we eat each day relates to, or affects, our health and longevity.

For instance, did you know that a person who eats an egg (or more) a day has a 25% increased risk of death in a 20-year period, compared to those who abstain from eggs and egg products? This was one of the findings of the Harvard's Physicians' Health Study I. For the diabetics who eat eggs, that risk is doubled (50%!). One egg yolk has about 215 milligrams of cholesterol, much more than many other common food items. And of course, eggs are animal proteins with a lot of saturated fats, which ravage our cardiovascular system and cause heart attack and stroke, to mention two ailments.

Animal proteins consumption also leads to a 32% greater risk of infertility among women, with just one serving a day. Those whose diet is mostly loaded with red meats (and eggs, as stated above), with high cholesterol, saturated-fat foods, have a 41% greater risk of ovulatory infertility, compared to those who eat the least animal proteins. Those who ate the highest amount of vegetable proteins had 22% reduction in the risk for infertility.

A diet rich in fruits and vegetables improves the brain functions in children and give them an academic edge over other kids.

Coffee, regular or decaf, four to six cups a day, has been shown to reduce the risk for the development of type 2 diabetes and Alzheimer's disease.

Soft drinks, cola—or uncola, diet or not, have been implicated in the causation of metabolic syndrome, characterized by high blood pressure, diabetes mellitus, heart disease, and possibly stroke. On the other hand, drinking about 8 glasses of filtered water a day helps hydrate the body and flush out toxins from our system.

It is worth repeating that eating processed meat (sausages, hot dogs, luncheon meats, etc.) has been shown to increase the risk of development of pancreatic cancer by almost 70%.

Americans in 2006 ate more than 1.5 billion pounds of hot dogs, an average of 32 pounds per year per person. There is 21% increased in the risk of colorectal cancers for every 50 grams processed meats ingested a day.

While the saturated fat in fresh (no preservative) red meat appears not to be linked to pancreatic cancer in this study, other studies have shown that people who eat red meat regularly have a higher risk for developing cancer of the colon, breast, and other cancers in general, compared to those who minimize eating red meat. Red meat also causes a quick rise in the cholesterol blood level, a condition that increases the risk for the development of high blood pressure, heart attack and stroke. Children are better off staying away from hamburger stores and other fast-food chains.

Today, the market abounds with "food supplements" claiming to be sexual "stimulants" and "libido-enhancing" concoctions and pills, which are actually useless, and may even be harmful.

In contrast to these expensive and ineffective "sex-enhancers" on the market, there are natural foods in the grocery stores, very much less expensive and healthier and safer that could boost libido, sex drive, and performance in both men and women.

Some of these sex "nutrients" from nature's own soil and water, include the following well-known and readily available items in most grocery stores: asparagus, avocado, banana, basil, bee pollen, celery, chili, fig, garlic, goji berry, maca, pumpkin seed, oysters, dark chocolates, soya beans like tofu, chick peas, carrots, cucumber, eggplants and other "phallic" vegetables and fruits, ginseng roots, and daily multivitamins and minerals.

Fish (rich in omega-3 fatty acids), fruits, and vegetables, in general, are essential parts of a healthy lifestyle, together with daily exercises. On the other hand, fried and rich foods, red meats, and other high-cholesterol and fatty foods increase our risk for developing cardiovascular diseases and cancer. Processed foods have also been linked to frigidity in women and diminished sexual stamina in men. Cigarettes, which cause cancer of the lungs and emphysema, also constrict the arteries, which reduces blood flow to our organs and diminishes libido.

Bee pollen, whose role is to help fertilize is supposed to boost the sperm count, and celery is purportedly a stimulator of the production of androsterone, an odorless "aphrodisiac" found in male perspiration. Chili is said to release endorphins, the "feel-good" hormone. Garlic has a high level of allicin, a substance which opens up small arteries and improve blood flow to various organs. Goji berries, which are good for those with arthritis, are dubbed as a "sexual tonic" also that is said to "increase testosterone, libido, youthfulness, and stamina." Maca has been reported to have the ability to increase testosterone and sperm count.

Pumpkin seed, which is a health food, has zinc, which is important in testosterone production. It is also a source of omega-3 fatty acids that is good our cardiovascular health. As reported in this column last week, the delicious and decadent chocolates, especially the dark ones, are great antioxidants and contain phenylalanine, an amino acid that increases endorphins in the body, a potent antidepressant, a hormone that provides a great sense of "high" and overall well-being, naturally and safely.

We have great choices and great trade-offs, depending on our philosophy of health, life, and longevity. Indeed, we are what we eat and how we behave. Our lifestyle and future significantly depend on our choices today. Health is really not a matter of luck but a matter of wisdom and of choice.

Eating Disorders

What is anorexia nervosa?

This is a "psychological" disorder where the person has a disturbed sense of body image. He/she has a morbid fear of obesity, refuses to maintain a minimally normal body weight, and has, in women, amenorrhea (absence of menstrual period).

What causes this condition?

The cause is still unknown, but it appears that social factors play a big role. In the Western society, there is a pervasive obsession among people, especially among the young females, to stay thin. Obesity is looked at as unhealthy, undesirable, and unattractive. Roughly about 85% of prepubertal children are conscious of these attitudes, and more than 50% of these children go on a diet themselves or practice habits to control their weight. But since not many of them develop anorexia nervosa, it is obvious that there are other factors that play significant roles.

What other factors could be involved?

Some undefined psychologic, genetic, or metabolic vulnerability might predispose some persons to develop anorexia nervosa. It is interesting to note that anorexia nervosa is most rare among the deprived sectors of the world, where there is food shortage.

Does peer pressure play a role?

Peer pressure and a sense of competition, especially among young girls, could play a role. The only chubby one in a circle of friends might feel uncomfortable and under stress to be "as shapely as all my friends."

The psychological impact of this could lead to misguided and unhealthy practice in dieting and weight control, more likely to happen among those with weaker personality and character.

Are females more prone?

Yes, roughly 95% of patients with anorexia nervosa are female. The usual onset is mostly during adolescence, much less often among adults. Majority of these people are in the middle to upper socioeconomic classes.

What are the symptoms of anorexia nervosa?

The manifestations could be mild and temporary, others severe and chronic. The classic victims are usually intelligent, high achievers, compulsive, meticulous, very conscious of how they look, and success-driven. The initial indication is their extreme concern about their weight (even if their weight is normal) and their religious diet control practices. They study diets, measure everything, and count every calorie consumed. There is an extreme anxiety and anger with any increase in weight, disproportional to the situation. There is lying and denial about what is going on and a great resistance to seeking medical treatment.

What is the treatment for this illness?

The two-phase management consists of short-term regimen to restore body weight and prevent death, followed by long-term treatment to cure the psychological dilemma and prevent relapses. In severe cases, hospitalization may be required or even crucial for survival. Individual psychotherapy, psychodynamic, cognitive, behavioral—and even family—therapy are essential. Some oral medications have been used after the weight loss has been regained.

How does bulemia differ from anorexia?

Bulemia is an uncontrollable and recurrent binge eating (2-3 times a week) where the individual consumes an enormous amount of food followed by remedial efforts to avoid weight gain, such as self-induced vomiting, vigorous exercises or fasting, use of diuretics and/or laxatives.

Only about 50% of anorexia nervosa patients have bulimia. The other half simply eat very little or not at all for fear of gaining weight. About 2% of young women have bulimia of varying severity. Bulemic patients have wide variation in their body weight. Because they frequently induce vomiting after binge eating, they have swollen parotid glands, scars on their knuckles and fingers, and dental erosion. Bulemic patients usually have normal weight and more revealing of their problem and more likely to seek medical care, compared to anorexia patients.

What is the treatment for bulemia?

Psychotherapy and use of antidepressant drugs are the mainstay of the therapy for bulimia. Experts now believe that the combination of cognitive-behavioral psychotherapy and antidepressants is the treatment of choice. While antidepressants and diet suppressants help a lot, psychotherapy is more effective with more lasting results. The patient should be under the care of a specialist in diet disorders and a psychiatrist.

Any preventive measures?

Family and friends can help minimize the development of these eating disorders by showering our children often with love and reassuring words as they grow up. This will reduce the social and environmental stress on these young individuals, making them feel loved, secure, and accepted. As they grow, children must learn that inner beauty and character are more attractive and more important than physical appearances. That while having a nicely shaped body is great, having a beautiful personality, good character, and brains is more admired and adored in today's society.

Egg Salmonella Outbreak

If you eat raw eggs, as a "health shake" with juices or as a cocktail mixed with alcoholic drink, or prefer them runny or sunny-side up, please read on about this important historical incident.

There was serious salmonella outbreak involving contaminated eggs in the United States; and the recall involved many states, including Iowa, Arkansas, Arizona, California, Colorado, Illinois, Georgia, Minnesota, Nebraska, Nevada, North Carolina, Oklahoma, Oregon, Texas, Utah, Washington, and Wisconsin.

The alert and egg recall started August 13, 2010, which resulted in more than 380 million eggs being recalled, according to the Centers for Disease Control and Prevention, which was working with the state health department. The initial recall was 228 million eggs (19 million dozen-egg cartons) by the company Wright County Eggs of Galt, Iowa.

The eggs were packaged under the labels Albertson, Boomsma's, Ducth Farms and Kemp, Farm Fresh, Hillandale, Lucerne, Lund, Mountain Dairy, Ralph's, Shoreland, Sunshine, and Trafficanda.

Some of the salmonella poisoning were in salad, pies, and puddings, besides fried (sunny-side up) or undercooked eggs. This salmonella bug could be in eggs from healthy-appearing chickens.

The commonest symptoms include abdominal cramps, diarrhea, and fever within 8-72 hours of eating the contaminated egg/egg products. In children, seniors, and persons with compromised immune system, the poisoning risk could include death.

If in doubts, dump them. Although this salmonella egg outbreak is in the United States, it is prudent for everyone, anywhere, to stay away from raw eggs, sunny side-up fried eggs, and egg salad that is more than 4 hours old. Fried egg is safer from contamination when it is hard-boiled, fried scrambled, or fried over hard (not over easy), making sure the yolk (yellow part) is fully cooked.

The Truth about Eggs

In this more health-conscious era, egg, a very popular standard items in most any breakfast around the world, has been a controversial food item because of its high cholesterol content.

Clinical reviews in various medical journals around the world the past five decades have pointed out the danger of dietary cholesterol for those at risk of developing cardiovascular diseases, like heart attack and stroke, metabolic illness such as diabetes, and even cancer. Most of these studies have considered the egg yolk as the worst offender when it comes to cholesterol.

Depending on the size of the egg, it could contain between 125 and 275 mg of cholesterol in its egg yolk. The recommended daily limit for cholesterol intake is 200 mg per day. So eating two eggs a day will more than exceed the limit by at least 25%. And since other foods we eat also contain cholesterol, it is easy to see that adding even one egg a day to our diet will greatly increase our cholesterol intake.

However, it is not cholesterol in the egg yolk per se that is harmful. It is the oxidized cholesterol that is atherogenic (causes hardening of the artery and eventual blockage in the circulation to the heart, brain, abdominal organs, or legs). Oxidation of cholesterol in eggs can be minimized by using less heat in the cooking process. Liquidy soft-boiled egg appears to be healthier than hard boiled or fried eggs in any style. When fried, eggs obviously provide higher level of oxidized cholesterol.

Other highly atherogenic food items include saturated fats from milk products, especially butter. Most butter substitutes, margarines, have hydrogenated vegetables oils, which produce unhealthy trans-fatty acids and are very atherogenic like saturated fats. Reading all food labels is a wise practice.

Margarines without trans-fatty acids are available in large grocery stores. While vegetable oils contain N6 fatty acids, fish oil (from salmon, mackerel, nonalbacore tuna, etc., or fish oil capsules) contains the healthy N3 fatty acids (omega-3), which are potent antioxidants, antiinflammatory, anticlot, and effective in lowering triglyceride, bad cholesterol, and blood pressure, and in preventing irregularity of the heartbeat. They slow down arteriosclerosis (hardening of the arteries) and thus, the aging process of the cells in our body.

A corroborative review of several studies involving hundreds of thousands of cases was done by Dr. David Spence, stroke prevention expert at the University of Western Ontario; Dr. David Jenkins, nutrition expert of the Risk Factor Modification Centre at St. Michael's Hospital in Toronto; and Dr. Jean Davignon, cholesterol expert of the Clinique de nutrition métabolisme et athérosclérose in Montreal, according to *The Medical News Today*.

"We wanted to put cholesterol into perspective as there's been a widespread misconception developing among the Canadian public and even physicians, that consumption of dietary cholesterol and egg yolks is harmless," says Dr. Spence, a professor and scientist at the Schulich School of Medicine and Dentistry, Robarts Research Institute. "Much of this has to do with effective egg marketing."

While two of those large studies reported no harm from egg consumption among healthy people, the authors stated that "in both studies, those who developed diabetes while consuming an egg a day doubled their risk of cardiovascular disease compared to those eating less than an egg a week . . . the studies also showed a significant increase of new onset diabetes with regular egg consumption."

The UWO researchers concluded, "There is no question that egg white is classed as a valuable source of high-quality protein. Egg yolks, however, are not something that should be eaten indiscriminately by adults without regard to their global cardiovascular risk, genetic predisposition to heart attacks and overall food habits."

Knowing some people who ate eggs daily all their life and not getting a heart attack or stroke is just anecdotal and a hardly scientific fact to prove eggs are safe for everybody over the long run. Due to variance in our genetic make-up, most of us, statistically, will be adversely affected by the high cholesterol and saturated fats in egg yolks, if eaten daily.

Egg white (egg minus its yellow yolk) is a highly nutritious source of protein in itself. The yummy but unhealthy egg yolk is not really an essential food item and actually deleterious to those who are at risk of cardiovascular, metabolic, or cancer disorders.

If only science could identify individuals who are at risk of developing high blood pressure, diabetes, heart attack, stroke, cancer, and a host of other diseases when they eat fatty foods, smoke cigarettes, drink alcoholic beverage in excess, and not exercise, then we would know who, among us may safely consume high cholesterol foods, be sedentary, smoke like a chimney, and/or drink alcohol to our heart's content the rest of our life and still be free from serious diseases.

Unfortunately, we still do not have a practical medical test to address this issue. Therefore, it behooves all of us to be wise and prudent, and indulge in moderation, since we've got only one body, one life, no spare, no backup.

Eight Don'ts after a Meal

There are many myths floating around concerning various subjects. Some of them are about what *not* to do after a meal. These were emailed to me by a friend for scientific verification. Myths are obviously the fruit of partial or total ignorance and speculations handed down from generation to generation. While many of them are totally false, some of them are true or partly true. Here are eight of them:

1. "Don't smoke after a meal because the bad effect (emphysema, cancer, etc.) of smoking a cigarette becomes ten times worse."

This is true in the sense that the natural bodily absorption rate following a meal is heightened, magnifying the ill-effects of tobacco (nicotine) on our system. One stick of cigarette, like one drop of any poison, is one too many.

2. "Don't eat fruits immediately after a meal because this will cause the stomach to bloat with air."

This is not true. Fruits improve our digestion. However, there are people who have some degree of intolerance to fruits (fructose intolerance), who will have the sense of bloating after ingestion of fruits. In general, eating fruits right after a meal is good and well-tolerated by the body. Diabetics should discuss this with their physician since fruits will be additional calories that must be taken into account when computing their "diabetic diet."

3. "Don't drink tea after a meal because tea is high in acid which will harden the protein and make it difficult to digest."

It is true that tea is high in tannin or tannic acid, but the rest of the statement is false. Tea, as a matter of fact, improves our digestion. It is a tonic that invigorates the brain, speeds up the circulation, and makes the stomach digest food easier.

4. "Don't loosen your belt after a meal because this will cause your intestines to twist and get blocked up."

The first part of the statement is a sound advice, but not for the reason given. Not loosening your belt after a meal makes you more conscious that your stomach is full enough, so you do not overeat. Also, the "normal tightness" of the belt provides one a natural "suck-in-the-abdomen technic" of controlling your waistline. It has been shown that sucking in the abdomen (as in the required military posture among cadets, etc.) does help prevent "bulging waistlines," since sucking in the belly is nothing but an exercise to contract the muscles of the abdomen. If one does it every moment of awareness, that is like exercising the bad muscles every few minutes to make them taut and firm. The part about intestinal twisting and obstruction is false.

5. "Don't bathe after a meal because this will weaken digestion."

While taking a bath (especially a warm one) will divert some blood from the stomach to the skin, taking a bath after a meal will not significantly impair digestion. The general rule is: after a meal, do not to do strenuous activities that will divert a lot of the blood away from the stomach, which needs "enough" blood for digestion. What's enough for one person may be different from another individual's physiologic need.

6. "Don't walk after a meal. The digestive system will be unable to absorb the food."

Walking or strolling after a meal is not bad at all. It will help burn up some calories without significantly diverting blood from the stomach. Only strenuous physical and mental activities are discouraged immediately after a meal.

7. "Don't sleep immediately after a meal because food will not be digested properly, and this will lead to gastric infection."

The first part is true: it is not healthy to sleep with a full stomach. Not that it will cause pancreatitis (as another myth claims), but gastric distention can lead to some heart irregularity in some people. Habitually sleeping immediately after a meal will also increase the tendency to obesity. As far as gastric infection is concerned, that claim is false.

8. "Don't eat again until after four hours or longer because this will make the stomach stretch and grow larger."

This is not a myth but a sage advice. The stomach grows larger the more often we eat and the more food we eat, stretching our stomach, and conditioning our brain to crave for more food with every meal. And this will inevitably lead to obesity and its dangerous implications and complications. Drinking a tall glass, or two, of water before each meal will distend the stomach somewhat and "fool" the brain and curb the hunger sooner, leading to less total caloric intake. A simple, cheap, and great dieting strategy.

Scary Electronic Fraud

The mind-boggling advances in wireless technology has ushered in great wonders to the world. Like any good discoveries that are benefiting humanity as a whole, some of these inventions, in the hands of crooks, could be used to victimize unsuspecting people. The criminal act could be so subtle and surreptitious that unless we are aware of the possibility of such a covert strategy, we won't even know what hit us till much too late.

Did you know that thieves can now buy an $8 RFID (radio-frequency ID) reader and steal your credit card or passport data without you even knowing it? If you have credit cards or passport with RFID, all the perpetrator has to do is to come very close to you, holding his RFID reader almost touching your purse or wallet, and bingo! All your credit card and/or passport data are instantaneously transferred to their laptop computer or possibly to their android or 4G cell phone.

The RFID reader is similar to the bar code scanners used in store checkout counters or at airport gates to scan boarding passes.

Criminals no longer have to steal your wallet or run away with ladies' purses. The thieves are now high tech and sophisticated. They now steal by electronic pickpocketing. The victims only discover what happened when they receive their credit card statement from their bank or a notice from the government that someone tried to use their passport.

For the past year or so, I have been locking and unlocking my car manually, either with my key or the keypad on the hand console by the door. I no longer use my remote control to lock or unlock my car. There is an electronic gadget available that could be used to "copy" the electronic impulse or sound wave from a remote control key as it is clicked in a parking area. The person with the gadget could be several yards away or in a car nearby. Once you have left the vicinity, the thief can easily unlock and steal items you left in your car and your car stereo. Worst, the person could hide behind your seat and surprise you.

Another sensor criminals use is one that could detect the electronic wave when you click your handheld garage door opener. This will give them access to your home.

ATM skimming is popular fraud. There was a time when thieves simply attached a small camera by the ATM units to videotape credit card data, including the PIN. Today, they want a much larger loot, so they get data from dozens of credit cards and consolidate them to be able to make much larger withdrawals.

Only about 30% to 40% of credit cards have RFID chip in them, and those without the chip are obviously safe from RFID readers. To be sure, check with your issuing bank.

One way to disable the RFID chip and still be able to use your card is to look for the RFID chip by putting your card against a bright lamp and puncture a hole thru it, with a large nail and a hammer or a drill. But it would be better to get a credit card without an RFID chip.

What I have done to protect my credit cards, driver's license, and passport was to improvise. It is easy to do. Get two business cards or cut two pieces of cardboard no thicker than your credit card. Put the two pieces end to end, with 1/4 of an inch space between them, on top of a foot of aluminum foil. Roll-wrap them "as one" in 3 layers of aluminum foil all around them, providing six layers of protection on either side. The credit cards and driver's license will be sandwiched between these two when they are put back in the wallet or purse. Do the same for the passport. Simple, practically free, and effective.

There are now vendors selling RFID protector sleeves or wallets on the Internet. Some of them use aluminum foil, others, thin metals, like stainless steel sheets. The government and banks are now well aware of electronic fraud and are finding ways to foil crooks. Hackers and scammers can also gain access to your personal data in your laptop when you connect to the Internet in public places.

The gravest is identity theft, which could ruin one's life.

Here are some helpful tips:

1. If you have RFID credit cards, driver's license, passport, etc., buy RFID shields or improvise RFID blockers using aluminum foil.

2. Each family member using the same credit card account must inform the others as to their purchases, amount, and date.

3. Thoroughly check your monthly credit card statements and ATM account, or call the customer service number printed at the back of the credit card to obtain purchases and balance updates.

4. When you get a call from "your bank," get the name and position of the caller and say you would call back later. Dial the customer service number at the back of the credit card to confirm.

5. Power off the garage door opener, especially at night or before going out of town. With the electrical switch off, the remote opener will not work.

6. It is more secure not to use remote control to unlock or lock the car.

7. Do not open and immediately trash all e-mails sent by people you do not recognize, no matter how tempting the subject might be.

8. When you receive an email from a familiar name telling you a sob story of being robbed of his wallet, stranded overseas penniless, and requesting you to send money, call and talk to your friend or relative to confirm. Chances are this is a fraudulent e-mail, using a familiar e-mail address to victimize you;

9. Never give out your username or PIN or password or key code to anyone, even if the call is from "your bank." Bank personnel and online vendor clerks are prohibited from asking for such confidential data.

10. When you receive an e-mail which states you won in a lottery or millions of dollars are awaiting transfer to your bank account, trash it right away. Do not even send a reply, otherwise you will only be giving them and confirming your email address.

11. When emailing, it is more secure for everyone concerned to use the "bcc," instead of the "send" or "cc," when typing down the email address(es) of your contact(s).

12. Facebook, Twitter, and other social network sites are dangerous sites to post private matters and personal data. They are not secure sites.

Constant awareness, vigilance, carefulness, and common sense are the most effective antifraud, antitheft "tools" we have at our disposal. A bit of "healthy paranoia" might also keep us more on our toes.

Emphysema

What is emphysema?

Emphysema is a condition where the alveoli (air sacks) of the lungs are overinflated as a result of the destruction of the walls of the alveoli. These air sacs are responsible for the oxygen transfer from the inhaled air from the atmosphere to the bloodstream of the person, as the alveoli gets the carbon dioxide from the bloodstream, to be exhaled and eliminated. These damages from emphysema reduce the respiratory function of the lungs causing severe (dyspnea) shortness of breath. With this disease, the lungs become very inefficient in oxygen diffusion and renders the blood low in oxygen content. Hence the shortness of breath.

How common is emphysema?

Emphysema is found worldwide, mostly among cigarette smokers, who have "burned" their lungs. In the United States alone, more than 2 million people have emphysema. Medical literature records that 70,000 to 100,000 Americans were born with a deficiency of alpha 1-antitrypsin (AAT), a special and important protective protein, which is responsible for the inherited form of emphysema. Among chronic illnesses, emphysema, which debilitates the person, ranks the 15th. Men with emphysema outnumber the women by 22%, but since women have also started smoking, the gap is becoming narrower.

What causes emphysema?

The deadly poison (smoke and chemical) from cigarettes is responsible for 82% of chronic lung diseases, including emphysema. Air pollution, irritating fumes, and dust are factors in the development of emphysema. Majority of lung cancers are from smoking.

How severe can the shortness of breath be?

Dyspnea (shortness of breath) and orthopnea (shortness of breath when lying down) can be moderate to severe, to the point that the person cannot breathe (nor survive) without oxygen. When the lungs are burned and destroyed by smoking, their capacity to absorb oxygen and oxygenate the circulating blood is greatly diminished. This explains why the person with severe emphysema is huffing and puffing, gasping for air, and is having a hard time coughing up collected phlegm in his lungs and throat.

How does emphysema develop?

The normal lungs function well with a remarkable balance between two chemical systems with opposing action. The lungs have elastic fibers that allow them to expand and contract as we inhale and exhale. When the chemical balance is affected by, say, cigarette smoking, fumes, etc., the lungs lose their ability to protect themselves against the damages to these elastic fibers. The walls of the air sacs become thin and fragile, get destroyed, and then become overinflated, losing their efficiency in oxygen-carbon dioxide diffusion. A small percentage of people have emphysema due to deficiency in AAT as we have alluded to earlier.

What is chronic bronchitis?

Chronic bronchitis is the frequent, long-standing inflammation of the air passages or bronchi (breathing pipes), causing frequent coughs. Among smokers, chronic bronchitis (and the so-called smoker's cough) is usually a prelude to the development of emphysema. The combination of bronchitis and emphysema affect more than 15.8 million people in the United States alone. More than 100,000 people die each year from COPD.

What effect do cigarettes have on our bronchi?

The local adverse effects of smoking on our breathing pipes and lungs include, among others, the destruction of the ciliary motion on the mucosa (wall lining) of our bronchi. Normally, this ciliary function acts like strands of brushes (hairlike structures that move in a wavy fashion) that moves secretion (phlegm) upward and outward, so the person could cough it out. With smoking, this action ceases to function, so that whatever phlegm is in the lungs remain there (causing more damages as it get infected), the person having great difficulty coughing it out without the help of the cilia. The constant irritation from the fumes is also carcinogenic (cancer-causing).

Can emphysema affect the heart?

Yes, when the emphysema is severe and the oxygen level in the blood is low as a result, then the heart will also suffer from lack of oxygen, besides being overworked by the lungs that are inefficient. The heart tries to compensate for the low oxygen level in the bloodstream by beating harder and faster.

Is emphysema curable?

No, once emphysema has developed and the lungs are "burned," they will not recover and be normal again. The destruction of the lungs and breathing pipes in emphysema is permanent. This is the reason why prevention of emphysema is essential.

How do we prevent emphysema?

Abstinence from cigarette smoking is an effective way to prevent emphysema. A healthy diet, regular exercises, a good sleep, on top of a smoke-free lifestyle, are almost a sure way to ward off emphysema. Those with AAT deficiency obviously can benefit a lot from avoiding tobacco. Also, stay away from air pollution and fumes whenever possible. When the ozone (smog) level is unhealthy, limit your activities to early morning or evening.

What is the treatment for emphysema?

The main objective of the treatment is to give relief of symptoms and prevent worsening of the disease. To accomplish this major goal, the recommendation include quitting smoking, brochodilators (to open up airway passages and ease breathing), antibiotics to prevent infection, breathing exercises, use of Alpha 1-Proteinase Inhibitor for those with AAT deficiency, lung volume reduction to remove the damaged lungs and allow the remaining healthier lungs to expand better, and lung transplantation for those who are otherwise beyond help.

Our Polluted Environment

The industrial age has gifted the world with great advances in science and technology. However, we humans have neglected to prevent the expected adverse side effects on our environment of this quantum progress. As a result, we have contamination of the air we breathe (industrial pollutants), the water we drink (heavy metals), the food we eat (pesticide residues), which cause debilitating and deadly diseases and destruction of the ozone layer, which increases our risk for the development of cancer, etc.

One latest study shows that the umbilical cord blood samples of newborns tested positive for a variety of toxic substances, obviously inhaled or ingested by the mothers throughout the pregnancy.

Our rivers, lakes, and oceans are used as "dumps" for garbage and toxic chemicals, destroying water life and coral reefs. Our irresponsibility and cruelty to our environment is ushering in global warming and the melting of the ice caps, resulting in grave weather changes and tsunamis around the world.

Each year, about 64,000 people in the United States who die prematurely from cardiopulmonary diseases associated with air pollution, according to the US National Resources Defense Council.

Air pollution constricts blood vessels and may even trigger heart attack. Global warming and air pollution are linked by combustion of fossil fuels. The burning of natural gasses, oil, and coal lead to "greenhouse" gasses and a variety of harmful air pollutants, like ozone, sulfur dioxide, nitrogen oxides, and airborne particulates. All these cause grave effects on health, such as respiratory, cardiovascular, and metabolic illness and even cancer of the lungs and other organs.

Ozone in the stratosphere (upper atmosphere) is a significant factor that makes life on earth possible. Chemical pollution caused by industry and by us, as individuals, erodes the ozone layer. With the depletion of the ozone belt that shields the earth from excessive ultraviolet rays from the sun, there will be increased health problems for us and disruption of the sensitive terrestrial and aquatic ecosystems. While ozone (a form of oxygen with 3 atoms instead of the normal 2) is protective in the stratosphere, it is most toxic near ground level, forming acid rain and photochemical smog that are dangerous to health.

Governments around the world, especially those of the rich nations, must control the pollution in the environment caused by the $1.5 trillion global chemicals and related industries and protect the health and well-being, not only of the nearly 7 billion people around the world, but of our friendly planet earth, the only home we've got.

"Erotic" Foods

In another article, we discussed the several health benefits from sex, a natural human activity that is psychologically and physically essential to well-being and the relative sense of youthfulness among most people.

For millennia, people have explored and experimented ways to improve their libido and sex life. The Chinese have extensively used the expensive rhino horns, the Romans, hippo snout and hyena eyeballs, as sex-enhancers. In the United States, people have spent about $1.4 billions in 2005, to treat male sexual dysfunction, reported the Amsterdam-based healthcare information firm Wulters Kluwer. This does not include the trillions of dollars spent around the world by the victims of fraud perpetrated by dozens of unscrupulous pharmaceutical companies.

Goaded by profit, manufacturers all over the world have introduced "sex beverages, lotions, potions, and pills" that are no better than fruit juices and sugar capsules, which are unreasonably expensive, victimizing the unsuspecting public, robbing people of their hard-earned money. Today, the market abounds with substances claiming to be sexual "stimulants" and "libido-enhancing" concoctions and pills, which are nothing but a legal way of stealing people's money and defrauding the consumers. Unfortunately, in spite of volumes of medical information available today attesting to the uselessness and possible deleterious side-effects from these "sex substances," we still have hundreds of millions of people out there who are wasting their money and risking their health and only enriching these unconscionable companies and vendors.

In contrast to these expensive and ineffective sex-enhancers on the market, there are natural foods in the grocery stores, very much less expensive and healthier and safer that could boost libido, sex drive, and performance in both men and women, in combination with various conducive factors we have listed near the end of this article.

Helping the mood for romance, besides a healthy lifestyle, are some foods that are claimed to improve libido. Some of these sex "nutrients" from nature's own soil and water, include the following well-known and readily available items in most grocery stores: asparagus, avocado, banana, basil, bee pollen, celery, chili, fig, garlic, goji berry, maca, pumpkin seed, oysters, dark chocolates, soya beans like tofu, chick peas, carrots, cucumber, eggplants and other "phallic" vegetables and fruits, ginseng roots, and daily multivitamins and minerals.

Fruits and vegetables, in general, is an essential part of a healthy lifestyle and the sex gourmet recipe. Fried and rich foods, red meats, and other high-cholesterol and fatty foods make us sluggish and "too full," sensations not good for romance. Processed foods have been linked to frigidity in women and diminished sexual stamina in men. Cigarettes constrict the arteries, which reduces blood flow to our organs and therefore bad for sex, and they dampen libido. And alcohol, more than a shot or two, according to Shakespeare, "increases the desire, but diminishes the performance."

Bee pollen, whose role is to help fertilize, is supposed to boost the sperm count; and celery is purportedly a stimulator of the production of androsterone, an odorless "aphrodisiac" found in male perspiration. Chili is said to release endorphins, the "feel-good" hormone. Garlic has a high level of allicin, a substance which opens up small arteries and improve blood flow to various organs. Goji berries are dubbed as "sexual tonic" that is said to increase testosterone, libido, youthfulness, and stamina; and maca had been reported to have the ability to increase testosterone and sperm count.

Pumpkin seed, which is a health food, has zinc, which is important in testosterone production. It is also a source of omega-3 fatty acids that is good our cardiovascular health. The delicious and decadent chocolates, especially the dark ones, are great antioxidants and contains phenylalanine, an amino acid that increases endorphins in the body, a potent antidepressant, a hormone that provides a great sense of "high" and overall well-being, naturally and safely. How these foods could help depends on various factors (lifestyle, belief, philosophy, attitude, etc.) among the sexual partners.

Obviously, the largest sex organ in the body, which is the brain, needs more than just sex foods or even pills, like Viagra, Cialis, or Levitra, to work maximally for a great romantic encounter. The love for, and attraction to, one another; good health and personal hygiene; the absence of fear or distraction; the romantic words spoken to set the mood even before foreplay; the ambiance; the privacy; and the concentration are all essential factors for lovers to have optimal romance. Naturally, the older the lovers are, the more important these factors are, since their hormonal levels are much lower compared to those in younger people. But medical data abound showing that healthy men and women, even in their 70s, can outperform people in their prime of youth who live unhealthy lifestyles.

Medically speaking, one thing is clear: the healthier the lifestyle one lives, the greater the person enjoys sex and maintain the ability and the pleasure longer, even in the ripe old age. After all, sex is not only for the young, but for all those young at heart with healthy mind and body.

Essential Health Tips

Flu and Humidity

While flu vaccines and the healthy habit of frequent hand washing significantly reduces the risk of catching influenza, humidity also plays a very important role in warding of this virus infection. Studies have shown that in dry environment 80% of the flu virus survived, while only 10% did in a well-humidified environment. A home or room humidifier will certainly help in preventing the spread of flu and making us breathe more comfortably.

Electromagnetic Risks

At what dose of repeated radiation exposure from medical imaging diagnostic devices, natural or artificial sunbathing, microwave oven, cell phone signals, radiofrequency (radio-TV) signals, extremely low-frequency power lines (said to be associated with childhood leukemia) can cause various forms of illnesses, including cancer, is still controversial. But we cannot simply ignore the warnings. In this current situation, the wise and prudent strategy is to minimize exposure to any of these electromagnetic forces as much as we can as we take advantage of the benefits provided by these advances in science and technology. Let's just be more conscious and careful.

Exercise Wonders

The amazing wonders of physical exercise are scientifically proven to keep the body and mind healthy, strengthen the immune system, improve cardiovascular fitness, and reduces heart attacks by 33%, lessen the risk of the development of type 2 diabetes by 91%, prevent, if not minimize high blood pressure by more than a third—all these for doing 30 minutes of exercise at least 5 days a week. Tai chi, tai bo, dancing at any speed, walking (moderate to brisk), swimming, bicycling, or any aerobic exercise. There is no age limit to doing exercises. My 93-year-old mother still does (at a moderated pace) daily 2-mile exercise following the Leslie Sansone's DVD aerobic exercise program. And she feels great for her age. Besides a proper diet, abstinence from smoking, and moderation in alcohol intake (red wine preferred), exercise is a major key to health and longevity.

Shaving Calories

A good strategy is reducing calories is by substitution or swapping: drinking an 8-oz bottle of water instead of a can or bottle of regular soft drinks saves you 100 calories; chicken sandwich instead of hamburger, 290 calories; one teaspoon mustard instead of mayo, 100 calories; apple slices instead of French fries, 270 calories; swap chocolate ice cream with strawberry slices, 115 calories; mixed salad with low-fat dressing instead of pizza saves you 2 slices about 300 calories; and one bagel replaced by sliced light whole grain bread, 269 calories; high-fiber cereal instead of granola, 110 calories. And brown rice is certainly healthier than white rice.

Pistachio Lowers Cholesterol

Studies at the Pennsylvania State University shows that pistachio nuts with its monounsaturated fatty acids and high antioxidant content have beneficial effects on cholesterol, body mass index (for weight reduction), and for hypertension control. With as little as 1.5 ounces of pistachios a day for one month reduced the cholesterol by 8.4% and the low density (bad) lipoprotein by 11.6%. Monounsaturated fats, as in pistachio nuts and green leafy vegetables, are cardio-protective and lessen the risk of cardiovascular diseases like heart attack and stroke.

A Dozen Reasons to Have Sex

The recent admission of Tiger Woods that he was unfaithful to his wife and revelation of the infidelity of several popular public personalities in the past "have given sex a bad rap," says a psychologist and sex therapist. The following have been cited as the health benefits from sex: (1) It relieves stress. (2) Sex improves the skin complexion. (3) Sex burns calories. (4) Sex heightens immunity. (5) Sex boosts self-esteem. (6) Sex maximizes cardiovascular health. (7) Sex improves intimacy and love. (8) Sex is an analgesic that reduces aches and pains. (9) Sex reduces the risk of prostate cancer. (10) Sex improves sleep and provides good rest. (11) Sex strengthens the pelvic floor muscles. (12) Sex adds "fire, fuel, and mileage" to a marriage.

Supplement Physicians Take

While not all physicians take supplements, many around the world are on any of the following: Daily multivitamins with minerals, vitamin B complex for stress, vitamin D3 for cancer prevention, lutein for the eyes, omega-3 fish oil, calcium, low-dose (81 mg) aspirin, a statin drug to lower cholesterol, and whatever prescription drug they may be on for high blood pressure, arthritis, diabetes, GERD, etc. This regimen is not for everyone, since various medications, no matter how common or popular they may be, may have some adverse side effects for some individuals. Consult with your physician before taking any medications, vitamins or food supplements, especially the so-called health beverages, hyped-up fruit juices, or herbals.

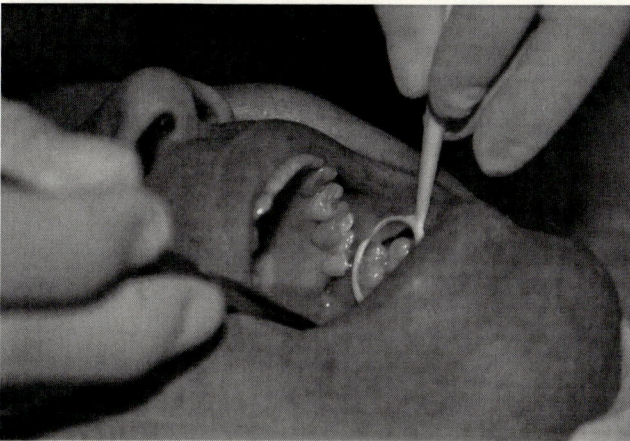

Intensive oral hygiene and regular visit to the Dentist are important part of a healthy lifestyle. Dental infections can lead to more serious diseases like heart attack and stroke. It is best for everyone, especially children, to stay away from candies, soft drinks, and other sugar-loaded food items.

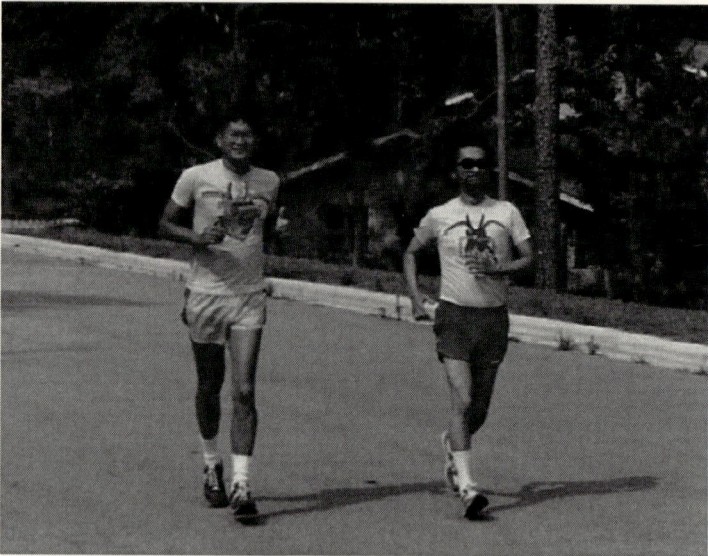

Regular exercises, like jogging or brisk walking for 30 minutes, at least 5 times a week, work wonders in reducing the risk of heart attack, stroke, diabetes, depression, and even cancer. They also boost the immune system.

Tai Bo aerobic exercise

There is no question at all that physical exercise, no matter how minimally strenuous, at least 5 times a week for those who medically fit, helps ward off diseases, from metabolic, cardiovascular, and even from many forms of cancer. For individuals already with essential hypertension (high blood pressure) and/or diabetes, hypercholesterolemia (elevated cholesterol in the blood), and heart disease, exercise also offers great benefits, making their treatment easier to manage and reducing the risk of these diseases. The morbidity and mortality of these illnesses are also lower among those who do regular exercises compared to those who are sedentary and not on any form of exercise regimen.

Athletes

Athletic prowess highlights how exercise can heighten one's health, speed, stamina, resistance to diseases, and even longevity.

Indeed, our body can be healthfully conditioned to maximize the integrity of our physical and mental state, our physiology, and our immune system and arm us with the necessary protection against daily stress and bodily insults from our environment and from diseases.

We have a lot of excuses and alibis why we do not exercise. They range from lack of time, exercise equipment for home or sports club membership being expensive, and a host of other reasons. The fact of the matter is most of us do not exercise because of plain laziness or lack of motivation.

But all this could change when we consider an exercise regimen that is very simple to do, anywhere you are, requiring no equipment except your mind and body, one that takes only 10-15 minutes of your time, and one that is free of any expense, except for perseverance and sweat. I am referring to the cardio-fitness exercise called tai bo, which is surging in its popularity, especially among busy businessmen, Hollywood celebrities, and young people in general.

Tai Bo for Body and Mind

This playful aerobic exercise regimen rose to popularity in the 1900s. The developer of Tai Bo was taikwondo expert Billy Blanks of Erie, Pennsylvania, who introduced the routine in 1976. This popular physical fitness trainer, one of the top in the USA, is a 7-time world champion in martial arts. Tai Bo was derived from the two words: taikwondo and boxing. Technically, the art is that of shadow kickboxing, modulated to one's physical capability, customized by the person exercising as far as the degree of forcefulness and speed are concerned.

The Health Benefits

Many of the choreographed kicks and punches in Tai Bo are similar to those in karate, basically intended as an aerobic exercise to provide cardiovascular fitness, bone health, muscular strength, flexibility, agility, balance, and endurance. The same moves, or variations thereof, have been practiced for centuries in the East for total body fitness. Exercise has been also shown to prevent or lessen anxiety and depression and improve self-esteem. Any form of physical exercise induces our body to secrete beneficial hormones and substances within our system, which help provide us mental-soothing serenity, lubricate our joints, firm-up our muscles, and boost our immune system. The exercise itself lowers bad cholesterol, increases good cholesterol, and lowers the risk of the development of high blood pressure, diabetes, heart disease, stroke, and even cancer, as we have stated above. While going thru the dancing-martial arts motion of tai bo, one's mind is allowed to peacefully concentrate on good and happy thoughts. I find this refreshing, relaxing, and at the same time energizing.

The dance moves in Tai Bo confers upon the entire body, joints and all, a high-energy workout at your own pace. It also provides improved mental coordination, self-confidence, and self-awareness. But the most attractive attribute of tai bo is its simplicity and practicality, which allows practically anyone at any age who are up to it to practice it. You can do tai bo anywhere in the house, in the backyard, even at work, without much hustle. You can even do it while lying down or in a chair. You can even invent your own moves and routine, with or without music, with or without inspiration from Pacman. With tai bo, you are the choreographer and the practitioner in one. And all the equipment you need is your mind and body. Of course, you have to pull in your resolve too.

Start Slow and Customize

Before doing Tai Bo or any exercise regimen, it is best to consult with your physician. As with any exercise, the best strategy is to do tai bo slowly, gradually increasing its intensity, not abruptly, until you modulate it to your own comfortable level and speed. Practiced 5 times or more a week, this aerobic exercise, which is better than jogging or the treadmill, can yield great dividends in terms of cardiovascular fitness and mental health for a minimum of investment.

Any more excuses?

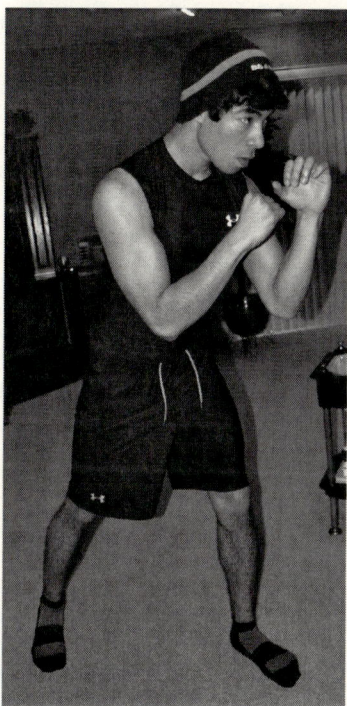

Tai bo, shadow kick-boxing, is a good form exercise for young and old. It can be done practically anywhere, even in a limited space, and needs no special equipment. This practical and inexpensive exercise regimen only requires determination and discipline. The intensity of the movements can also be "adjusted" to suit the individual's need and capacity.

Exercise for Fitness

Is physical activity important to health?

Yes, very much so. To illustrate a point, let us exaggerate and consider a situation that is extreme: a person who is bedridden, a stroke victim or a quadriplegic, someone practically unable to move. What happens? The muscles all over the body atrophy and in most instances are replaced with fats, become flabby, and lose bulk; the heart and lungs deteriorate; the circulation slows down; metabolism becomes impaired; the immune system declines; and the brain and all other organs function poorly. Humans, animals in general, were not meant to be vegetables. Physical activities are essential for cardiovascular fitness, fundamental to a healthy lifestyle.

What benefit do we get from exercise?

Medical literature is replete with documented studies showing increased levels of physical activity and fitness are associated with a decreased incidence of heart attack and hypertension (high blood pressure) and a fortified immune system, making the individual more resistant to infections and diseases. Regular exercise also makes one look better physically by improving muscle tone. The person who exercises regularly also has increased stamina, energy, and capacity for work and leisure activities, superior ability to lose body fats and maintain a desirable weight, and has greater resistance to stress, fatigue, and anxiety. They also have a more positive outlook on life. Those who are sedentary are twice more prone to develop heart attack.

What type of exercise is good for fitness?

Practically any form of physical activity helps; but a regimented exercise of half an hour to one hour, done at least 3-4 times a week, confers the greatest cardiovascular benefit. The exercise could be walking (leisurely to brisk), dancing, aerobics, bicycling, swimming, running, playing tennis, jogging, etc.

Why is brisk walking better than jogging?

In the '60s and '70s, jogging was very popular as a form of exercise. However, there were significant attendant complications resulting from jogging, like injuries to feet, ankles, knees, hips, spine, etc. Studies in sports and cardiovascular medicine two decades later showed that the cardiovascular benefits from brisk walking were the same as those derived from jogging, minus the injuries.

What is target heart rate?

When exercising, the heart rate normally speeds up. The heart rate that one wants to achieve with exercise is called target heart rate (THR). Reaching this heart rate when exercising means maximum benefit is being derived from the physical activity. To compute your THR, subtract your age from 220. Example: the THR of someone who is 50 years old is 220 minus 50, or 170. When exercising, one tries to reach his/her THR, so long as no symptoms occur, like chest pains or tightness of the chest, dizziness, or fainting. Some expected shortness of breath is normal, which should subside with rest. Among the elderly and those on medications, adjustments need to be made. The best thing to do before embarking on an exercise regimen is to consult your physician, who will advise you accordingly and prescribe what is best for you.

How fast should the heart rate go down after exercise?

Your heart rate should go back down to your normal rate (preexercise heart or pulse rate) within 15 minutes after ending your exercise. Therefore, it is advisable to always take your pulse rate before you start your exercise. If it takes longer than 15 minutes, you should reduce your pace. It is prudent to take a 5—to 10-minute warm-up, such as leisurely walking before engaging in brisk walking, or slow dancing before going into fast dancing, etc. After exercise, whatever it is, end the session with a 5—to 10-minute cool-down period that includes gentle stretching.

How much calories are burned by exercise?

For a 150-pound (about 68-kilo) person, doing the following for one hour burns the corresponding amount of calories indicated here: walking, 2 mph, 240 calories; walking 4.5 mph, 440; jogging 7 mph, 920; bicycling 6 mph, 240, 12mph, 410; jumping rope, 750; running in place, 660; running 10 mph, 1,280; swimming 25 yards per minute, 275; tennis, singles, 400. For half an hour of nonstop fast dancing (like swing or boogie), 200 calories; and in contrast, for a 30-minute foreplay and sex, only 90 calories are burned, as we have stated before.

What are the three kinds of exercise program?

They are those that promote endurance, muscle strength, and flexibility. Any complete program for cardiovascular fitness should include all three. Components of endurance exercise include type, duration, frequency, and intensity.

Does exercise improve sexual libido?

Minus any medical problem and all other factors being equal, yes, a daily exercise regimen does improve sexual libido and also endurance for both the males and the females.

How about for those who already had a heart attack?

Properly prescribed exercise regimen after a heart attack can help reduce the risk of having another heart attack and also improve the chances of survival, besides improving the quality of life. It is routine practice for the cardiologist to recommend post-heart-attack cardiac rehabilitation exercises as a part of a comprehensive management for heart attack or coronary artery disease.

What are the benefits of a well-conditioned heart?

The heart of a well-conditioned person, beating at 50 beats per minute, pumps the same amount of blood in the circulation as the heart of a less conditioned (inactive) person beating at 75 beats per minute. The average heart pumps about 36,000 more times per day or 13 million more times a year, compared to the heart of a well-conditioned individual, which do not beat as fast, thereby having more reserves. The well-conditioned heart also has stronger and more efficient ventricles (muscles).

What is the minimum exercise recommendation?

The American College of Sports Medicine has the following minimum exercise recommendation for healthy men and women—frequency: 3-5 days a week; intensity: Target heart rate; duration: 20-60 minutes of continuous aerobic activity depending on intensity; method: should use large muscle groups (walking, hiking, running, cycling, dancing, rowing, swimming, etc.); resistive strength training: at least one set of 8-12 repetitions of 8-10 exercises that condition the major muscle groups at least two times a week.

Is there such a thing as overexercising?

Everything depends on the individual and his/her objective in doing the particular exercise regimen. Beyond one hour of daily moderate or vigorous exercise will result in little added cardiovascular/pulmonary fitness and may only increase the risk of injuries attendant to the physical activity. But if the aim is to lose weight, and if the person's condition and endurance allow it, increasing the duration of the exercise may be done. However, remember that cutting the caloric intake, on top of the exercise, is the most effective way to lose the extra pounds.

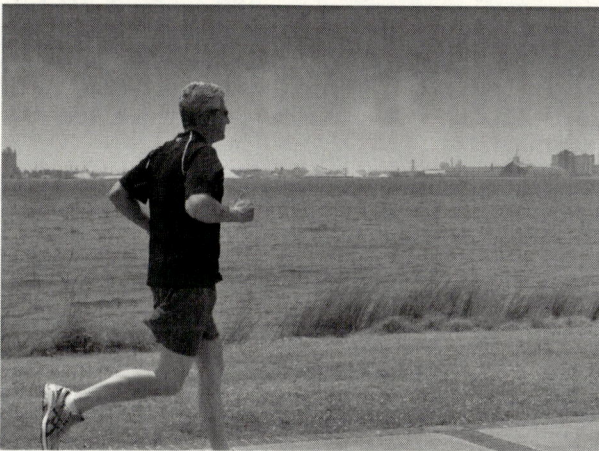

Exercise can ward off high blood pressure, diabetes, heart attack, stroke, even cancer.

Fibromyalgia

What is myalgia?

Myalgia means muscle aches and pains. There is a condition called fibromyalgia, which is a disorder that causes achy pain, tenderness, spasm, and stiffness of the muscle, areas of the tendons, and ligaments. These tender points are common around the neck and shoulders, in the front of the knees, elbow, hip joints, chest, low back, thighs, and calf (lower leg) muscles.

What is primary fibromyalgia syndrome?

Abbreviated as PFS, the typical pattern of this condition is generalized, idiopathic (of unknown cause) fibromyalgia accompanied by anxiety, fatigue, impaired sleep, and irritable bowels, with no evidence of underlying diseases contributing to the symptom complex. PFS afflict healthy young or middle-aged women who are anxious, stressed, tense, depressed. Children and adolescents (usually females) and older adults who have PFS may also have osteoarthritis of the spine. Men usually have localized fibromyalgia, which is related to recreational or occupational strain.

How common is PFS?

About 5% of the population, including children, have fibromyalgia; and some of this may be hereditary, with similar symptoms among family members.

What are the symptoms?

The onset of the pain and stiffness is gradual and diffuse. The pain may be a deep ache or burning, is worsened by straining and overuse, and may be constant but varies in severity in response to weather changes, stress, and activity. The pain may move around the body. There may be spasms or muscle tightening. Most sufferers feel fatigued or out of energy, have problem sleeping, and a few may have diarrhea/ constipation, difficulty swallowing, gas, heartburns, and abdominal cramps. There may be sensation of tingling or numbness in various parts of the body. Many patients have super sensitivity to odor, loud noise, bright lights, or even to medicines. Headache and pains in the jaws may also be present. Sometimes, they have dry eyes or problem focusing on objects that are near, imbalance, or dizziness. Others may have palpitation or shortness of breath. Women with fibromyalgia may have urinary complaints, pelvic pains, painful menstrual periods, or even painful sexual intercourse.

Could fibromyalgia be due to some illnesses?

Yes, the following may cause the same symptoms: generalized osteoarthritis, rheumathoid arthritis, polymyalgia rheumatica, polymyositis, and other connective tissue diseases and hypothyroidism. A minority of fibromyalgia cases may be caused by psychophysiologic abnormality.

Does any permanent damage result?

No permanent damage to any organ in the body results from fibromyalgia. The condition, while chronic and causing many bothersome symptoms, is not life-threatening either.

Does exercise aggravate fibromyalgia?

No. As a matter of fact, exercise is one of the best therapies for fibromyalgia. Starting with gentle, low-impact stretching exercises, like walking, bicycling, and aerobics.

So what is the treatment for fibromyalgia?

The comprehensive management of fibromyalgia includes ruling out or treating diseases causing the symptoms, reassurance from the attending physician that the condition is benign and not hopeless, stretching and aerobic exercises, local application of heat and gentle massage, improvement in sleep, and medications.

Aspirin and NSAIDS (nonsteroidal anti-inflammatory drugs) may be tried but they are usually not sufficient. Tramadol, a prescription drug, has been found to help ease the pains. For severe persistent tenderness, local injection with 1% lidocaine (alone or in combination with hydrocortisone) has been effective. Antidepressants (Duloxitine, Milnacipran, Fluxetine, etc.) and antiseizure drugs (Gabapentin, Pregabalin, etc.) have also been found useful for fibromyalgia, under the supervision of a physician. Physical exercise and counseling are vital part of the regimen in the management of fibromyalgia.

What are the side effects of these drugs?

Some of the side effects of these medications include drowsiness, dryness of the eyes and the mouth, increased appetite, constipation, and nightmares. These symptoms are usually worse at the beginning and diminish with time. The best is to discuss the details of the treatment with the attending physician.

What is the prognosis?

Functional prognosis is usually very good with aggressive and comprehensive treatment. Fundamental in the success of therapy is patient motivation, involvement, and discipline. Armed with these three, persons with fibromyalgia are soon on their way to a more comfortable, happier, more productive, and a fulfilling life.

The Wonders of Fish Oil

Fish oil, which contains essential substances scientifically known as omega-3 fatty acids, started to gain public interest and popularity in the late 1990s when the results of large clinical trials (like the GISSI study) showed that omega-3 fatty acids provided great benefits to the human cardiovascular system. The objectionable fishy taste of the original fish oil supplement, when it was first introduced, had turned off consumers. However, improved molecular distillation processing of today has enhanced fish oil's purity and flavor to its present well-accepted, much-sought after omega-3 gelcap supplement. Nonetheless, eating fish daily is still the more natural and better way to get omega-3 fatty acids.

What are omega-3 fatty acids?

Omega-3 fatty acids, like those in fish oil, are essential polyunsaturated fatty acids (PUFA), which cannot be synthesized in the body *de novo.* They must come from the food we eat or supplement we take. One of their counterparts, linolenic acid (LNA) is an 18-carbon n-3 essential fatty acid, the major sources of which are canola, soybean, wheat germ, flaxseed, and walnut oils. The other, linoleic acid (LA), is 18-carbon n-6 essential fatty acid and found in safflower, soybean, cottonseed, and corn oils. Meat products are a source of arachidonic acid (AA), while the 20—and 22-carbon PUFA are from fish and fish oils, which are the most beneficial oils for our cardiovascular health and more. Those found in fish contain highly polyunsaturated EPA (eicosapentanoic acid) and DHA (decosahexanoic acid) and those found in dark green vegetables have alpha-linolenic acid, all of which are considered "good fats." Omega-3 fatty acids are indeed "essential from womb to tomb."

How do fish oils do it?

In simple terms, fish oils, following their metabolism in our body, produce eicosanoids (prostaglandins, thromboxanes, leukotrienes, etc.) whose actions result in lowering cholesterol-triglyceride levels, decreasing blood pressure, maintaining and stabilizing normal rhythm of the heart, stimulating endothelial-derived nitric oxide which causes vasodilatation (opening of arteries), decreasing platelet aggregation (reducing blood clot formation that blocks arteries), and counteracts the pro-inflammatory actions of some harmful substances in the body.

Are there studies to support these?

Yes, there are a number of studies that showed the benefits of fish oils to our body. Besides the GISSI study, there is the DART (diet and reinfarction trial), which found 29% reduction in total mortality among those heart attack survivors who consumed more oily fish (equal to 500-800 mg/day of omega-3 fatty acids). Those patients with low baseline level of the essential acids (omega-3; eicosapentaenoic acid, or EPA for short; and decosahexanoic acid, or DHA) have a greater risk of sudden death. The subgroup in this study who chose to take fish oil capsules (450 mg EPA and DHA) had a 62% reduction in cardiovascular deaths and 56% lower death rate from all other causes. One of the latest was from the Institute of Human Nutrition at Columbia University College of Physicians and Surgeons in New York, which had a symposium titled "Omega-3 Fatty Acids: Recommendation for Therapeutics and Prevention," highlighting the glowing beneficial values of fish oil.

Are omega-3s really good for our health?

Yes, omega-3s are necessary for our health. They are a natural blood thinner which prevents thickening of blood and blood clot formation, thus reduces hardening of the artery, including coronary arteries of the heart and carotid-brain arteries, thereby lessening the risk of heart attack and stroke. They also play a role in preventing depression and some diseases, like diabetes and cancer, and in improving conditions like asthma and allergies, arthritis, migraine, menstrual cramps, etc. How significant a role they have, science at the present has no way of quantifying exactly.

What are the other sources of Omega-3s?

Walnuts, butternuts, canola oil, and especially flaxseeds and flaxseed oil, which contain a lot of omega-3 in the form of alpha-linolenic acid (LNA), which our body converts to EPA and DHA. Purslane, a low-growing plant, has been found to have the highest level of omega-3, vitamin C, and vitamin E among green leafy vegetables. Fish and shellfish contain only small amount of LNA but a large amount of omega-3s in the form of EPA and DHA, as in seaweeds. Flaxseed is richest in nonfish LNA. Other sources include macademia nuts, olives, soy protein (tofu), oat and wheat germ, bean sprouts, hickory nuts, spirulina, and lamb.

How about peanuts and cashew nuts?

These very popular nuts have very little omega-3 in them. Per 100 grams, peanuts contain 44.2 grams of fats, 23.6 grams of carbohydrate, 26.9 grams of protein, and yields 559 calories. They contain 0.3 mg of Vitamin B, 0.74 mg calcium, 1.9 mg iron, 393 mg phosphorus, and 337 mg potassium. One hundred grams of cashew nuts contain 48.2 grams of fats, 27 grams of carbohydrates, 18.5 grams of protein, and yields 578 calories. They contain 0.63 mg of vitamin B, 46 mg of calcium, 5 mg of iron, and 428 mg of phosphorus.

What can one with ApoE4 gene do?

Like the age factor, having ApoE4 gene is not a modifiable risk. The two other major risk dynamics (homocystine and DHA) can be managed. Prospective studies showed that eating at least one fish serving per week decreased the risk of Alzheimer's by 60%. The recommendation is to have at least 3 serving of fish per week, but eating fish (especially the belly part) daily would be ideal in minimizing the risk of cardiovascular diseases and Alzheimer's.

Are fish oil capsules any good?

Fish oil capsules, manufactured by reputable pharmaceutical companies, can provide the required level of essential fatty acids to raise the level of DHA and EPA in the blood plasma to normal. One oil capsule (gelcap or softgel) has 850 mg of natural fish oil concentrate and usually provides about 180-200 mg of DHA and EPA, sufficient to raise their levels to normal. This is supplemented by vitamins B6, B12, and folic acid, or by vitamin B complex or the so-called super B vitamins, to reduce the homocystine level. This combined therapy has been shown to decrease the incidence of dementia. But eating fish daily is superior to taking fish oil capsules. Fresh and properly prepared sushi provides a bit higher potency fish oils than cooked fish, but the omega-3 fatty acids from either of them, together with the B vitamin supplements, confer significant protection against cardiovascular ailments and Alzheimer's.

Does fish oil also prevent Alzheimer's?

It has been shown in epidemiologic studies that the 3 major risk factors in dementia or Alzheimer's, besides the age of the person, are ApoE4 genotype, elevated level of homocystine in the plasma, and decreased DHA plasma level. Data from the Longitudinal Framingham Study reported that ApoE4 carriers had about 2.5 times increased risk of dementia. Homocystine is deemed to be a direct vascular toxin that hastens arterial blockages, not only to the coronary arteries of the heart but also to the arteries to the brain, leading to almost 2 times higher risk of dementia.

Can omega-3 prevent cancer?

Researchers claim that fats high in Omega-6 promote tumor growth and fats high in omega-3 blocks tumor growth. They also reported that omega-3 creates a roadblock, which slows down distant spread (metastasis to other organs) of cancer cells. Omega-3 boosts the immune system, making the body less vulnerable to diseases. Having said these, we have to emphasize the (obvious) medical fact that to prevent cancer, we must stay away from potential carcinogens, which includes tobacco, red meats, and fatty foods, chemicals, radiation, excessive alcohol ingestion, to name a few. If we continue to "injure" and abuse our body with these potential carcinogens, no amount of omega-3, antioxidants, or any medications, will help. It is plain common sense.

Which seafoods contain the highest level of DHA and EPA?

These omega-3 fatty acids are highest in salmon, mackerel, tuna, herring, sardines, bluefish, trout, whitefish, and striped bass. Per 100 gm of this fish, one gets about 1 gm of EPA and DHA. Moderate sources are carp, flounder, mullet, smelt, cod, catfish, perch, halibut, pike, and pollock. Shellfish, squids, octopus contain little EPA and DHA.

Warning: Flu Can Kill!

A recent report from the Center for Disease Control and Prevention of the United States stated that an annual average of 36,000 Americans die from complications of influenza. This has surpassed the death toll from AIDS. Records show that the mortality quadrupled during these periods: 16,263 deaths in 1976-77, and 64,684 in 1998-99. The remarkable decrease in deaths is attributable to the greater acceptance of the flu vaccine, but general compliance is still lacking. In the flu pandemic of 1918, more than 20 million people died all over the world, half a million in the United States.

What is influenza?

Commonly known as "flu," "grippe" or "grip," influenza is a specific acute viral respiratory disease characterized by fever, chills, coryza (cold), cough, malaise, headache, inflamed respiratory mucous membranes, and some muscle aches.

What causes influenza?

The viruses that cause flu are called orthomyxoviruses, tiny "germs" whose sizes vary from 80-120 nm. They are classified into types A, B, and C. Type A is the most common single cause of flu. Type B causes epidemics about every five years. Type C is not a very prevalent virus. The influenza pandemic of 1918 left more than 20 million people dead.

How does it spread?

Flu is a very contagious illness. It spreads by person-to-person contact. Airborne droplet spray (from sneezing or coughing) into the atmosphere infects people and contaminates objects that can transmit the infection. This is why persons who have the flu are advised to cover their nose and mouth. Washing hands frequently is highly recommended to limit the transmission of the virus.

Who has the greatest risk?

Persons of all ages are afflicted, but school children are most prone to catch the flu. People at highest risk of developing severe disease are those with chronic lung disease and valvular heart disease and those with lung congestion. The elderly, the very young, the bedridden, and women in their third trimester of pregnancy are also at great risk. About 90% of deaths have been reported following a bout of flu in this group, especially those who are old and bedridden.

Which type kills more people?

Type A influenza is associated with significant morbidity and deaths during epidemics, higher than type B, which could also cause severe disease but not as bad. Type C is the most benign of the three. This admonishes us not to take flu lightly.

How long does it take for the symptoms to show?

From exposure, the incubation period is about 48 hours. During this period, asymptomatic viremia (virus flooding the bloodstream) occurs with replication of the virus in the respiratory tract. The, "suddenly" chills and fever up to 39 to 39.5 °C (102-103 °F) develop over 24 hours. Body aches and pains (back and legs) and malaise follow. Headache and sensitivity to light (pains in the back of the eyes) are most common. There is accompanying watery eyes, scratchy throat, dry cough, and a lot of nasal mucus discharge. The face is warm and flushed. The throat and tonsils might be sore and reddened. Nausea and vomiting may be present. After 48 to72 hours, the acute symptoms rapidly subside and fever disappears, but weakness and fatigue may linger another few days.

Are there severe cases?

Yes. In severe cases, complications could set in, like hemorrhagic bronchitis and pneumonia could set in within a few hours. Fulminant and fatal viral penumonia can occur, with severe shortness of breath and spitting up blood and death following in 48 hours. This happens among patients with pulmonary, heart, or neurologic problem and among the elderly or the very young with impaired or weak immune system.

How is influenza diagnosed?

A specific diagnosis may be made by isolating the virus by immunoflourescense technique or serologic tests, but the condition is so common just about any lay person can make the diagnosis. The important thing is to make sure it is "only the flu" and nothing more serious, especially when the symptoms persist for more than 5 days. In this case, a physician should be consulted.

Is there a pill for preventing the flu?

Yes. Amantadine 100 mg orally (for adults) has been used for prophylaxis against influenza type A. It is not effective against type B. This is recommended for those who are at high risk of developing complications. During the Amantadine treatment, those persons who have not been vaccinated should receive the flu vaccine, and Amantadine may be discontinued after 2 to 3 weeks. If, for any reason, vaccine cannot be given, then the pill should be continued for 6 or 8 weeks.

Does Amantadine have adverse side effects?

Yes, among them are nervousness and insomnia in about 7% of patients. These side effects are more prevalent among elderly persons and those with impaired kidney functions and brain dysfunction. A newer drug with lesser side effects is Rimantidine.

Is chicken soup good for the Flu?

There is no curative value of these foods, but they do make persons with the flu or cold feel better. They are light and warm, and warm liquids in general are soothing to the person with the flu. Taking liberal amount of oral liquids also prevents dehydration and helps bring the fever down. Regular or heavy meals make most patients feel bloated and nauseated.

Why is aspirin unsafe for children?

Aspirin was once used among children like water. However, since about 1963, a fatal condition known as Reye's syndrome was discovered and was linked to the use of aspirin, which increases the risk of having the syndrome by as much as 35-fold. The cause is still unknown but viral agents (influenza A or B and chicken pox virus) have been implicated and so with aspirin ingestion among children under 18 years of age. Children develop acute encephalitis and go into coma and die. Today, pediatricians no longer prescribe aspirin and prefer acetaminophen (Tylenol) for fever and aches and pains in children.

What is the treatment for the flu?

Generally, the treatment is symptomatic: bed rest to conserve energy and minimize malaise. To reduce fever and body aches, antipyretic-analgesic (antifever, antipain) pills (Tylenol) is given. Ensure hydration. Sponge bath or cold compress over the forehead, if fever goes above 39 °C (102 °F). If fever persists, especially in infants, young children, and the elderly, medical consultation is highly recommended. The physician might prescribe an antibiotic if he/she suspects a superimposed bacterial infection and antiviral drugs for those who are at high risk of developing complications. As always, prevention is most essential.

How does one prevent the flu?

Having a healthy lifestyle helps a lot in warding off many forms of illnesses. This includes high-fiber (vegetables and fruits for the phytochemicals in them), low-fat diet, no smoking, daily exercises, taking multivitamins daily, including Vitamins B, C, and E and the mineral zinc. Most one-a-day multivitamins already include these. Flu vaccines are now available and are recommended to be taken by adults September-November 15 each year. This annual flu shot, which takes two weeks to take effect, has been found to be 75% effective in preventing the flu. It also reduces the severity of the disease and can even be lifesaving for some people. Both the person with the flu and those around him/her should be careful to prevent airborne droplet transmission of the virus and infection by contaminated items. Kissing, handshaking, or any form of physical contact can transmit the virus.

Covering the face with your hands when you sneeze or cough could spread the flu virus to others you touch. Again, simple, old-fashioned hand washing that we learned in kindergarten can prevent infection.

What is the FDA drug warning about?

The Yale University Hemorrhagic Stroke Project researchers found in May 2000 that a common ingredient in many cold, flu, and diet medications called phenylpropanolamine hydrochloride (PPA) increases the risk of hemorrhagic stroke (caused by bleeding in the brain). Many of these drugs are sold over the counter, and some of them are prescription drugs, which physicians have prescribed over the years until the recent FDA warning about the dangers of PPA.

What are these medications in the United States?

Any medication containing phenylpropanolamine hydrocholoride, or diet aid ephedra *(ma-huang*, which is converted to PPA when ingested), can potentially cause brain hemorrhage and death, according to the Yale study. Some products with PPA include Dimetapp, Vicks DayQuill Sinus caplets, Robitussin CF, Comtrex, Tavist-D, some Triaminic products, Contac 12-hour, some Alka Seltzer Plus cold medications, appetite suppressants like Acutrim and Dexatrim.

Remember, influenza is nothing to sneeze at!

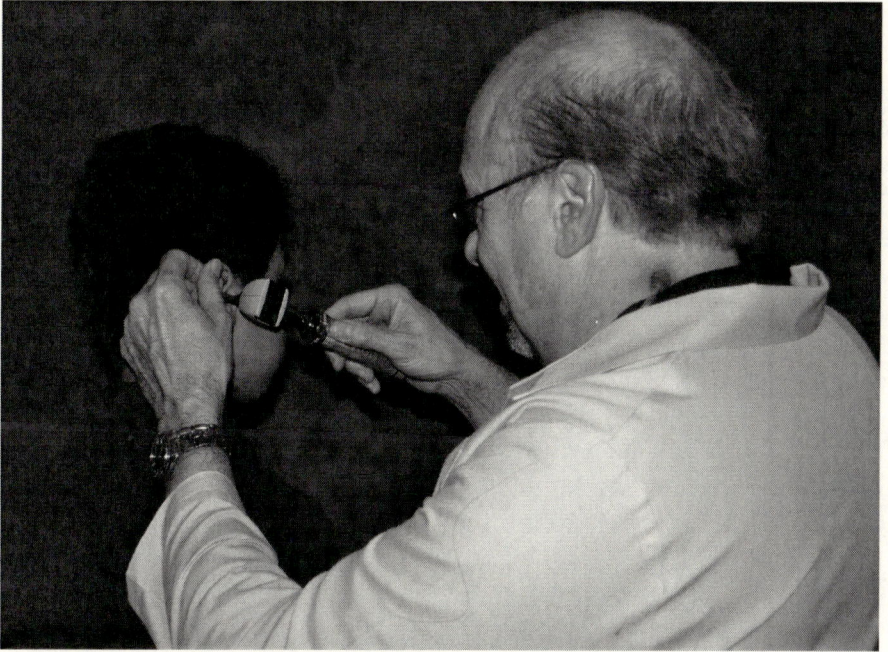

Any infection, even of the ears, can cause more serious health problems, which may not be immediately obvious, the reason why we must "listen" to our body.

Folic Acid, Vitamin E, are out!

The progress in medical science is ever evolving as man's battle against diseases and his quest for better health and longevity continue to inspire him. Advances in medicine almost invariably result in changes in previously held concepts, dogmas, and therapies in the arena of clinical practice. The standard of medical care today may be archaic tomorrow. Rather than defaulting to a stagnant status quo, the constant transformation in medicine is a welcome upgrade that positively translates to unceasing improvement in the quality of medical care for mankind as a whole.

Our consultant for this article is Luisito C. Gonzales, MD, FACC, a board-certified interventional cardiologist, Director of the RiverPointe Cardiac Catheterization Laboratory and director of Cardiopulmonary Rehabilitation Program at Elkhart General Hospital in Elkhart, Indiana.

We have chosen the following interesting and most frequently asked questions from our readers for Dr. Gonzales to discuss in this issue:

Why are folic acid and vitamin E no longer recommended?

It was previously thought that folic acid, by lowering homocysteine levels, was able to reduce the risk for heart attacks, strokes, cancer, and lower the need for revascularizations. Vitamin E, acting as antioxidant and mild blood thinner, was considered beneficial in lowering the risk for cardiovascular diseases, like stroke and heart disease.

However, a review of all the major clinical trials (CHAOS-2, VISP, WAFACS, HOST, HOPE-2, WENBIT, NORVIT, and SEARCH studies) involving 37,485 individuals did not show any benefits from taking either supplements; and if taken beyond the recommended dose, folic acid and vitamin E may even be harmful. The take-home message from all these trials is that nothing can replace a balance nutritious diet, regular physical activity, and abstinence from smoking and alcohol abuse to preserve health.

How much aspirin is safe?

The US Preventive Services Task Force has recommended that low-dose aspirin (81 mg) is all that is needed and is as effective as higher doses, both in men and women, to prevent coronary heart disease. Following consultation with their physician, men are usually advised to start taking low-dose aspirin at age 45 years to prevent a heart attack and women to start at age 55 to prevent a stroke. Women who are still menstruating release estrogen, which protects them somewhat from developing heart disease. In general, higher doses of aspirin (greater than 81 mg) may increase the chances of bleeding from the stomach. For those aged 80 and beyond, there is paucity of available data to tell us how safe aspirin is. In this age group, we advise extra caution and vigilance while taking low-dose aspirin under their physician's supervision.

What has my thyroid problem to do with heart attack?

The association between hypothyroidism or under functioning thyroid and heart attacks and deaths was seen in several studies. The possible explanation could be due to the effects of the thyroid hormone itself leading to a stiff blood vessel (increased systemic vascular resistance, arterial stiffness, altered endothelial function, increased atherosclerosis) and a thicker blood that seems to clot faster. These are the usual associated factors among those with thyroid problem that cause heart disease. When the thyroid hormone is also not working properly, it can lead to very high cholesterol levels that could deposit in the walls of the blood vessel and eventually cause blockages and heart attack. Hypothyroidism can also cause a weakening of the heart muscle called cardiomyopathy that will improve with treatment of the thyroid gland.

Can stem cell help people with cardiomyopathy?

Genetic modulation of the heart function may offer hope for treatment of heart failure. Cellular cardiomyoplasty involves directly injecting cells, such as stem cells, that may become new heart muscle cells into the diseased heart after a heart attack. This has been used during the acute heart attack setting. There was some short-term benefit with improvement in exercise treadmill time. However, it was found that in some angioplastied patients with heart stents, there was an increased rate of the stent being plugged up (in-stent restenosis). Stem cell therapy has also been studied in ischemic cardiomyopathy (heart muscle damage related to previous extensive heart attacks). The result showed significant increase in the heart function. This technique, which is still investigational, may have potentials in reducing the size of heart muscle damage and leading to improvement of heart muscle function in patients with cardiomyopathy. Presently, experience with this approach is still limited to a few small trials and the potential risks of dangerous heart rhythm problems (ventricular tachycardia), and possible increase in in-stent restenosis should be taken into account.

Food Children Eat

What children eat greatly determines their growth and development, the integrity of their immune system, their body's ability to ward off infections and diseases, and their morbidity and longevity. The other essential factors are their daily physical activities, abstinence from harmful substances like tobacco and illegal drugs, and disciplined intake of alcoholic beverages. While genetics play a role in all this, it has been proven that a healthy lifestyle can significantly benefit even those individuals with some of the so-called "bad" genetic trait.

Dieting must really start in the crib. Babies are taught discipline this early, whether we realize it or not. Giving them their formula at a set amount, at a scheduled interval, teaches the baby about the rules of feeding. And their young brain soon learns this.

When the baby is 4 to 6 months, pediatricians usually recommend starting solid foods, like a teaspoon of semiliquid iron-fortified rice cereals and other grains, like oats or barley, mixed with breast milk or formula and gradually increasing it to a tablespoon twice daily. At age 6-8 months, pureed or strained fruits (banana, pears, applesauce, peaches) and vegetables (squash, well-cooked carrots, sweet potato, avocado).

It is at this age and 2 to 3 when it is best to teach children to love and eat healthy food like vegetables, fruits, fish, white chicken meat, instead of pork and beef and other red meats, which are all high in unhealthy animal saturated fats and cholesterol. When bad habits have settled in at age 2 or older, they are hard to break. This where we, as parents and as a society, have failed our children, the future leaders of our country.

And since effective teaching is by example, we, parents and grandparents, must practice what we preach. The "do what I say, not what I do" command will never work.

Those children whose parents eat a lot of vegetables, whole grains, nuts, and fruits, who stay away from red meats, who do daily exercises, who do not smoke and drink only socially and in moderation, grow up to develop the same healthy habits and preferences.

Menu for school lunches in the United States, by and large, is a social injustice, according to chef Ann Cooper, known as the Renegade Lunch Lady, who is "transforming how US children eat, one federally subsidized school lunch at a time." I could not agree more.

The fatty red meats and carbo-loaded (sugar-loaded) and processed food lunches are out, and salad bars, whole grains, organic milk, and fish are in.

As Cooper says, "When we feed children with diet high in sugar and corn syrup, they just can't think, and if kids are not well-nourished, they can't excel."

Around the world, it is not rare to find kindergarten student with type 2 diabetes, or kidney stones among preteens, and teenagers with high cholesterol and clogged arteries. This is terrifying and unfortunate, because these are all preventable to a significant extent.

At least 32% of children and teenagers in the United States are overweight or obese. And Asians, especially Filipinos, are not lagging far behind in this pandemic. Obesity leads to increased risk of developing diabetes and other metabolic illness, hypertension, heart disease, stroke, Alzheimer's, and even cancer.

In this day and age of lightning speed telecommunication, public media, and rapid Internet access, we simply have no excuse to remain ignorant of scientific data on how to live a healthy lifestyle for maximum longevity and productivity and protecting our loved ones along the way, especially the young children.

Having said all that, there is really no such thing as too late in our quest for healthy lifestyle, no matter how old we are. Simple changes in diet and institution of exercise, for instance, even among those who are older than 50, have been shown to positively affect the control of, if not prevent, metabolic diseases, such as arthritis and diabetes and hypertension, heart disease, stroke, and cancer.

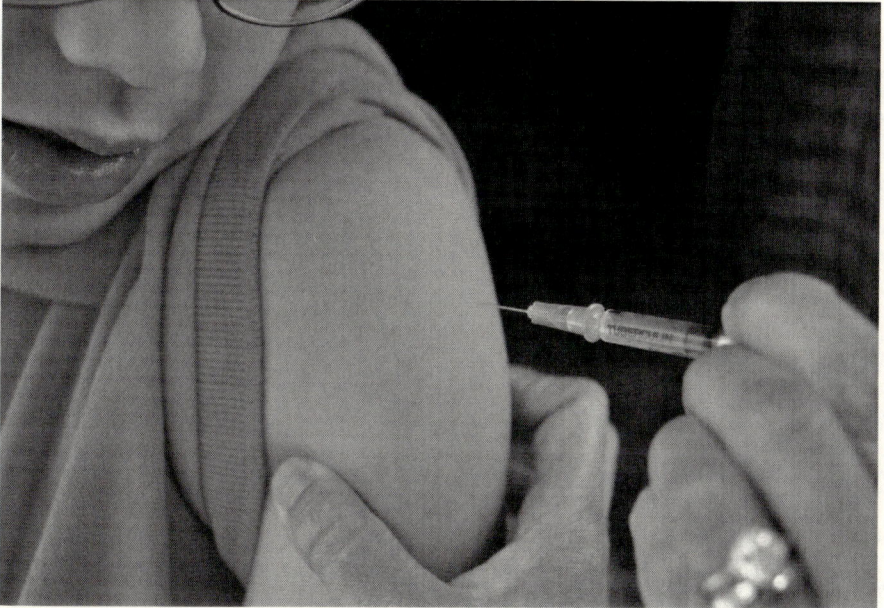

Allergy among children, as in adults, can cause more than just skin rashes and itching. Untreated, it could lead to shortness of breath, fall in blood pressure, or even loss of consciousness. The immediate use of EpiPen (pre-measured epinephrine shot for self-injection), or of a syringe to administer ephinephrine, can be a life-saver.

Food Ingredients and Labeling

The clamor for a healthier lifestyle has transformed society into more conscious, more intelligent, and more discriminating consumers of food and food ingredients. Truth in food labeling is a law that is strictly implemented, especially in the United States. Here are some of the most frequently asked questions on this subject, with very informative answers from Trader Joe's of Monrovia, California.

Why are some meats irradiated?

Some companies irradiate their meats to prevent food-borne illnesses. At the legally prescribed level, irradiation is effective and safe. However, some people are uncomfortable about it. In the United States, the Radura symbol (international symbol for radiation) must be on the label of foods that are irradiated, together with the wording "treated by radiation" or "treated with radiation."

Does MSG have to be listed too?

Yes, monosodium glutamate food taste enhancer must be printed on the label of food items containing such ingredient. Some people are allergic to MSG; and some others may react to it with headache, sensation of chest tightnes, and/or warm flushing sensation all over. MSG is commonly used in Chinese restaurants, where a special request from the diner to the waiters should preclude its use in the cooking of the food ordered.

How long can an unopened can of food be stored safely?

Canned low-acid foods, like meats, pasta, spinach, corn can be safely stored in a dry, cool, pantry for two years, while high acid foods (foods packed in vinegar based marinades, fruits, and tomato products), one year to 18 months. One caveat: if in doubt, throw it out!

Do yogurts contain live cultures?

Most yogurts on the market do, in varying amount, but the average is about 10 million *Lactobacillus acidophilus*, 10 million Bifid cultures, and over 10 million *Lactobacillus bulgaricus* and *Streptococcus thermophilus* cultures, per gram.

Why are soybeans good for us?

Soybeans are the richest natural source of isoflavones, phytochemicals that are also found in tofu, vegetables, fruits, nuts, seeds, legumes, some herbs. Isoflavones are phytoestrogens and beneficial to the body when consumed regularly by lowering the incidence of certain forms of cancer and heart diseases.

What is flash pasteurization?

This is a process used in food "sterilization" to kill food-borne pathogens, utilizing 170-180 degrees Fahrenheit for about 20 seconds.

If the label says fat-free, is it really cholesterol-free?

No, when the food label says fat-free, and you see oil in the product, it only means the product has less than one half gram of fat per serving. This is in consonance with the official FDA labeling definition of fat-free. This is the reason we should all be familiar with the system.

What are trans fats?

Adding hydrogen to unsaturated vegetable oil results in trans fat. The hydrogen crosses the chemical bond, and the liquid oil becomes solid in room temperature, like lard. This is also found in foods with hydrogenated oils and naturally seen in meat and dairy products.

What is the source of canola oil?

Originally, canola oil came from Canada, as an altered form of rapeseed oil. Canola has less saturated fats compared to olive oil and is a great source of omega-3 fatty acids and is high in monosaturated fats that have been proven to lower the bad cholesterol (LDL, low-density lipoproteins). Canola oil is the preferred cooking oil, and safflower is next. The other so-called vegetable or corn oils are not as good as canola oil.

What are essential fatty acids?

These are fatty acids that are important for our body but which our body cannot produce, unlike fats, cholesterol, and triglycerides which our liver can synthesize. We must therefore get our essential fatty acids from the food we eat. The two types are linolenic acid, an omeg-3 fatty acid, and linoleic acid, an omega-6 fatty acid. Safflower, sunflower, and corn are rich in linoleic acid, while sardines, salmon, albacore tuna, herring, and flaxseed oil have abundant linolenic (omega-3 fatty) acids.

Is oatmeal really good for us?

One of the healthiest breakfast foods is oatmeal, better and healthier than eggs and bacon/ham/sausages, etc. Together with fruits in the morning, oatmeal, like wheat and bran cereals, are health food items that lower our cholesterol, make our bowels regular, and reduce the incidence of heart diseases and malignancies, like cancer of the colon.

How about the "flake" cereals?

The various "flake" cereals (cornflakes, rice flakes, choco-flavored ones) are high in sugars and much less on fiber. These are carbohydrates with high glycemic indices and not recommended. Wheat, bran cereals, oatmeal are the best. And the same thing with wheat bread being better than regular white bread and brown rice superior to white rice.

Is sugar-free food devoid of sugar?

The name would make one think so, but unless the label says "zero" sugar, the product could have sugar in it, in spite of the label. The official FDA rule says if the product contains less than one half gram sugar per serving, it may be labeled sugar-free.

What are malitol, sorbitol, xylitol, and manitol?

These are sugar alcohols (not related to alcoholic drinks), which are used as artificial sweeteners, used by many, especially diabetics. They are absorbed by the body more slowly (lower glycemic index), which is good. They also promote lesser dental carries compared to regular sugar. These are also used in sugar-free chewing gums or mouthwashes, etc.

Why are soft drinks unhealthy?

Soft drinks of any kind are not healthy because of their very high sugar contents and their link to the development of metabolic syndrome. They are the worst enemies of overweight people trying to control their poundage. Children are especially advised not to drink pop beverages, not only for its effect on blood sugar and body weight but for its bad effects on their teeth. The most refreshing beverage is filtered water.

The "Food Supplements" Scam

The United States Food and Drug Administration (FDA) issued a public alert on May 1, 2009, warning consumers to "stop using Hydroxycut Products, dietary supplements used for weight loss as fat burners, as energy-enhancers, as low carb diet aids, and for water loss under the Lovate and MuscleTech brand names."

The FDA reported that "thus far Hydroxycut has been linked to at least one death and twenty three reports of serious health problems; consumers who use the products are at risk of serious liver injury. Some of the health problems associated with the Hydroxycut products include jaundice, elevated liver enzymes (an indicator of potential liver problems), seizures, cardiovascular disorders, rhabdomyolysis (a type of muscle damage that can lead to other serious health problems such as kidney failure) and liver damage requiring liver transplant."

The report stated that "Hydroxycut, Lovate and MuscleTech products are manufactured by Lovate Health Sciences Inc., of Oakville, Ontario and distributed by Lovate Health Sciences USA Inc. of Blasdell, N.Y.Â." All 14 Hydroxycut products are being recalled.

While the Hydroxycut products were obviously legitimate products, the chemical formulation produce dangerous side effects that make them unsafe for consumption. Hence, the recall.

On the other hand, there are hundreds of products marketed as "food supplements" that are nothing but a scam, victimizing the unsuspecting, innocent, uninformed, and gullible consumers. The manufacturers of these items hide under the name "food supplements" to be exempt from the stringent scrutiny of governmental agencies like the US-FDA, and similar agencies in other countries. As food supplements, these products are then *not* considered as *drugs* and do not have to pass the superstrict and extensive laboratory and clinical investigation by these agencies.

However, while they advertise them as "food supplements," these manufacturers claim or infer that their products have medicinal or health benefits, or even effective against various diseases. As such, they should be considered as drugs and not food supplements.

But the sad part of it all is that, while the manufacturers and merchants of this deception enrich themselves with trillion dollar sales around the world each year, the poor consumers are duped into thinking that the very expensive version of the "food supplements" ("designer" vitamins, weight-loss products, beauty aids, immune system boosters, whiteners, sex enhancers, etc.) are better than the regular over the counter and cheaper versions. Most of them have no proven good effects or advantage over the conventional household products people have been using five decades ago. The hype is so much, because of the tremendous marketing blitz (print media, TV and via Internet) that uninformed or misinformed people easily fall victims to them.

In the infomercials, some manufacturers or dealers even promise a "100% satisfaction or money back" guarantee. What these companies do is to deposit all sales proceeds in the bank, which earn interest. By the time they refund the customer's money, if ever, and perhaps after a lot of hustle, it will be at least 8 weeks, after they have already earned the bank interest on the money of millions of customers. And this translates to hundreds of millions of dollars in "extra" income for these companies.

A good example of the scam is the so-called Oxygen Bar that is seen in many shopping malls and airports. For $10-$15 dollars, one can sit on a stool and breathe in oxygen flowing through colorful fluid (whose cleanliness and sterility are suspect since the liquid is not changed from customer to customer). This is terrible and unhealthy. The ambient oxygen we breathe in is just right, healthy, and also free. Too much oxygen is even bad for our lungs.

Another is the popular Slim Tea or weight-loss tea. If that tea is all one drinks in a day and not eat, then one would lose weight. But if one does not diet and controls the food intake and simply drink the Slim Tea, the result is obvious. The other diet control beverages could also have chemicals in them that are unsafe for the kidneys or liver, etc.

Then there is the breast enlarger cream or lotion, or the penis-enhancer pill or lotion. These are all ineffective, useless, and nothing but a scam. Let us be thankful for whatever we were blessed with and not mess around with Mother Nature too much. Unless one is an insecure person and has low self-esteem, these enlargers and enhancers are not necessary. They are the character and the personality of the individual that truly count and matter.

Worse is the cure-all tablets or beverages, which are claimed to be good against several diseases, from acne to high blood pressure, immune diseases, allergies, diabetes, heart disease, stroke, to athlete's foot . . . and on and on.

But the most despicable of them all are those "food supplements" that infer or suggest that they are effective cures against cancer. They are not only baseless and unfounded claims but lies that rob cancer patients of their dignity by giving them false hope.

The sage strategy for a healthy lifestyle is doing daily exercise, eating a diet low in saturated fat, cholesterol, and carbohydrates; maintaining a desired weight; abstaining from tobacco and excess alcohol; taking regular time out to relax; and perhaps taking a multivitamin with minerals daily and whatever prescription medications, if any, as ordered by the physician.

We do not really need those "food supplements" to be healthy, attractive, and happy. These products are not only expensive but useless and a waste of money and expectation. As we have reported in the past, a few of them could also have harmful side effects, some serious or even fatal. Unfortunately, it may take time before these adverse effects or organ damage/failures become manifest or evident.

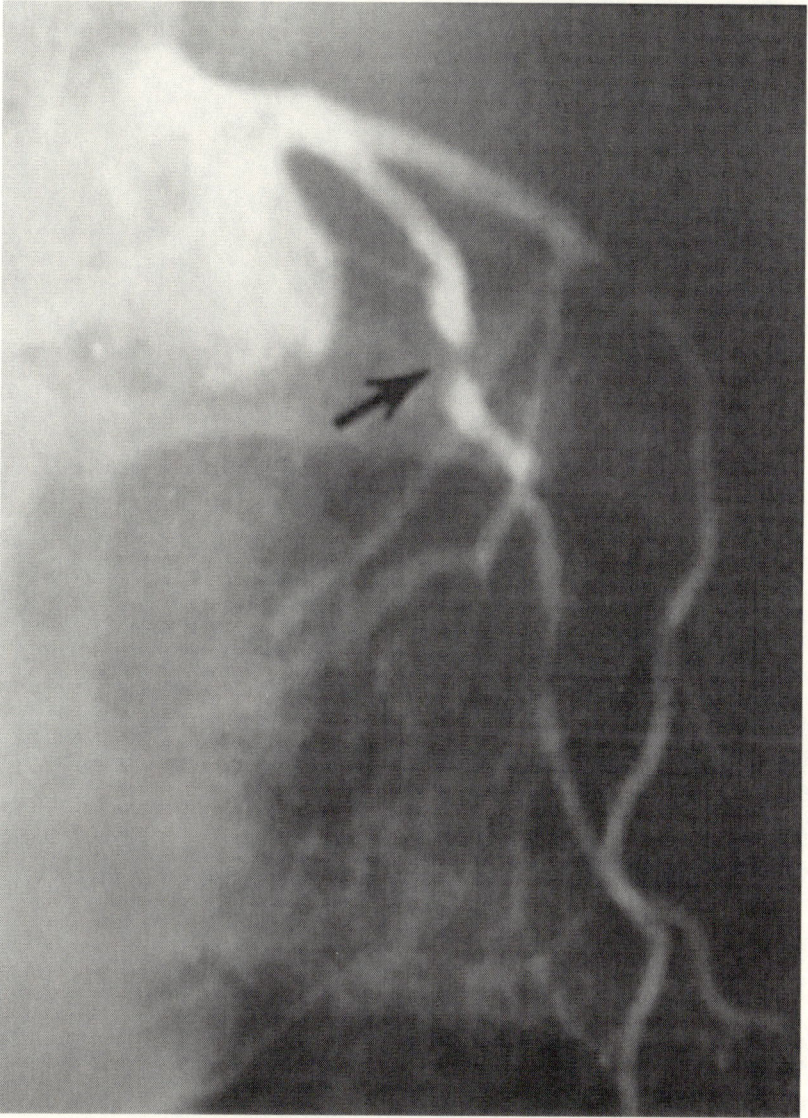

Claims that food supplements can dissolve arterial blockage and unclog the heart arteries are simply false. The coronary angiogram film above shows the arrow pointing to the severely narrowed coronary artery that could cause heart attack. Only proper diet, daily exercise, weight control can prevent arterial blockage and reduce or open the narrowing among those already with mild or moderate obstruction. Severe blockages need either angioplasty or coronary bypass surgery.

Foods to Avoid

Unlike beef which could be eaten rare or medium, pork is safe only when fully cooked, especially in barbeque. Improperly cooked pork could lead to a microworm infestation called trichinosis, where the tiny roundworms enter the muscles, even in the eyelids, the heart, etc., and pose a danger not only to health but to life. Eating raw seafoods, like oysters, mussels, shrimp, and fish can also cause bacterial infection, like salmonella, not to mention hepatitis. Unhygienic food handlers (including all of us) can contaminate the food and cause staphylococcus food poisoning, Shigella, and *E. coli* infection (from fecal contamination of food and or water), leading to severe diarrhea, nausea, vomiting, and abdominal pains. Even leftover rice, if not refrigerated and if it is kept covered airtight in a warm environment, can cause *Bacillus cereus* to thrive, multiply, and produce chemical toxins, resulting in food poisoning. Rice is best consumed within 24-48 hours. When leftover rice appears moist or sticky, and/or smells spoiled, it should be discarded.

Microwave Popcorn

A recent UCLA study reports that chemicals (one of them perfluorooctanoic acid—PFOA) in the inner surface (lining) of the bag are compounds that may be a culprit in the development of infertility in humans. The findings also stated that these chemicals vaporize with high temperature and seep into the popcorn and can cause cancer of the liver, pancreas, and testicles as they accumulate in the body over time until they reach the toxic level years later. Manufacturers, like Dupont, have promised to phase out PFOA by 2015 under the US EPA (Environmental Protection Agency) voluntary plan. In the meantime, pop your own corn in a skillet.

Canned Tomatoes

Bisphenol-A (BPA), a synthetic estrogen, is in the resin linings of tin cans. The acidic nature of tomatoes causes this chemical to leach into the tomatoes. BPA has been linked to heart disease, obesity, diabetes, and suppression of sperm production and chromosomal damage.

Corn-fed Beef

To fatten cattle for better profit, commercial farmers feed them corn and soybeans. A new comprehensive study by the US Department of Agriculture and Clemens University found that "compared with corn-fed beef, grass-fed beef is higher in beta-carotene, vitamin E, omega-3s, conjugated linoleic acid, calcium, magnesium, and potassium; lower in inflammatory omega-6s; and lower in saturated fats." Better option: beef from grass-fed cattle, stipulated on the packaging label.

Nonorganic Fruits and Vegetables

The same chemical contamination is found in nonorganic fruits and vegetables. Those with skin or rind are better protected. After washing them, peel the skin, like in apples, bananas, papaya, oranges, pineapple, carrots, radish, squash, etc. Those which are eaten as a whole, fruits like the various berries, prunes, grapes, and vegetables like lettuce, beans, etc., obviously contain more contamination and should be thoroughly washed. Again, organic, where possible, is the choice.

Milk with Artificial Hormones

To increase milk production, producers treat their dairy cattle with recombinant bovine growth hormone (rBGH or rBST), which exposes the cow to have udder infection and even pus in the milk. At the same time, it also leads to higher levels of insulin-like growth hormone factor (IGF-1) in milk, which, in some people, might "increase the risk for the development of cancer of the breast, prostate, and colon," according to Rick North, former CEO of the Oregon Division of the American Cancer Society and now an advocate for food safety. While this quoted statement is still not proven 100%, IGF-1 in milk is banned in industrialized countries.

Genital Herpes

What is genital herpes?

Genital gerpes is an infection caused by herpes simplex virus (HSV). Type 1 HSV causes oral herpes, involving the lips and mouth. Oral herpes could manifest as cold sores or fever blisters. Type 1 HSV can also cause genital herpes, but most cases of genital herpes are caused by type 2 HSV. Oral herpes, which is very common, and which could spread to just about anyone, does not have the negative sexual implication like genital herpes. There are many children with oral herpes.

How does the infection spread?

Kissing and oral sex transmit the type 1 virus. The type 2 virus is usually transmitted by vaginal and anal sex and can be spread from one person's genitals to another individual's mouth, causing oral herpes. HSV-1 can likewise cause genital herpes. Since the virus can't survive on nonliving surface, one cannot get the infection from a toilet seat, hot tub, etc. The infection is not life-threatening, but HSV infection makes it easier for HIV to enter the individual's body and which could lead to AIDS.

Who gets infected?

In the United States, roughly about 20% of all people 12 and older have HSV-2 infection, and 90% of these cases do not even know they have it. The infection is more common among women, because of the anatomy of their genitals. Twenty five percent of women have the infection compared to 20% of men. Multiple sex partners increases the risk of infection. As far as oral herpes is concerned, about 50-80% of adult Americans have oral herpes. About 30% to 50% of newly infected pregnant mothers transmit the HSV-2 to their newborns.

What are the signs of herpes?

The classical signs and symptoms are cluster of small vesicles (fluid-filled) blisters that break, resulting in painful sores that heal and crust over a period of days. These lesions may be found on the vagina, penis, vulva, scrotum, urethra, anus, thigh, and buttocks. Some of these sores may be mistaken for razor burns, or pimples, jock itch, ingrown hair, vaginal yeast infection, or bug bites. Many people with the infection do not have symptoms or sores. If they do, the symptoms disappear after the infection has set in but may recur from time to time. Some people may have only two "outbreaks" in their lifetime unless reinfected with a new sexual contact.

How can one reduce the risk or prevent infection?

1. The use of condom or "dental dam" during sex is one way, so long as the "latex protective gear" covers the area which sheds the virus. Those with sores on the genitals should avoid sex, and those with oral sores should not have oral sex. Even if there are no symptoms, HSV-2 infection is very contagious.

2. Since those with a history of sexually transmitted diseases (STD) are more likely to have genital herpes, ask your partner as delicately and as sensitively as possible if he/she has ever had STD. It can be an awkward situation, but it is most important for the partners to be honest with one another.

3. Sexual history is important because those with multiple partners are more likely to have the infection, albeit without obvious sores or symptoms. Limiting the number of sexual partners is essential.

4. Do not have sex with a person who has sores on the genitals.

5. Abstain from receiving oral sex from someone with sores on the mouth.

6. Illicit drugs and/or alcohol impair judgment, so do not have sex while intoxicated.

7. To reduce STD, sex therapists recommend mutual masturbation (avoiding genital-genital or oral-genital contact) for those who want a safer form of sexual intimacy, until the individual finds a life partner and live a clean, monogamous life.

A comedian once said, "The difference between love and herpes is that herpes is forever." HSV infection is indeed a life-long condition that does not have a cure. It comes and goes. It is best to avoid HSV.

Pills vs. Surgery for GERD

Good news for those with gastro-esophageal reflux disease. A recent open, parallel-group, multicenter randomized controlled study in Sweden (LOTUS—Long-Term Usage of Acid Suppression Versus Antireflux Surgery) showed that drug (Esomeprazole) is equally effective, if not more, than surgery for reflux, according to the September 2008 issue of *GUT*.

What is reflux/heartburn?

Reflux heartburns is a milder stage of reflux esophagitis, which is an inflammatory condition where hydrocholoric acid, normally produced by the stomach to aid in the digestion of food, regurgitates (goes back up) to the lower end of the esophagus (food pipe) which is connected to the stomach. In most cases, the lower esophageal sphincter ("valve") is incompetent (loose) and allows stomach acid and food to back up to the esophagus, a disease medically known as gastroesophageal reflux disease (GERD).

Why is acid reflux bad?

The stomach mucosa (lining) normally produces the digestive acid and tolerates it much better than the esophagus does, which has a different cell lining that is less resistant to the acid. Reflux of stomach acid into the lower end of the esophagus, therefore, causes esophagitis (irritation, inflammation, swelling, ulceration), which, if allowed to continue untreated, could cause esophageal stricture (scarring) and narrowing, making the channel connecting the food pipe to the stomach too small for food to pass through.

Is this condition common?

Yes, very common. Most patients complain of burning discomfort in the pit of the stomach after meals or at night, while lying down, allowing stomach acid to flow back to the esophagus. Many times the burning disappears when the person gets up. The symptom could also be that of indigestion or "sour stomach." People who take antacids, like Alka-Seltzer, Maalox, Tums, etc., could have GERD.

What are the possible complications of GERD?

Uncomplicated gastroesophageal reflux responds well to medical therapy and may be tolerated for many years. However, some people on treatment may still develop complications, like esophagitis, esophageal ulcer, hemorrhage, esophageal stricture, and Barrett's metaplasia (cell changes in the esophagus that could transform to cancer).

What is the first step treatment of GERD?

The initial management of patients with persisting symptoms of GERD consists of (1) changing diet (avoiding spices, caffeine, chocolate, alcohol, cola drinks); (2) quitting cigarette smoking; (3) avoiding tight, binding clothing, especially after a meal; (4) refraining from lying down immediately after a meal and elevating the head of the bed when lying down to keep gastric acid and contents in the stomach by gravity; and (5) taking medication like esomeprazole under the close supervision of your physician.

Is surgery for GERD passé?

While these promising findings from the clinical research at the Karolinska University Hospital in Huddinge, Sweden, and its partners in the other dedicated centers in 11 European countries show that GERD responds very well to medical treatment, with even lesser post-op residual symptoms than those treated with surgery (laparoscopic anti-reflux surgery, LARS, fundoplication), surgery still has a role in managing resistant cases and those with complications of chronic GERD.

What is the final verdict?

In consonance with a caveat in medicine, positive findings like this one will have to be confirmed and reconfirmed by other clinical studies before it becomes accepted as a standard convention in medical practice.

As for this wonderful news about the preference today for pills instead of surgery, for GERD, these cohort studies are significant enough to warrant further clinical application by the physicians, since H2 blocker (acid pump inhibitor) drugs are presently an integral part of the management for GERD anyway. Any new treatment where drugs are found to be equal to, or better than, surgery is a boon to medical therapeutics, a preferred regimen and, obviously, better for all of us.

Gastric ulcer used to be a surgical disease, where an operation (to cut a part of the stomach out) was necessary to manage the condition. Today, thanks to the progress in science, it is a medical disease, where effective modern drugs are the accepted mainstay of therapy. Tuberculosis used to kill millions by spreading like wild cancer, destroying most organs in the body, the lungs, bones, brain, liver, kidneys, spleen, etc., literally acting like cancer. Today, majority of TB is cured by medications alone.

As an eternal optimist and a physician who has great faith in medical science, I look forward to the day when cancers could be cured by medications or, better yet, prevented by a healthy lifestyle plus a vaccine. That day will surely come, and hopefully, for the sake of mankind, it would be soon.

GI Endoscopy

Endoscopy is a medical procedure where the gastroenterologist (specialist in diseases of the food pipe, stomach, and intestines) inserts through the mouth a thin, flexible, lighted, fiberoptic tube with a mini TV camera (for direct viewing by the physician performing the test, or displaying the color video image on a TV screen) into the esophagus (foodpipe), stomach, and (usually the duodenum, the first part of the) small intestines to do what is known as UGI (upper gastrointestinal) endoscopy. The same examination done through the rectum to view the rectum and the colon (large intestine) is called LGI (lower gastrointestinal) endoscopy. Besides being an outpatient diagnostic procedure, endoscopy could also be therapeutic (a treatment), like excision of polyps or removal of a foreign body, cauterizing to stop a small bleeder, etc.

Historical records show that it was Aranzi, in 1585, who first used a light source for an endoscopic procedure; but technically, it was Hippocrates, the Father of Medicine, who lived 400 years before the birth of Christ (born in 460 B.C., died in 377 B.C.), who first performed an endoscopic procedure where he inserted a speculum to examine the rectum. That was the exact principle and concept of endoscopy, which advances in technology today have impressively refined to its current state of awesome sophistication.

Endoscopy is done to examine and view the inner lining of the entire upper and lower gastrointestinal (digestive) tract for possible cancer, polyps, ulcers, bleeding, diverticulum (outpouching), hiatal hernia, varices, etc. The UGI endoscopy also frequently detects signs of GERD (gastroesophageal reflux disease), a very common condition where the acid from the stomach "regurgitates" upward to the lower end of the esophagus, causing esophagitis (inflammation of the foodpipe) and symptoms of heartburns. This test also checks for Barrett's esophagus, a condition that increases the risk of the development of esophageal cancer. Cancer of the GI tract is one of the commonest fears why these two procedures are very popular and frequently performed.

This prevalence of stomach cancer varies among countries and by sex. Per 100,000 Japanese population, for example, it is about 80 men and 30 women; white American men, 11; white American women, 7; British men, 18; and British women, 10. There has been an impressive decline in incidence in North America, New Zealand, and Australia since 1930; but the reduction has been slower in Europe. The incidence also seems higher among those with Type A blood. In the USA, cancer of the stomach is relatively more common among Japanese American and Hispanic groups. The death rate in the USA for gastric cancer is between 14,000 and 15,000 a year. Sixty to 70 cases of these are men.

Besides the routine practice, prophylactic colonoscopy is recommended for those with FAP (familiar adenomatous polyposis) of the colon. Upper GI endoscopy, also called esophagogastrocopy, is recommended for those with UGI symptoms, unexplained anemia, a history of UGI disease, or even for individuals with a history of FAP of the colon.

We are luckier in this era of advanced and sophisticated medical science compared to the generations before us. All we have to do is to take advantage of these state-of-the-art and cutting-edge healthcare technology that modern medicine offers.

Ginseng: Sex Aid?

What is ginseng?

Panax ginseng, or ginseng for short, as it is popularly known, comes from Asian plant roots that have been used for its "medicinal" value for more than 2,000 years in China. Literally, the word *ginseng* in Chinese means "man-root." Asian Ginseng in English is *Panax ginseng*, and the American ginseng is *Panax quinquefolius*. Since the word *panax* means "panacea," this has led to a lot of confusion and misunderstanding. While some quarters report it as a miracle "cure-all" panacea, official Chinese publications on herbal therapeutics do not make such a claim at all.

What is the main element in ginseng?

The active ingredients in ginseng are saponins called gensinosides. There are at least 19 of them, and to date, scientists still do not know which of them are the essential ones that have the beneficial pharmacologic value. Ginseng reportedly contains vitamins, minerals, insulin-like protein called maltol, which is also claimed to be antiaging. At the recommended dose, ginseng is a central nervous system stimulant, but at high doses it acts as a sedative.

Is ginseng an aphrodisiac?

Contrary to popular belief, ginseng is not an aphrodisiac (a substance that induces or stimulates sexual desire). It is supposed to increase energy and improve the general health of the person taking it, which could indirectly improve overall performance in any activity. This was why Chinese traditional armamentarium has ginseng as a "treatment" for sexual dysfunction.

Can ginseng really help sexual dysfunction?

Probably yes. Investigators at Hamilton's McMaster University have scientifically shown that ginseng contains chemicals that are vasodilators (they open up arteries and veins, resulting in improved blood flow to all parts of the body, including the pelvic region and sexual organs). Congestion in these areas is associated with sexual arousal.

Is ginseng as potent as the ED drugs?

No. Erectile Dysfunction drugs, such as Viagra (scientifically known as sildenafil citrate) is 100% more potent and more predictable in its effectiveness than ginseng.

Can ginseng be taken safely with Vitamins?

Taking ginseng, together with vitamins and minerals, has been practiced for decades by millions of people around the world and appeared to be safe. There are even preparations now that are marketed as a combination capsules.

Is ginseng harmful or toxic?

In itself, ginseng, in recommended dose, has not been found to be toxic or harmful. If ingested in excess of the recommended dose (not more than 2 Grams a day), the most common side effect is mild diarrhea, high blood pressure, insomnia, and nervousness. However, American ginseng capsules, which are processed products and not 100% ginseng, contain preservatives, stimulants, filters, and other unidentified substances, which could be harmful.

What is ginseng claimed to do?

Ginseng is believed to alleviate exhaustion, fatigue, amnesia, headaches, and the debility of aging, acting as an antioxidant, neutralizing free radicals in the body, and therefore allowing natural cell repair and self-healing. Some studies also revealed that ginseng reduces platelet adhesiveness, making blood thinner, thus helping prevent blood clots. There are many laboratory studies done on ginseng, and some medical reports have shown this substance does have some beneficial medicinal value. One thing that is also comforting is the finding that ginseng has not shown serious adverse side effects. As with any medications or the so-called "food supplements," they are the short-term and long-term serious side effects that one should always be concerned about.

What is "GAS"?

Ginseng abuse syndrome (GAS) is a condition resulting from a combination of a large dose of ginseng (up to 15 grams a day) and a lot of caffeine (coffee). This syndrome was first reported by Siegel in 1979, characterized by elevated blood pressure, insomnia, anxiety, nervousness, skin rashes, and diarrhea in 105 of the 133 Ginseng users in his study. Manufacturers recommended dose is 1.5 Grams to 2 Grams per day in divided doses. Those taking ginseng should cut back on their caffeine (coffee, cola drink) intake. Most commercial preparations of ginseng in the market only have insignificant traces of ginseng in them.

Glaucoma and Blindness

Our guest glaucoma expert for this column today is Emily Chua Greenlee, MD, Clinical Assistant Professor of Ophthalmology, University of Iowa Department of Ophthalmology and Visual Sciences, and director of the Glaucoma Service at the Iowa City Veterans Administration Medical Center, who provided us vital information about this dreaded visual malady.

Next to cancer and heart disease, blindness ranks third as a major fear among people. Everyone is possibly at risk for glaucoma. One in 30,000 babies in the United States is born with this condition, and about 120,000 Americans are blind from glaucoma, roughly 10.5% of all blindness. Only half of the 2 million Americans with glaucoma know they have it. According to the World Health Organization, this eye disease is the second most common causes of blindness in the world. There are about 65 million people with glaucoma worldwide.

What is glaucoma?

Glaucoma is a disease of the optic nerve (optic neuropathy). Damage to the optic nerve leads to vision loss. This loss tends to be peripheral (side vision), which is why people tend not to notice it until it is very advanced. Vision loss can also be central. People with central vision loss come to medical attention much earlier because they notice their vision problem.

What causes optic nerve damage?

The optic nerve may be damaged by various causes. These are called optic neuropathies. The causes may be due to a lack of blood flow (ischemic optic neuropathy), inflammation (optic neuritis), infection, trauma (traumatic optic neuropathy), and toxic/metabolic causes. Glaucoma is one type of optic neuropathy.

Are there different types of glaucoma?

Yes. The main two types of glaucoma are open-angle and closed-angle glaucoma. These terms refer to the drainage angle of the eye which is located at the juncture of the cornea and iris. A person with glaucoma does not effectively drain this fluid (aqueous humor) from the eye.

In open-angle glaucoma, the angle is visualized to be open; but for some reason, it is not draining aqueous humor effectively. This could be due to a problem with the angle. It could be ineffective from genetics, trauma, or something blocking the angle, such as blood or pigment.

In closed-angle glaucoma, the angle is blocked by the iris being pushed forward. This tends to happen in people with smaller eyes (farsightedness) or those developing cataracts. A cataract is the lens of the eye which becomes cloudy over time. As it progresses, it becomes thicker; and since it is located behind the iris, it can eventually block the drainage angle. Treatment is based on the type of glaucoma.

What are the signs and symptoms?

Usually, there are no signs and symptoms in open-angle glaucoma until vision loss becomes advanced. This is the reason why it is prudent to have a regular eye exam, especially among those 40 and over. Early diagnosis is essential to prevent optic nerve damage and blindness. Closed-angle glaucoma may present much more dramatically with sudden decreased vision and eye pain due to the sudden rise in intraocular pressure.

Who gets glaucoma?

The following are risk factors for open-angle glaucomas:

1.) Genetics plays a part. Patients with a family history of glaucoma are at risk for developing the disease.

2.) African descent. People of African descent are more likely to develop glaucoma and have more severe disease, which is harder to treat.

3.) High eye pressure (intraocular pressure, IOP). Those with a high eye pressure are at risk for developing glaucoma. Most people without glaucoma have eye pressures < or = 21 mmHg. A high intraocular pressure is only a risk factor for glaucoma but is not required for the disease.

4.) Age > 40. As people age, the likelihood that they will develop glaucoma increases. Although there are some congenital (present at birth) and juvenile forms of glaucoma, most cases are adult.

5.) Thin corneas. The clear front part of the eye, or cornea, is what is touched when eye pressure measurements are made. If this is unusually thin, it may be easier to push against which creates an artificially low eye pressure reading.

The following are risk factors for closed-angle glaucomas:

1.) Hyperopia (farsightedness). People who are farsighted, or hyperopic, tend to have smaller eyes which puts them at risk for angle-closure.

2.) Age. As people age, their lenses of their eyes tend to develop into a cataract. As the cataract matures and thickens, it can cause angle-closure.

3.) Asian descent. Asians tend to have smaller eyes with the possibility of developing closed-angle glaucoma.

4.) Women. Women also tend to have smaller eyes, which predisposes them to this type of glaucoma.

What is the treatment for glaucoma?

Treatments for open-angle glaucomas aim toward lowering eye pressure since high eye pressure is a risk factor for the development of glaucoma. Numerous eye medications exist which lower the eye pressure by either lowering aqueous humor formation or facilitating its outflow from the eye. In addition, laser (Argon laser trabeculoplasty, selective trabeculoplasty) or incisional surgery (trabeculectomy, glaucoma drainage implantation) may be performed to increase aqueous outflow and lower eye pressure.

The treatment for closed-angle glaucoma is different, however. In this case, the treatment is aimed toward relieving the blockage of aqueous outflow. A laser procedure is performed, which creates a small hole in the iris. This allows aqueous to come forward and prevents it from pushing the iris into the drainage angle. This laser procedure is called a laser peripheral iridotomy (LPI).

While there is no cure for glaucoma, it is essential that it be treated to prevent loss of vision.

Is Glutathione Safe?

The glutathione craze seems to have spread around the world, inspired mostly by women's desire for a fairer complexion and people's quest for the fountain of health and youth.

Knowing that any substance or drug we use, including "simple" aspirin, is associated with possible adverse side effects, the concern about the safety of long-term use of glutathione comes into question.

What is glutathione?

Popularly known as GSH and nicknamed glute, this substance is a protein (a tripeptide) made up of three amino acids: cysteine, glutamic acid, and glycine. It is normally produced by our body and found inside every cell in our body, including the cells of the immune system. GSH is a detoxifying agent, an essential scavenger and neutralizer of the bad free oxygen radicals and peroxides that destroy cells. Our body glutathione is really a potent antioxidant that enables the cells to maintain intracellular health and also helps repair damaged DNA.

Which foods contain glutathione?

This substance is found in fresh fruits, vegetables, walnuts, fish, and freshly prepared meats. Dr. Dean Jones, PhD, professor of biochemistry and director of nutritional health sciences at Emory University, stated that people who eat well probably have enough glutathione from their diet. Under normal situation and in general, there is really no need for any glutathione or any other food supplement.

What conditions can lower GSH?

Low levels or deficiency in glutathione have been seen in people with diabetes, high blood pressure, HIV/AIDS, low sperm count, cataracts, among smokers and those with cancer. However, most of these individuals, except those who are unable to eat properly and are emaciated because of their illness, will still not have glutathione deficiency.

Who, then, should take glutathione supplements?

Scientifically speaking, only those with proven glutathione deficiency by blood test should receive glutathione supplement. Oral glutathione pills are destroyed by gastric juices in the stomach and are not absorbed. Hence, the pill form of glutathione is useless. This substance can also be given by intravenous injection. It also comes in aerosol nasal spray, but its effectiveness and the practicality of its application in adequately boosting the blood level of glutathione for those with deficiency is still uncertain.

What happens if GSH is used by healthy persons?

Healthy people, with no evidence of deficiency of glutathione, as we intimated earlier, do not need glutathione supplement. The glutathione derived from food will, as a rule, be enough for them to maintain healthy cells, unless they abuse themselves by smoking, excessive alcohol intake, using illegal drugs, etc. When healthy individuals use glutathione anyway, intravenously or by nasal aerosol, their body will not have any added protection or benefit. They will just be wasting money and subjecting themselves to yet undefined potential health risks associated with long-term use of the exogenous (laboratory-produced) glutathione.

Are GSH whitening skin cream safe?

In the market today, there are dozens of bleaching or whitening products for the skin. One of them is glutathione facial cream/lotion, and the others are facial soaps with glutathione as bleaching/whitening agent. While anything substance applied to the skin is absorbed by the body into the bloodstream (like dermal medication patches), we have not found any information on the adverse side effects of GSH in these cosmetics for the skin. People allergic to milk protein and organ transplant patients are advised against using any form of glutathione.

How does GSH whiten the skin?

One side effect of topically (locally) applied glutathione as a cosmetic slows down the production of melanin (a protein manufactured by melanocytes in our skin that gives the skin the brown color), and as a result, there will be less melanin pigment and the skin becomes whiter. While this particular side effect of topical glutathione on the complexion is good, factual information is not available on the safety of chronic use of glutathione, even as a skin bleaching agent.

Does GSH cure autism, Parkinson's, or cancer?

Commercial ads claim glutathione is effective in the treatment and cure of autism, Alzheimer's, male infertility, Parkinson's, and even cancer. Unfortunately, there is no scientific evidence to support these claims. Some people consider GSH and the other cure-all "food supplements" as scams and the snake oils of the present.

Does GSH have any role in cancer therapy?

There is no scientific evidence that glutathione prevents, cures, or aggravates any form of cancer. In one study it was observed that women with ovarian cancer who were undergoing chemotherapy, "those given the glutathione (intravenously) not only had fewer side effects from the chemotherapy but also had better overall survival rates."

Are drug makers liable for adverse effects of their products?

Unless it can be proven that the drug manufacturer had lied to, or hid vital safety information from the US Food and Drug Administration when it applied for the drug approval and patent, or neglected to appropriately apprise the US-FDA of any life—or health-threatening complications caused by the drug after its wide circulation and clinical use, the manufacturer, in general, cannot be held legally liable for the side-effects of its product.

As long as the company acted in earnest, in good faith, and had complied with all the rules, regulations, and stringent criteria of the US-FDA, it is may not be held liable. This is especially true when the manufacturer voluntarily withdraws the drug from the market upon discovery of the danger. In reality, though, more often than not, the issue becomes convoluted and much more complex as greedy ambulance chasers come to the picture. This is especially common in large cities in the United States, where lawyers advertise on giant billboards and on TV commercials egging people on to sue healthcare providers for drug or surgical complications, "totally free legal service if you lose."

A time-honored sage advice perhaps older than civilization itself: *caveat emptor*! Let the buyer beware!

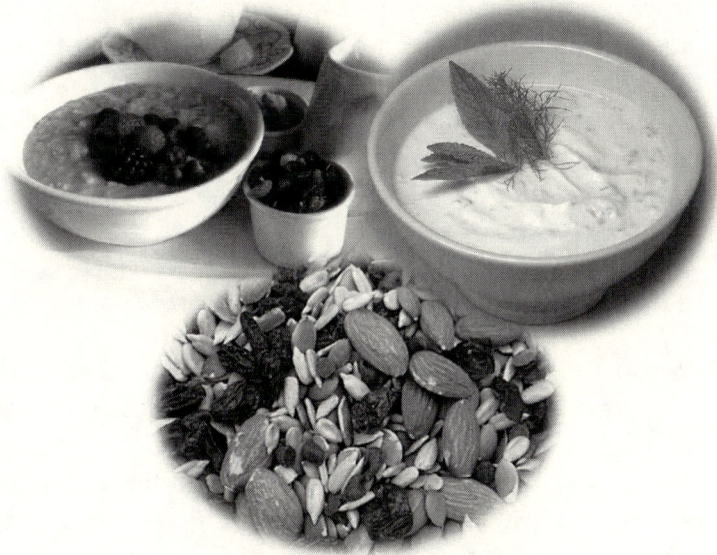

Oatmeal, yogurt and nuts are wholesome ingredients in our diet.

14 Ways to Good Health

1. Less Alcohol, More Tea

Alcohol is the cause of more than one-third of all the illnesses known to man, directly or indirectly, including some forms of cancer. Tea, on the other hand, especially the green variety, is a well-known antioxidant that is good for the body in more ways than one.

2. Less Meat, More Vegetables

Red meat (pork, beef, etc.), like the yellow yolk of the egg, is high in saturated fats and cholesterol. The medical literature is replete with countless studies that prove saturated fats and cholesterol are the prime causes of arteriosclerosis (hardening of the arteries) that lead to arterial blockages, heart attack, and stroke and even cancers, like cancer of the colon. Vegetables, on the other hand, contain phytochemical antioxidants that protect the cellular structures of the body, strengthen our immune system, not to mention providing the fiber and roughage our gastrointestinal system needs to ward of cancer of the colon. Vegetarians, in general, have lower risks of developing heart attack, stroke, and cancer.

3. Less Salt, More Vinegar

We eat too much salt today. And excess salt raises our blood pressure and causes our body to swell up, inside and outside, no matter how subtle or undetectable this may be. Low-salt diet, in general, is good for us. Before putting the salt-shaker into action, taste the food first. Chances are we do not need more salt. And easy on the salty condiments also. The impact of excess salt on our cardiovascular system is adverse, even if we are healthy. You can imagine what it does to those with high blood pressure and other cardiovascular diseases. Vinegar is a better alternative to salt, if the salt substitute (potassium) does not appeal to you. Vinegar also prevents spikes (the sudden rise and fluctuation) of blood insulin and glucose level after a meal, even among healthy people, and more so among diabetics. Vinegar itself, or as a salad dressing (oil and vinegar) or even in pickled vegetables, have been found to help in weight reduction, besides in diabetes control.

4. Less Sugar, More Fresh Fruit

Low carbohydrate diet is in, for better health. Less sugar, less sweets (candies, ice cream, rice, bread, cakes, etc.) is better. This is medically proven. Most of our food and food products, which basically contain protein and vegetables, also have carbohydrates in them. So eating meals with two only tablespoon full of rice, or even without rice, is healthier for us. The more carbs we eat, the greater the chances of gaining weight and developing diabetes. Fresh fruits provide fructose, the healthier form of sugar, and also give us fiber, which is beneficial to our colon in the prevention of GI diseases, like cancers. Diabetics will have to consult with their physician/dietician when adding fruits to their diabetic diet regimen.

5. Less Eating, More Chewing

Most of us eat more than we should. My former mentor in medical school told us her "secret" for health and longevity: "Push yourself away from the table a little less than full." This might sound overly simplistic or even impertinent, but she is right. Medical science has shown that people in general today eat more than what the body needs to stay healthy and that eating less than what we consider "enough" is healthier. We really eat too much. This is why there are more than 18.2 million Americans who are diabetics. Chewing the food well is also healthier than gobbling the food down in a hurry. Drinking a lot of water before each meal, or while eating, is also a great way to control our appetite and our weight.

6. Less Couch, More Exercise

A couch potato "addict" holding the remote control, watching the television, munching on carbos is a most likely target for obesity, diabetes, hypertension, heart attack, and stroke. The human body was made to be physically active for better performance and efficiency in the maintenance of good health and well-being. The more exercise we reasonably do daily, starting from our teenage years, the better is our health. This explains why athletes, in general, are well-conditioned, fit, and healthy, even when they reach their 80s and 90s.

The following are the additional 8 simplified ways to good health, which are not only philosophical but scientifically proven to be medically sound in the successful pursuit of physical, mental, and emotional health:

7. Less Driving, More Walking

8. Less Words, More Action

9. Less Greed, More Giving

10. Less Politics, More Religion

11. Less Worry, More Sleep

12. Less Frown, More Smiles

13. Less Crying, More Laughter

14. Less Anger, More Love

Gout—Foods to Avoid

What is gout?

Gout is a condition where there is abnormally high level of uric acid in the blood caused by the kidneys' failure to excrete uric acid through the urine efficiently. Uric acid is derived from purine, which comes from food and also produced by the body. This diminished ability results in the accumulation of very high level of uric acid in the blood. This then induces uric acid crystal formation in the kidneys and in the joints, resulting in kidney stones and painful inflamed gouty joints.

How common is gout?

Gout is very common, affecting more men than women. Among men, the first attack of gout usually happens between the ages of 30 and 50, while in women, it is usually after menopause. Twenty 20% of gout is familial. Gout is common among Pacific Islanders and affects about 1% of people in western countries.

What foods are rich in purine?

Meat and meat products—fatty foods in general—contain high levels of purine. These include pork, beef, and other red meats, poultry skin, liver, tripe, kidneys, and even fish skin. Canned sardines, salmon, tuna, mackerel, shellfish (shrimps, mussels, crabs, etc.), chocolate, cocoa, cola drinks, herrings, anchovies, scallops, fish roe are likewise high in purine. Sweets increases uric acid level also. On the other hand, vegetables, vitamins B and C, and cherries are good for people with gout. Chicken, minus the skin, and fishes other than those mentioned above, are likewise suitable.

What is the goal of therapy?

The fundamental objective of the treatment is to lower (normalize, as much as possible) the level of purine in the blood to minimize acute gouty arthritis (inflammation of the joints), chronic gouty pains, and the disability gout can cause. Prevention is the key, the first step in the management of gout, and complemented with prescription medications as needed. The way to prevent the level of purine in the blood from rising to an abnormal level is by avoiding purine-rich foods.

Is alcohol allowed?

Gout patients, in particular, should abstain from alcohol, especially beer. Alcohol dehydrates the body, making the level or uric acid higher and more concentrated. Alcoholic beverage also stimulates the body to produce more uric acid. On top of this, alcohol further diminishes the ability of the kidneys to excrete uric acid. Red meats, alcohol, and cigarettes are poisons for persons with gout or tendency toward gout.

How about fasting?

Fasting is bad for gout because it leads to an abnormally fast metabolism of fat cells, which produces ketone bodies that inhibit excretion of uric acid. On the other hand, the opposite is also true: feasting and gluttony can result in gout attacks.

What are some general dietary tips?

The standard regimen for patients with gout includes avoiding red meat, meat products, all fatty foods, shellfish, and other purine-rich foods listed above and drinking 8 or more glasses of unsweetened and nonalcoholic liquid, preferably water, daily. The total calories from daily meals may be divided into small frequent (5 or 6 times) a day. A lot of vegetables and a helping of fruits (except for diabetics) are beneficial. If overweight, the person should control the calorie intake and do daily exercises until the goal is reached. Diet and eating habit changes are a fundamental part of the therapy, but not a substitute for competent medical care.

H. pylori Infection

What is *Helicobacter pylori*?

Helicobacter pylori, or *H. pylori*, is a bacterium found in the stomach which is the commonest cause of chronic gastritis (inflammation of the stomach), stomach and duodenal (small intestine) ulcerations, and implicated in the development of B-cell gastric lymphoma and distal gastric cancer.

Aren't ulcers caused by eating spicy foods?

Prior to the discovery of the *Helicobacter pylori*, conventional medical thinking was that stomach and small intestinal ulcers were caused by hyperacidity (increased hydrochloric acid production) in the stomach, precipitated by ingestion of spicy foods, alcohol, coffee, and other items (like some medications) that led to hyperacidity. Medical science has since proven that gastritis and peptic ulcers "are not a chemical disease," but a bacterial infection . . . with H. pylori. This discovery led to a revolution in the overall treatment of chronic gastritis and gastroduodenal ulcerations, which has resulted in more effective and faster cures.

Who discovered this "new" bug?

J. Robin Warren, a pathologist from Perth, Australia, who made the initial observation, and Barry J. Marshall, a young clinical fellow, collaborated in the clinical studies that proved Warren's theory as correct. The story goes that when they first proposed the theory, they were the laughing stock of the medical community and were mocked and ridiculed at meetings because "their theory that peptic ulcer disease was caused by a bacterial infection was absurd and preposterous." Subsequent independent clinical studies all over the world eventually confirmed their findings. In 2005, they were awarded the Nobel Prize in Physiology or Medicine, "for their prepared mind and tenacity to challenge the prevailing dogmas."

When does the infection start?

This *H. pylori* infection is usually acquired in childhood, without any obvious symptoms, or may present as mild stomach discomfort. The infection persists as the child grows. In most cases, the symptoms become more manifest in adulthood.

How prevalent is the infection?

The incidence varies in well-developed countries according to year of birth and social class. Among persons born before 1950, the prevalence is much higher (50-80%), compared to those born after that year where it is less than 20%. In poorer nations, the *H. pylori* infection rate is about 80-95% regardless of year of birth. Those who did not get the infection as a child usually do not get it later in life.

What are the risk factors?

Poverty during childhood is one of the main risk factors, especially overcrowded conditions and poor hygienic practices. These result in greater transmission and higher incidence. Reinfection in adults is very low, lower than 1% per year.

What are the symptoms of HPI?

Frequent stomach discomfort or pains, or sense of indigestion, are most common. When severe, there could be nausea or even actual vomiting. Many have symptoms of varying degrees that are persistent for years, some of them so mild and nonspecific as to be considered as indigestion. When gastric or duodenal ulcers form and they bleed, anemia (low blood count) and black tarry stools will be present. Fortunately uncommon, there could be perforation (deep ulcer becoming a hole in the stomach) and massive bleeding, among the neglected cases.

What are the diagnostic tests?

C13 urea breath test, stool antigen, and serology are tests for HPI. Serology is an indirect way of detecting *H. pylori* bacteria. The more accurate one is the C13 urea breath test, with sensitivity and specificity higher than 95% and diagnostic of an active infection, unlike serology which is not that accurate and diagnostic. In some centers, stool antigen tests are now available, which are as good as the C13 urea breath test.

How about endoscopy?

Gastroendoscopy is an examination, where a thin, flexible, lighted telescope (about 4 to 5 millimeter in diameter) with a camera at the tip, connected to a viewing monitor, is introduced through the mouth and advanced to the stomach to directly view its mucosa (inner wall) looking for any inflammation, ulceration, tumor, or any other abnormality. It is also used to collect specimen and gastric juice for laboratory examination, including culture for *H. pylori* and other bacteria to aid in the diagnosis. Endoscopy should never be delayed in patients at risk of cancer.

What is the treatment for HPI?

Before the discovery of HPI, gastrectomy (surgical removal of a part of the stomach to treat peptic ulcers) was very common. Today, it is done infrequently, only for the complicated ones. Medical therapy has taken over. The so-called quadruple (drug) therapy has been found on randomized clinical trials (outcomes study) to be no more effective than the triple regimen. The systemic review showed that "a triple regimen of metronidazole plus clarithromycin plus ranitidine bismuth increased eradication at 5-7 days compared with a triple regimen containing amoxicillin plus clarithromycin plus ranitidine bismuth." The attending physician can modify, "custom-tailor" and titrate the regimen according to his findings and the patient's response to therapy.

What is the prognosis?

Around 15% of individuals with *H. pylori* infection will have peptic ulcer, and about 1% will end up with gastric cancer in their lifetime. In 16 studies in 1,625 persons showed that a higher incidence (41.7%)

of peptic ulcer among those taking nonsteroidal anti-inflammatory drugs (NSAID, for arthritis, etc.), when they also had *H. pylori* infection, compared to those who did not have it (25.9%). There is very limited evidence that the observational studies which claim that 60-90% of those with localized, low-grade B-cell lymphoma had regression following eradication of the *H. pylori* infection.

The discovery of *H. pylori* has most tremendously improved the outcomes in the management of peptic ulcer disease caused by HPI, benefiting millions of people around the world, by transforming a formerly surgical disease to a medical one, where drugs, instead of the scalpel, are now the accepted standard of care.

Health Trends in Homes

In a previous column, we cautioned the public about the risks lurking within our own homes, where at least a dozen toxic chemicals are found in the form of common household cleaning agents, deodorizers, carbon monoxide emission from our cars, and potential gas leaks.

Besides the chemical risks in our own homes, we also have bacteria, molds, spores, dust mites, animal dander, mildew, (bed bugs in some homes), pollen brought in from the outside, odors and smokes from our cooking, and cigarette smoke that pollute the air we breathe in. The synthetic materials used in our carpet, furniture upholstery, curtains, etc., also slowly "emit" chemicals that contaminate the air we breathe in.

Since we spend between 50% and 90% of our time at home, all these affect our health, especially those with asthma, allergy, or other forms of upper respiratory disease. In the case of allergy and asthma, the effect could be immediate and obvious; but the complications of chronic chemical exposures could take years before they show, like impairment of the immune system, metabolic illnesses, cancer, etc. Common sense tells me that anything that is poison to our body when swallowed should be toxic to our health when inhaled.

To preclude the need for donning on a decontamination suit before we enter our home to protect ourselves, new concepts in future home building to address the health issues we raised above are being explored. This will be a super high-tech home building design, incorporating "protective" materials and gadgets to build and maintain healthy and safer homes.

One of the pioneers in this new technology and trend in future home design and construction is a company called Battelle. The Battelle scientists and researchers have cited the top ten trends in healthy homes for this year, in the following excerpts, in their sequence of importance:

Indoor Air Quality—What you're likely to see on the market and in homes are products for advanced air venting, air filtration, and biosensors that help fight humidity, mold, and other indoor pollutants.

Home-based Medical Monitoring, Diagnosis, and Care—Healthy lifestyles and disease prevention have never been more important than they are today. This will be easily achievable with the use of the Internet and wireless communications with attending physicians, nurses, and clinics. Rising medical costs and the health care industry's increasing reliance on home-based care and outpatient procedures will go far toward making this a reality.

Monitoring-Sensing for Home Safety and Personal Protection—Ever wonder if you left the iron on or forgot to close a window? Or if a water pipe has burst while you're on vacation? People often worry about their homes when they're not there. Those worries will be easily put to rest with remote home-security monitoring through home sensors and cameras that can transmit pictures and information to you via the Internet and other wireless devices. Computers can be trained with data and software to match the correct home motions with disruptions to normal activity. Members of the "Sandwich Generation" also will welcome these monitors in their efforts to care for children, the elderly, and the ill. Affordable biosensors also will be able to alert you to the presence of potentially harmful bacteria and viruses.

Absolutely Reliable and High Quality Power—What's the answer to this dilemma? Home power generators, especially highly efficient microturbines and engines that run on natural gas. Fuel cells also are a solution that will grow in popularity over the next decade. Equipment that generates both heat and electricity—known as microcombined heating and power—is already used in Europe and is likely to be popular in the United States.

Whole-house Water Quality—Pure water has become important to most people—witness the $22 billion bottled water industry and the interest in faucet filters. When the public water system is accidentally compromised by *E. coli* or cryptosporidium, people can become seriously ill and die. In the future, homes will have whole-house water safety systems—new appliances not yet developed—to supply the best water for all home uses.

Food Quality and Safe Handling, Storing, and Cooking—The risks involved with eating these days can be scary. Households will shift back to traditional, tasty, and high-quality foods that can be prepared quickly. Food safety comes to the forefront, and homes are likely to have tools for the detection of bacteria in food and water. Waving a wand over your countertop or cutting board will tell you if you have removed bacteria from uncooked meats. Foods of the future also may be engineered to have disease-preventing qualities.

The Baby Boomer Don't Want to Get Old—The health and grooming-conscious baby boomer generation of 78 million people is a built-in market for healthy home products and services. Witness the popularity of home gymnasiums, teeth-whitening home treatment kits, and antiaging skin creams. It's probably not too far-fetched to predict that if there is a way for baby boomers to perform minor plastic surgery at home, they'll do it.

Battling Mites and Molds in Bedding, Furnitures and Carpets—These buggers are hard to get rid of and increasingly are being blamed for a host of different major allergies. Researchers today are exploring the ways to kill mites using light and to fight mold by reducing humidity. This work will be stepped up in the coming years as the government and companies declare war against mites and mold.

Drudgery-free Housecleaning?—Super products and services can make the crucial difference in the hygiene of a home. Some of those might include a single cleanser for all surfaces and one appliance that will clean all fabrics. Laundry time may be greatly reduced with machines that might wash and dry in the same appliance.

Sterile Surfaces—Germ-resistant Materials, Coatings, and Fabrics—Homeowners are looking for new cleansers that provide lasting protection on kitchen and bathroom surfaces. This protection from disease-causing microorganisms might be built into surfaces with disinfectant treatment and materials.

An exciting future awaits all of us!

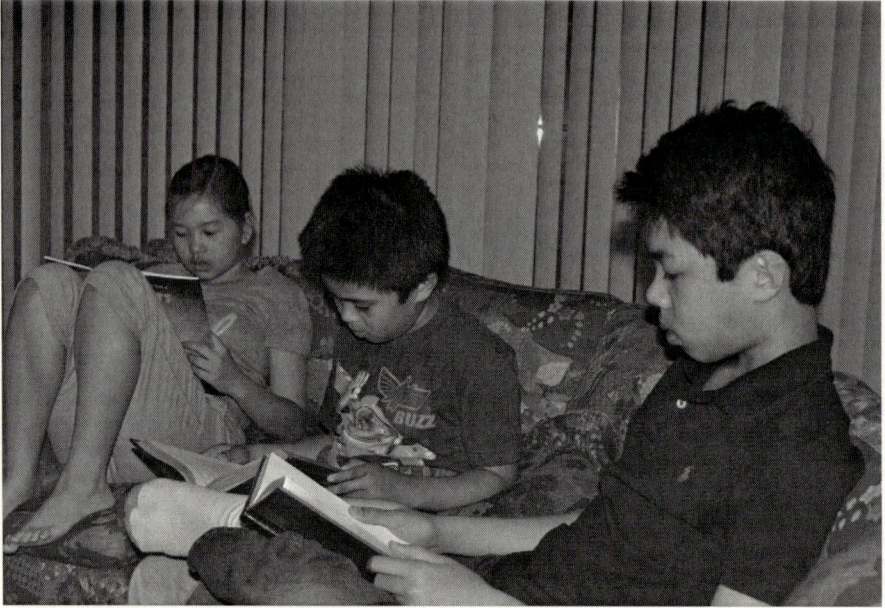

Research shows that the rate of drop-outs, smoking, and drug use are dramatically lower among children who love to read and spend more time with books.

Are You at Risk?

One person dies of heart attack in the United States every 20 seconds; statistically 3 a minute; 4,320 a day; or 1,576,800 a year! Since 1900, heart attack has been the number one killer of man in the European and Asian countries as well. These deaths are included in the global statistics of about 60 million who die each year from various causes around the world.

The number of deaths (2007 study, USA) from the other leading causes are as follows: cancer: 562,875; stroke (cerebrovascular diseases): 135,952; chronic lower respiratory diseases: 127,924; accidents (unintentional injuries): 123,706; alzheimer's disease: 74,632; diabetes: 71,382; influenza and pneumonia: 52,717; nephritis, nephrotic syndrome, and nephrosis: 46,448; and septicemia: 34,828.

The highest death rates from heart attack are found in the Soviet Union, Romania, Poland, Bulgaria, Hungary, and Czechoslovakia. Those with the lowest death are Japan, France, Spain, Switzerland, and Canada.

Diseases that Increase the Risk

The incidence of disease risk factors found in a 2005-2006 study showed lack of physical exercise as the most major one, followed by overweight and others: inactivity-39.5%, obesity-33.9%, high blood pressure-30.5%, cigarette smoking (or exposure to second-hand smoke)-20.8%, high cholesterol-15.6%, and diabetes-10.1%.

Together with the family history of heart disease, those 6 risk factors listed above are the main ones. Added to these heart-attack "boosters" are the following: (1) lack of sleep, getting only 5-6 hours a night, doubles the risk; (2) stress at work causes the risk to go up by 40%, and unemployment leads to high blood pressure, elevated cholesterol and overweight; (3) psoriasis, a chronic skin condition that causes inflammation in the body, almost as damaging as smoking; (4) periodontal disease, bacterial infection of the gums doubles the risk of a fatal heart attack, and unfortunately about 75% of people have them without even knowing it; (5) preeclampsia (high blood pressure and protein in the urine among those pregnant) doubles the risk of heart attack later in life and increases the risk of developing diabetes by 70%. Male-pattern baldness is also tagged as an incidental risk factor.

The significance and actual effects of those conditions in their impact on the predisposition to heart attack will vary somewhat in their gravity according to the genetic predisposition of the individual. Example: cigarette smoking could be the most major risk factor, as high as 50% in some people, while obesity could be in others. But there is no question that daily physical exercise, even simple brisk walking, at least 5 days a week, can ward off coronary artery disease and heart attack by 50%. Those who do not exercise double their risk of heart attack, compared to those who do.

The cost of heart disease alone in the United States in 2010 was $316.4 billion, which included health care services, medications, and lost productivity and income.

The Cholesterol-lowering Statins

About 30 million Americans have high blood cholesterol and are on cholesterol-lowering drugs called statins, like Lipitor, Zocor, Crestor, which block a liver enzyme that helps produce cholesterol. It is so effective in most persons taking any of them that their bad cholesterol (LDL, or lower-density lipoprotein) goes down by an average of 40%. Statins are consistently useful in bringing down cholesterol levels to reduce heart attack, and they even lower the mortality rate among those who suffer one.

The side effects of statins are actually low. Among the 7.5% of individuals on statin who might develop muscle pains, mild memory problem, and numbness, these symptoms stop within a few days or weeks after they are off the drug. The great health benefits from statin outweigh these temporary possible side effects.

Not a Vaccine or a Panacea

People should realize, though, that statins or any other drugs used to lower the risk of coronary artery disease or actual heart attack are not a vaccine that will totally prevent heart attack or a miraculous "cure" for this cardiovascular disease and other CV conditions.

The medications we have today in the treatment of coronary artery disease and its ultimate end result called heart attack are not, in themselves, the magic therapy that will make coronary artery blockages and heart attack disappear.

The fundamental strategy must include, not only the work of the attending physician, but greater efforts on our part. Our role as a person wanting to maintain health and prevent diseases requires discipline, determination, and sacrifices.

How to Reduce the Risks

A healthy diet and a lifestyle conducive to health are our greatest weapons against cardiovascular and other illnesses. Our life is literally mostly in our hands. The choices are ours. Children should be appropriately guided by the adults, who are supposed to be more experienced and wiser.

For diet, a lot of fish and some seafoods, a ton of vegetables (especially the green and leafy ones) fresh fruits, nuts, high-fiber foods (beans, whole grain, bran, etc.) are recommended. In general, low-fat, low-cholesterol, low carb diet is healthier. Red meat, if eaten at all, should be lean, and poultry without skin, prepared without added trans fat or saturated fat. For dairy products, fat-free, low-fat or 1% fat are healthier. Cut back on carbohydrates (rice, bread, ice cream, candies, and other foods with added sugar), and stay away from soft drinks of any kind as these pop beverages (cola or uncola, with or without caffeine, regular or diet) all increase the risk for the development of metabolic syndrome (high blood, pressure, diabetes, heart attack, and possibly stroke).

Besides the quality (the kind or type of foods), quantity is essential to maintain or achieve the proper weight, so watch your portion closely. Read food labels for the calorie, salt, fat, cholesterol, protein contents. Total abstinence from tobacco and moderation in alcohol intake are a part of healthy lifestyle, together with daily disciplined physical exercises. Rest, relaxation, and embracing our faith to achieve inner peace are all vital in the overall scheme for the maintenance of our spiritual, mental, and physical health.

Know Your Heart

Heart, the symbol of love, of Valentine's Day, even of religious adoration, is always fascinating but still a mystery to most of us. The amazing facts about our most loyal and dedicated heart are mind-boggling and a constant source of wonderment. Winning hearts, stealing hearts, breaking hearts, and for us cardiac surgeons, mending hearts, are easier to understand and do than to comprehend fully the wonders of this hardworking, ceaselessly pumping, untiring, and unique muscle in our body.

How large is our heart?

The size of the adult heart is about the volume of two hands clasping each other, with the fingers intertwined. In children, it is the size of the kid's one fist. The heart is located, not to the left, as often thought of, but in the middle of your midchest, enclosed in its own compartment, an envelope called pericardial sac, and located between the left and right chest cavity, where the left and right lungs are, respectively. Its tip is pointed slightly to the left.

Does the heart ever rest?

The heart beats about an average of 70 beats per minute, 4,200 an hour or about 100,800 times in one day, roughly about 36 million times in a year. In an average lifespan, the human heart will beat about 2.5 billion times. But contrary to what seems obvious, the heart rests for a split second in between beats. This happens between contractions, when the heart relaxes to accept more oxygenated blood from the lungs, and prepares to pump blood out of its chambers again.

How powerful is the heart contraction?

The heart contraction is so powerful that it approximates the force one needs to give a tennis ball a hard and full squeeze with all your might. The cardiac muscles work twice as hard as the leg muscles of a person running full speed. The hydraulic force generated is necessary to propel rapidly the blood that circulates about 13 kilometers per minute, or 780 kilometers per hour, about four times the speed of the fastest racing car there is.

Will an isolated heart beat on its own?

The muscle of the heart is a specialized one that beats on its own (automaticity) and one that has its own rhythm (rhythmicity), even when cut off from the body and lying on a surface. The isolated heart in this situation will beat continuously until its own residual energy is used up, which is within about 4 minutes. It then ceases movement.

What is the normal heart rate?

This varies from individual to individual, depending on the age, condition of the body, and the health of the person. A well-conditioned athlete may have a heart rate of 35 a minute and feel great, but this rate would cause almost all of us, nonathletes, to feel faint and pass out, or in the very least, feel very dizzy and weak. On the average though, the normal resting rate (medically speaking) is from 60 to 100 beats per minute. Anything below 60 is called bradycardia (too slow heart rate) and a rate higher than 100 is tachycardia (too fast a heart rate). Among children the range is between 90 and 120 beats a minute.

How much blood does a person have?

The adult human body has about 5.6 liters (6 quarts) of blood in the circulation. These 6 quarts completes a full round of circulation throughout the body about every 20 seconds. The blood travels a total of about 19,000 kilometers (12,000 miles) in 24 hours, which is about four times the distance from California to New York, or roughly five times the air miles from San Francisco to Asia. About one million barrels of blood is pumped by the heart in an average life span, a volume enough to fill more than three super tankers.

Where does the blood go?

The blood pumped by the heart goes out through the ascending aorta, the largest artery in the body (about half the size of an average wrist) that is connected to the heart, and circulates through the various arterial branches and capillaries to the brain and to all other vital organs (liver, pancreas, kidneys, adrenals, intestines, sex organs, etc.). The capillaries are terminal or end arteries, the size of which is about one-tenth the size of the human hair. These are the tiny vessels that actually bring blood to the tissues and cells of the various parts of the body.

How does blood get oxygen and nutrition?

The nutrition and oxygen in the blood are used up by the tissues and cells. The used blood (now containing much less oxygen and more carbon dioxide, lactic acid, and other "waste products") travels back from the tissues and cells to lungs for oxygenation. Then blood goes to the heart for pumping to all organs, like the liver where toxins will be detoxified, to the kidneys that will filter the waste products and passed out through the urine, to the stomach and intestines where it will be replenished with new nutrition. The used blood then flows back to the lungs. After the oxygenation, the blood flows into the heart, ready to be pumped back into the circulation once again. And the cycle goes on.

How strong is our heart?

A healthy heart can take a lot of beating (no pun intended). It is one of the most powerful pumps in the world, even when compared to the mechanical ones built by man. Self-contained, self-propelled, energy-efficient, the heart works without stopping and can survive grave insults and abuses we humans subject it to day in and day out.

Is mechanical heart better?

Certainly not. Not yet, anyway. The man-made hydraulic-driven artificial or mechanical heart prosthesis available today is still no match to the one we were born with. Besides being a bulky foreign body and made of hardware not as soft and tender as our body tissues, it also requires electrical energy from outside the body and the use of anticoagulants to prevent thrombosis (blood clots, which can cause stroke). The mechanical heart is also prone to infection and not as durable as a natural heart. At the present, the artificial heart leaves too much to be desired.

When is artificial heart used?

Mechanical heart is helpful as a bridge to heart transplantation, implanted temporarily (for a few weeks or so) while a transplant patient waits for a human donor heart, but not as a long-term, permanent, heart replacement. Obviously, of course, a suitable permanent mechanical heart with as close inherent features as those of the human heart is the ultimate goal of ongoing researches around the world. When that day comes, a dying cardiac patient would not have to wait for a compatible donor to die before getting heart transplant. The cardiac surgeon then would simply ask the operating room nurse for the appropriate size artificial heart from the shelves (much like asking for a pacemaker today) to be implanted on the patient. By then too, coronary bypass, heart valve surgery, and most cardiac surgeries would be a thing of the past; and the millions of lives lost annually around the globe today from severe and end-stage heart diseases would be saved. As a cardiac surgeon, I can't wait for that dream to come true.

Is Heart Attack Caused by Bacteria?

Conventional wisdom, even within the medical community, tells us that heart attack, stroke, and related blockages in the arteries are caused by arteriosclerosis (hardening of the arteries) which, in turn, is caused by high-cholesterol diet, obesity, diabetes, and lack of exercise.

A team of investigators, headed by Dr. Emil Kozarov at the Department of Surgery and the Herbert Irving Comprehensive Cancer Center, Columbia University College of Dental Medicine, were able to identify particular bacteria which may play a vital role in causation of hardening of the arteries, the leading cause of death in the United States and other countries around the world. This study was published in the latest edition, volume 18 of the *Journal of Atherosclerosis and Thrombosis.*

Could Infection Be the Culprit?

This new postulate about bacteria (infection) as the probable cause of hardening of the arteries is a welcome news. The discovery of *H. pylori* changed stomach ulcer from a surgical disease to a medical one, today amenable to treatment with pills instead of surgery. Hopefully, if Dr. Kozarov and/or other investigators are able to prove that hardening of the arteries is due to infection by a bacterium or bacteria, then prevention of heart attack, stroke, bowel, leg gangrene, and other diseases due to clogged arteries would be feasible with a trip to the drugstore. When that happens, coronary heart bypass surgery, carotid (neck) artery surgery to prevent stroke, and leg arterial bypass surgery will be replaced by antibiotics for the bacterial culprit.

Other studies are also focusing on infection or bacteria as the cause to Alzheimer's, metabolic conditions like diabetes and thyroid disease, even in the pathogenesis of the various forms of cancer. These investigations are still in the research laboratories around the globe and will take years before we hear about the results.

Cell Transplantation for Hearts

Cell transplantation to promote growth of new heart muscles was first done in the United States in 2002 through cardiac catheterization as a stand alone treatment for heart failure secondary to scarred heart muscles due to a heart attack. This was performed during coronary bypass surgery or among patients with left ventricular assist device (LVAD), which is a machine that helps the failing heart to heal and pump better.

Cardiac catheterization is a minimally invasive procedure that is used to inject dye into the coronary arteries to diagnose blockages in the coronary arteries. Using the same simple technique, cardiologists recently transplanted muscle cells from the thigh by injecting them into the heart's scar tissues. The transplanted cells regenerated part of the scarred (noncontractile) heart muscles, resulting in new heart muscles tissue formation, improving the contractile function of the heart muscles.

The study, conducted in five patients who had severe heart failure following heart attack, was published in the December 17, 2003, issue of the *Journal of the American College of Cardiology.*

Heart attack occurs when the heart muscles are deprived of blood (which is the source of oxygen and nutrition), due to blockages of the coronary arteries caused by arteriosclerosis (hardening of the artery). This condition results from high-serum cholesterol levels, especially abnormally high levels of the low-density lipoprotein (LDL, the bad cholesterol) and abnormally low levels of the high-density lipoprotein (HDL, the good cholesterol).

When the heart muscles suffer from lack of oxygen and nutrition, the muscles die and become scarred tissues, losing their ability to perform its normal function of contracting effectively to eject blood out of the ventricles of the heart to circulate all over the body.

The heart muscles have an insignificant ability to repair itself; and when so affected by a heart attack, the heart muscles become weak, then scarred and ineffective in its pumping ability. And heart failure ensues.

The cell transplantation procedure included harvesting the donor muscles (in these cases, the thigh muscles), and loading them in a catheter, which was threaded through the heart vessels (coronary arteries), much like a diagnostic cardiac catheterization or angioplasty and injected into the scarred muscles of the heart. These cells grow and generate muscle "production" which become part of the heart muscles, enabling them to regain their effective contractility.

Patients who had the cell transplantation done had improved left ventricular ejection fraction (LVEF), which is a measure of the heart's ability to pump effectively and eject oxygen and nutrition-rich blood into the circulation.

While the preliminary study is exciting and shows promise, more extensive studies by different heart centers and investigators are needed to confirm or negate these current findings.

Heart Bypass

What is Heart Bypass?

Heart bypass or coronary bypass surgery is an operation that reroutes blood circulation, using arteries behind the breastbone (internal mammary) and veins from the leg (saphenous veins) as "new conduit pipes" through which blood is carried around the blocked coronary arteries to the muscles of the heart that are not receiving enough blood because of obstruction.

What is this surgery done for?

Coronary bypass is done for patients who have heart pains (angina pectoris) that are resistant to medications and who have been found to have significant blockages in the coronary arteries by a dye test called coronary angiogram.

Are all chest pains angina pectoris?

No, not all chest pains are heart pains. Other conditions that can cause chest pains include muscles aches, skeletal pains, referred pains from pinched nerve in the neck, lung conditions, and many others. But since angina pectoris could lead to a heart attack, or even sudden death, any chest pains must be taken seriously and investigated without delay.

How about a normal EKG?

Just like many other medical tests, a resting EKG with negative finding does not totally eliminate the presence of blockages in the coronary arteries. Sometimes, we hear of someone dropping dead who had normal EKG a few days or so before the fatal event. Resting EKG (taken while the person is lying on his back) is helpful only if the findings are positive or abnormal. The more accurate test is a stress test (treadmill EKG), where electrocardiogram is taken while the patient walks on a treadmill. The stress challenges the heart to reveal any abnormality, if present, which at rest will not be evident. It is just like a car engine, which, while on idle, may not reveal any problem, but when running, starts to knock, if it has a problem.

Besides angina pectoris, what are the other symptoms?

Heart attack or coronary artery blockage could have other symptoms than the classical or usual chest pains. Other less obvious symptoms include any of the following: feeling of indigestion, chest tightness, pains or tightness at the front base of the neck, pains and or numbness of either arms, upper-back pains, dizziness, generalized weakness. If any one of these symptoms occurs, coronary blockage or impending heart attack should be suspected and ruled out. This is especially true when physical exertion or stress or exposure to cold temperature brings about the chest discomfort and any of those symptoms above. The prudent thing to do is to see your family physician or cardiologist promptly.

What causes the blockage of coronary arteries?

There are many factors that contribute to the formation of arteriosclerosis (hardening of the arteries), which lead to eventual obstruction of these arteries. Smoking, eating red meat, eggs, high-cholesterol foods, obesity, lack of daily exercise, inability to manage stress, heredity, thyroid disease, impaired cholesterol metabolism, uncontrolled hypertension and/or diabetes mellitus.

How much role does heredity have?

Contrary to the popular belief, heredity plays a less major role than lifestyle and environment. Children of parents who had coronary heart diseases will not necessarily have significant coronary problems if they did not live and misbehave like their parents did. If they live a healthier lifestyle, these children (as medical studies have shown) will not "inherit" their parents heart problems. At least, we now know that these children are not inevitably "doomed" to have the same fate as their parents. Medical data show that 98% of us do not really have a good excuse to have coronary artery blockages or a heart attack.

If the stress test is positive, what then?

If the stress test is positive, it is a very strong indication that coronary arteries are stenosed (blocked) and that the heart muscles suffering. In this situation, the next step is coronary angiogram to confirm with 100% certainty the location, nature, and severity of the blockages. This will also help the cardiologist decide whether drugs, angioplasty, or coronary bypass surgery is the best mode of treatment for the patient.

Is coronary bypass safe?

In trained and experienced hands, coronary bypass surgery is safe and effective. Today, this surgical procedure is one of the most commonly performed surgery in the United States and all over the world. Since its introduction in the mid-'60s, heart bypass has saved millions of lives and tremendously improved the quality and longevity of people. It has also brought back to the mainstream of life majority of these patients, who would otherwise be dead or having heart attacks or intractable debilitating chest pains. One of the medical wonders of the last third of the 20th century was the introduction of coronary bypass surgery and angioplasty. The diagram below shows two coronary bypass grafts.

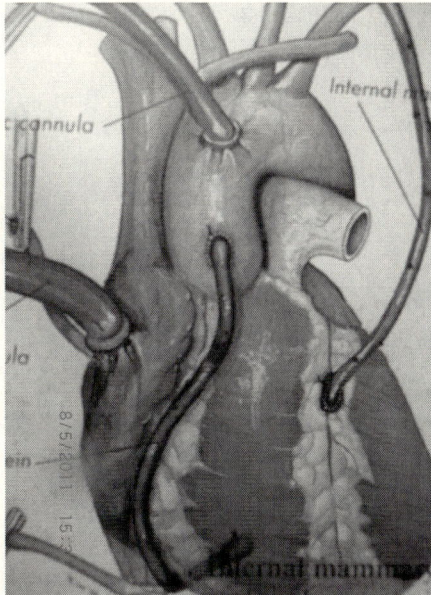

The Heart Connection

Did you know that any chronic (long-standing) bacterial infection, including dental problem like gum disease (gingivitis), can indirectly cause heart disease, like coronary heart disease that could lead to heart attack or blockage in the neck (carotid) arteries and potential stroke?

The underlying precipitating pathology in arteriosclerosis (hardening of the artery) is inflammation. And bacterial infection (like infection of the skin or other organs in our body) is now being suspected by scientists as a possible "initiator" of hardening of the arteries that causes arterial blockages in the heart (leading to heart attack), in the brain (causing stroke), in leg arteries, especially among diabetics (resulting in leg gangrene).

An important part of the healthy lifestyle we have been vigorously campaigning for in our column for decades for disease prevention are regular medical and dental checkups for overall health maintenance.

Hypertension

Hypertension (high blood pressure) also causes some injury to the intima (inner lining) of the arteries all over the body, including those to the brain and to the pumping chambers (muscles) of the heart. Those with hypertension are at an increased risk for heart attack and stroke; and controlling hypertension with a healthy diet, daily exercise, and medications reduces the risk and mortality from these two top killers. Therefore, managing hypertension is vital in preventing stroke and heart attack.

Diabetes Mellitus

Type 2 diabetes is very common harbinger of a variety of complications and pathologies in the body of the diabetic. They range from lowered resistance to infection (they heal poorly) to visual impairment and kidney disease, from elevated risk for heart attack and stroke, to foot gangrene. Persons with diabetes have 2 to 4 times greater risk to develop heart disease than non-diabetics.

Thanks to medications for diabetes (pills and insulin shots), diabetics around the world today have a better chance of living a life as normal as possible. Before these treatments were discovered, the morbidity and mortality among diabetics were of pandemic proportion. Only those who were truly disciplined with their diet and daily exercise lived with less morbidity and complications. A significant number of people, including children of diabetic parents, have prevented the onset of diabetes by dieting, watching their weight, and exercising daily.

Hypothyroidism

The thyroid gland produces vital hormones, thyroxine (T4) and triiodothyronine (T3), which are primarily the regulators of body metabolism, including that of the cardiovascular system. In hypothyroidism, the cardiac muscle contraction and relaxation both become weakened, impaired. To maintain the integrity of the heart and other organs in the body, normal levels of the thyroid hormones are necessary.

Homocysteine, Folic Acid, B12, and E

Elevated homocysteine was implicated a few years back in the causation of arteriosclerotic heart disease and the use of folic acid and vitamin B12 was tried. However, the results of the subsequent studies showed that, while the homocysteine levels were effectively reduced by folic acid and B12, the risk and mortality for heart attack among those patients were not reduced. Hence, these two supplements are today no longer recommended, just like vitamin E, which was very popular decades before for cardiovascular health, had been proven to be "of no benefit and was probably even harmful."

Migraines and Heart Attack

Studies on almost 12, 000 subjects published recently in *Neurology* revealed that "4.1% of people who had migraines had a heart attack compared with 1.9%" of those without. Those who experienced migraine with aura had nearly 3 times higher risk for heart attack.

The More Popular Connections

Some of the more notorious contributing factors to heart disease are cigarette smoking, high intake of saturated fats and cholesterol, lack of physical exercises, obesity, alcohol abuse, inadequate stress management, besides hereditary predisposition. However, as far as the last one is concerned, a healthy lifestyle has been proven to outweigh and outsmart the genes in the general population. Children of parents who have hypertension or heart attack or stroke are not necessarily doomed or "fated" to have these illnesses, provided they live a healthy lifestyle unlike their parents.

Happiness and Attitude

Bad attitude, pessimism, unhappiness, discontent, and other negative feelings also increase the risk for the development of heart disease. People who have positive attitude in their daily routines or especially in the face of adversities or calamities are less prone to heart attacks in general. These are usually people with natural happy countenance, hopefulness, who believe that the future will be brighter. Happy people sleep and rest better, are more content and have inner peace, and healthier overall. When flooded with the happy hormones, the mind and the muscles are more relaxed and the heart pumps easier, because the stress hormone (adrenalin) is lesser and outweighed by these soothing hormones naturally secreted by the endocrine glands of our body when we face the world with a positive attitude each day.

Individuals with a good attitude are 22% less likely to develop heart disease compared to the difficult and grouchy individuals. Negative persons are usually depressed, angry, anxious, malcontent, and hostile, and as such, have greater risk to develop, not only heart disease, but stroke and other illnesses, including cancer.

Indeed, it pays to have a positive outlook in life.

Myths About Heart Disease

Sex is bad for the heart

On the contrary, sex is good for the heart. The morphinelike opiates and other feel-good hormones our own body secretes during sex or during any happy activities or thought processes we have, the physical exercise during sex, and the healthy outlet it provides both partners actually benefit the heart. Only those with untreated coronary artery disease or heart failure could get into trouble during sex. With proper treatment and medical guidance, these patients can indulge in sex safely.

Heart disease is inherited

Rarely, certain congenital (inborn) structural defect of the heart may be genetic; but in general, we cannot blame our ancestry for the heart diseases that are very common today, like coronary artery disease (cause of heart attacks) or heart valve diseases (due to rheumatic fever). Although some families seem to be more prone to heart attacks and the traits could be a part of the genes, the important causative factors in this situation are mostly not hereditary but environmental—the lifestyle of the family members. These significant etiologic factors include smoking, eating red meats, eggs, and other high cholesterol foods, lack of exercise, obesity, unmanaged stress, hypercholesterolemia (elevated cholesterol blood level), untreated hypertension, diabetes mellitus (especially the poorly controlled ones).

Children of heart attack victims will have the same fate

This is not true. Even if both parents had heart attacks or coronary artery disease, their children are not necessarily condemned to same fate, provided the children live a healthier lifestyle, unlike their parents.

If these children stay on low-cholesterol diet, eat fish (instead of red meat), a lot of vegetables, fruits, and high fiber foods, do not smoke, exercise at least 5 times a week, maintain a normal weight, know how to relax and manage stress, they can escape significant coronary artery disease.

Women rarely have heart disease

Wrong. As one of the old cigarette commercials stated "You've come a long way, baby." Since today's modern women have entered the "men's world," working, smoking, drinking, competing, hustling like men, they have indeed "come a long way," approximating men in most respects, even in the incidence of coronary artery disease and heart attacks among them. Young women as a rule have greater resistance to coronary artery disease because of the protective effects of the female sex hormone called estrogen. However, women with unhealthy lifestyle negate the benefits of estrogen and suffer heart disease like men. The 2-to-1 (male to female) vulnerability has been narrowing the past 3 decades.

Executives are prime victims of heart attacks

Not so. We used to believe that top job responsibility and stressful executive positions led to higher incidence of heart attacks. Recent studies have proven this to be a fallacy. In a study, bartenders were found to be more vulnerable to heart attacks than barbers, and barbers more prone than physicians. In another series, blue-collar workers were found to be more susceptible to heart attacks than supervisory personnel and executives. It is obvious that lifestyle and not the line of work, position, or rank is more of the determinant factor in heart attacks.

Persons younger than 40 do not get heart disease

Another myth. The youngest patient we did coronary bypass surgery was a 28-year-old diabetic Caucasian female, who had very high cholesterol level, high blood pressure, and a cigarette smoker. Coronary artery disease does not respect any age, gender, or any person who abuses himself/herself with an unhealthy lifestyle.

Exercise damages the heart

Definitely does not. The heart can take a lot more challenges than one can imagine. It is one of the strongest muscular organs in the human body. Exercise has beneficial effects on the heart. Even heart attack patients who have recovered from the acute phase are prescribed an exercise regimen. Exercise dilates (opens wider) coronary arteries that supply the heart muscles with oxygen and nutrition. The benefits conferred by regular moderate exercise are "cumulative and lasting." If in doubt about your fitness to do exercises, consult your physician.

High blood pressure is due to heart disease.

This is another misinformation. The reverse is true: untreated or poorly controlled hypertension can lead to coronary artery disease. High blood pressure is, in most cases, idiopathic (cause unknown), but definitely not due to heart disease. High blood pressure taxes the heart and makes the cardiac muscles work harder, and in many cases, this causes cardiac hypertrophy (enlarged heart).

Heart attack victims should be sedentary

Nothing is farther from the truth. Heart attack patients who have recovered should resume normal activities as prescribed by their physicians. It is most essential for these people to be active again as soon as they are medically allowed to. A sedentary life for these patients would only lead to deterioration of the heart and to vegetation. Those who bounce back to as normal a life as possible following a heart attack will fare much better physically and mentally than those who resign themselves to invalidism.

Longevity is shortened by heart bypass

This is another myth. Coronary bypass surgery not only improves the quality of life by eliminating chest pains but also increases the life span of patients, whose life will otherwise be reduced by heart attack. More and more clinical studies are showing this to be the case.

Heart bypass patients are unable to work

Wrong. One of the goals of coronary bypass surgery is to allow the patient to go back to the mainstream of society. After adequate recovery, patients who were working prior to surgery can usually go back to their original job, with some initial restrictions. Very rarely are postbypass patients unable to resume previous work activities. These exceptions are among those with severe and neglected coronary artery disease where the heart muscles have already been damaged before the patients agreed to have bypass surgery.

Red meats and eggs are good for children

A very dangerous myth! A high cholesterol diet of red meat and eggs is bad for children as it is unhealthy for adults. Fish, vegetables, whole grain, nuts and fruits are much healthier choices.

How to damage your heart in just 8 easy steps!

Some may already be doing a good job at wrecking their heart, besides other organs in their body; but for the others who may not be as innovative and cunning, here are eight easy and simple ways to accomplish the job more efficiently and effectively.

(1) If you are not a cigarette smoker, start smoking or inhale as much secondhand smoke as possible. If you are, continue this very dangerous and expensive (moneywise and healthwise) habit. Out of the 1.3 billion smokers around the world, one dies from smoking every 6.5 seconds. Smoking kills 5.4 million each year. This is projected to rise to 6.5 million by 2015 and 8.3 million by 2030. One billion will die from tobacco use in this century alone. Besides heart disease, smoking causes cancer of the lungs and other organs, besides causing emphysema and air-hunger. Secondhand smoke is no less a brutal killer. People who quit smoking lower their risk of heart disease to the level of nonsmokers in just 2 years and also protect their loved ones from secondhand smoke.

(2) Binge daily, 3 times a day or more, on saturated animal fats like red meats (pork, beef, processed foods like bacon, hamburgers, ham, hotdogs, sausages, etc.), eggs. French fries, junk foods, and foods with trans fats. Do not eat any vegetables, fruits, nuts, oatmeal, bran, and other hi-fiber foods, because these lower cholesterol, are good for our immune system, and lower our risk for cancer. Besides, these are health foods, good for our body. They will not damage but protect our heart, colon, brain, kidneys, liver, etc.

(3) Throw away the scale. Just take in all the calories you can grab, especially carbohydrates (rice, bread, cookies, candies, ice cream, sweets, and especially the megasugar-loaded softy drinks, which I call

the liquid candy). Allow yourself to put on weight. Forget about the gorgeous body curves, ladies. The fatter, the heavier, the faster we can damage the heart. So do not read food labels and learn about the calorie, fat, sodium, and trans fat contents. Just don't watch your diet, because losing 10 pounds alone will lessen the risk for heart attack by 50% and help lower cholesterol, blood pressure, and the risk of cancer too. So stay heavy. Fat is cute, anyway.

(4) Be a couch potato. Live a sedentary life. Do not exercise. Do not move a muscle, except the fingers needed to click on the TV remote control as we gorge on junk foods while watching the soaps, sports, or game shows. Lack of exercise weakens not only our body but our heart and brain. Believe it or not, it also impacts our psyche. For those who are overweight, dieting and counting calories would be more effective with daily exercise in achieving the target more effectively. So why exercise? It will only help lengthen our life.

(5) Eat more salt. Don't listen to your doctor. Add salt to everything you eat, even before tasting the food. Just keep on shaking. This will raise your blood pressure and cause damage to the arteries in your body, including those that supply blood to your heart. The higher the blood pressure, the greater the risk for stroke and heart attack. If you lower the salt intake, it will help lower your chances of developing high blood pressure; and among those already with hypertension, it will greatly help in maintaining a normal blood pressure. For flavoring, go the natural way and use pepper, garlic, onion, oregano, and other no-sodium food seasoning. But I want to warn you that this will NOT damage your heart.

(6) Sleep and rest as little as possible. The TV shows are exciting and worth the time. You can nap while you drive anyway, and you can also snooze on the job. If you want to harm your heart, why even have rest and relaxation, which are simple and natural pleasures that are healthy? Those who lack sleep are prone to heart attack, high blood pressure, and stroke. These conditions and diabetes become harder to manage and control when sleep and rest are not adequate.

(7) Do not pay attention to stress or depression. Both of these have adverse impact on the heart, besides the mind and, actually, on the

whole being. The earlier they are managed, the easier they are to cure. Stress and depression increase the risk for heart attack by more than 30% and also lead to weakened immune system, which predisposes these people to other illnesses as well.

(8) Don't waste time bothering about ecology, about helping save Mother Nature or being kind to planet Earth, and simply continue to pollute our air, water, and soil, which negatively impacts our health and contributes to heart disease and other illnesses. Do whatever your heart desires. Never mind about living a healthy lifestyle. Life is too short; let us make it even shorter by wrecking our heart in these eight easy and simple steps.

Almost 1.6 million people die from heart attack, or 3 every minutes, 136,000 from stroke; about 75,000 from diabetes; and about 263,000 from cancer, each year.

Those seemingly effortless 8 steps are, indeed, very tempting. But since they are obviously dangerous alternatives that only guarantee sickness and misery, the more prudent and wiser "one-step" option is living a healthy lifestyle.

This may not sound that inviting and exciting to the young and those still healthy. But once health deteriorates, especially among those with severe shortness of breath from heart failure, those losing their eyesight or legs from diabetes, those with stroke, those with cancer that has spread all over the body, the priceless value of health becomes clearer. At that point, the adage "Health is Wealth" ceases to be a cliché and becomes a more convincing and a more powerful reality. By then, it could be too late to bring back health.

So why even wait?

Automatic Heart Shocker!

Is there an implantable device that shocks the heart?

Yes, it is called automatic implantable cardioverter defibrillator, or AICD for short. It is a computerized unit a little larger and thicker than a silver dollar that is implanted under the skin by the left upper chest or abdominal area, programmed to detect any dangerous rhythm of the heart. These so-called fatal arrhythmias (ventricular tachycardia, ventricular fibrillation, or cardiac arrest) result in death, among persons with serious heart rhythm problem, who would otherwise look "quite healthy" and active, but who are prone to sudden cardiac death.

Are these rhythm problems the same as atrial fibrillation?

No, atrial fibrillation is a very common type of heart irregularity (with skipped heartbeats) where the atria (upper chambers of the heart) are the ones which are beating irregularly. This is generally well-tolerated, and many of patients are treated with digitalis, among other medications. Most of them are otherwise healthy and grow old with their atrial fibrillation, but those with heart valve disease and atrial fibrillation are more prone to form blood clots inside the heart.

Why is ventricular fibrillation fatal?

If not electrically defibrillated (shocked) within 2-3 minutes, a patient who develops ventricular fibrillation will rapidly deteriorate to cardiac arrest and die. This type of heart rhythm problem involves the left ventricle, which is the main pumping chamber of the heart. When the left ventricle fibrillates (quivers instead of beating normally), blood in the heart chambers and all over the body does not circulate and stagnates because the "pump" is not pumping. As a result, the brain and all other vital organs are deprived of fresh blood that carries oxygen and nutrition, etc. Brain cells and all body cells suffer from "suffocation" and die.

When the heart stops, how much time is there to save the person?

As a rule, we say no more than 3 minutes by the clock. The brain is most sensitive to hypoxia (lack of oxygen). If ventricular fibrillation or cardiac arrest is left untreated beyond 3 minutes, the brain deteriorates, is irreversibly damaged, and the person strokes out and dies. That was the very reason why AICD was invented.

How does AICD work?

After AICD has been implanted in a person, it constantly "analyzes" the heart rhythm of the patient and is "on guard" at all times. This tiny computer is programmed to detect serious or fatal arrhythmias. Once it senses ventricular tachycardia or ventricular fibrillation or cardiac arrest, it instantly sends out a premeasured (18-20 joules) electric shock from the AICD unit through the lead (insulated wire) to the electrodes (contact points) which have been inserted and positioned to lie in contact with the inner walls of the heart. This shock will jolt (convert) the heart back to normal rhythm, much like the external handheld defibrillators emergency room physicians use to shock the patients in cardiac arrest. The only difference is that AICD is small and implanted in the patient, with no exposed wires, etc. Besides "shocking" the heart, the AICD unit is also a pacemaker and paces the heart in the event the heartbeat is too slow, which happens in more than 50% of these patients.

Is this the same as a pacemaker?

No. A heart pacemaker only paces the heart to correct bradycardia (heart rate slower than 60 beats per minute) to make it beat at a higher chosen rate, but it does not have the capability or feature to defibrillate (shock) the heart and convert a fatal rhythm to a sinus (normal) rhythm. An AICD has these capabilities and at the same time it functions (on demand) as a pacemaker as well.

Who are candidates for AICD?

Candidates are those patients who pass out and are diagnosed with ventricular tachycardia, ventricular fibrillation, or cardiac arrest. They are potential victims of what is called sudden cardiac death syndrome. An electrophysiologic study is done on these patients for definitive diagnosis. Once the diagnosis is established, prompt implantation of AICD is recommended. AICD implantation, without any doubt, is lifesaving; and the best alternative today for patients with any of these fatal arrhythmias.

Will AICD trigger airport metal detectors?

Yes. And so with a cardiac pacemaker, a metal heart valve, artificial metal joints, etc. These patients usually carry a medical device ID card with them.

Is the AICD shock transmitted to a dancing partner?

No. When the AICD fires a needed shock, the dancing partner of the patient will only feel a sudden jerk, but not feel the electrical jolt. The patient will feel a bit weak and wobbly for a moment, and very tired after this defibrillation. Had the patient not have an AICD in this hypothetical instance, he/she would have most likely died.

Are AICD patients allowed to drive?

AICD patients are advised not to drive, for a very obvious reason. They are also advised against climbing tall ladders or working on the roof and similar "dangerous" situations. But most of these patients are otherwise active, feeling well, healthy looking, and working normally. Unless they tell you they have AICD on them, even physicians would not be able to tell. These individuals simply have to be more careful and change their lifestyle a bit. However, the extra medical security and the benefits are certainly worth it. Compared to the general population, patients with AICD are better protected against cardiac arrest.

Beware of Hepatitis B

What is Hepatitis B?

Hepatitis B is inflammation of the liver caused by hepatitis B virus (HBV), a lifelong infection that could lead to cirrhosis (scarring) of the liver, hepatoma (cancer of the liver), liver failure, and death.

How does one catch hepatitis B?

HBV is transmitted by receiving blood transfusion from a donor infected with the HBV, by unprotected sexual contact with a person with the infection, by using HBV contaminated needles among patients or by sharing HBV contaminated needles or drugs among drug addicts, and by maternal-fetal (mother to baby during birth) transmission.

How about thru food, water, etc?

No, hepatitis B virus is not spread through water, food, eating utensils, pots and pans, sneezing, coughing, holding hands, hugging, kissing (no matter how passionate), or by casual contact.

How prevalent is HBV infection?

Roughly 2 billion people worldwide are infected with the virus and about 360 million are chronic carriers, 78% in Asia, 16% in Africa, 3% in South America, 3% in Europe, North America and Oceana combined. Roughly 600,000 die each year. About 25% who were infected during childhood later die of liver cancer or cirrhosis. Hep B is 50-100 times more infectious than HIV. Mass HBV vaccination in many Asian countries showed the EPI (Extended Program on Immunization as a public program) has led to a drastic reduction in the prevalence of HBV infection. Notwithstanding these great strides, HBV infection rate in this region of the world is still the highest. In the USA, in 2003 alone, there were 73,000 people infected with HBV, and about 5,000 Americans die each year from the infection or its complications.

How is the diagnosis made?

Only a blood test can confirm for sure if a person has hepatitis B or not. After a person is exposed to the HBV, it takes about 4 weeks (range: 1-9 weeks) for the blood test (HBsAg) to show if a person has acquired the HBV infection or not.

How soon after the exposure do symptoms occur?

After exposure to HBV, the symptoms, if they occur, will manifest on the average of 12 weeks (9 to 21 week range). Only 70% of patients will have symptoms, the 30% will be symptom free although infected. Adults are more likely to show clinical symptoms than children.

When is the HBV patient infectious?

About half (50%) of the persons with hepatitis B will no longer be infectious (not "contagious") seven weeks after the onset of their symptoms. The other half will still be able to spread the infection even after 7 weeks. All patients with HBV who do not stay chronically infected will test negative for HBsAg 15 weeks after the start of their first symptoms.

What symptoms do HBV patients have?

Not all patients develop symptoms, especially among adult and older patients. One might have hepatitis B infection and spread it around without even knowing he/she had the infection. If symptoms show up, they might include: jaundice (yellow discoloration of the skin and the whites of the eyes), anorexia (loss of appetite), fatigue (tiredness), nausea, vomiting, arthralgia (joint pains), abdominal discomfort, chalky-white bowel movements, dark yellow urine.

What are the risk factors for HBV?

You have a higher risk of getting HBV infection if you (1) have sex with a person infected with HBV, (2) have sex with multiple partners,

(3) shoot drugs, (4) are a homosexual, (5) have a housemate(s) who has chronic (long-term) HBV, (6) have hemophilia, (7) work with, and in contact with human blood, (8) live in a home for the developmentally disabled,(9) travel to countries where HBV infection is common, (10) have parents who were born in Southeast Asia, the Amazon Basin in South America, Africa, the Pacific Islands, or the Middle East.

Who should be vaccinated?

The following should be vaccinated: all babies, at birth; all children up to 18 years who have not been vaccinated before; and people of any age whose job or behavior puts them at a high risk for HBV.

Is there an oral treatment for chronic Hep B?

According to an article in the *New England Journal of Medicine* in July 1998, use of oral antiviral Zeffix (lamuvudine, 100 mg per day) for Hep B led to 98% reduction in hepatitis B DNA (a marker of viral replication) and a very high rate of seroconversion (predictor of long-lasting remission). Today, there are at least 5 antiviral drugs available for the treatment of chronic hep-B (Adefovir, dipivoxil, interferon alfa-2b, pegvlated interferon alfa-2a, lamivudine, and entecavir), but there is no drug that prevents hepatitis B infection or treats recently acquired (acute) hep-B infection. The best strategy is still prevention, especially for hepatitis B which could lead to liver cancer, liver failure, and death.

Hepatoma is Deadly

What is hepatoma?

Also known as hepatocellular carcinoma, hepatoma is the most common (70% to 85%) primary cancer of the liver. The rarer ones are cholangiocarcinoma, hepatoblastoma, and angiosarcoma. The word *primary* means the cancer originated in the liver, in contrast to secondary or metastatic liver cancer, which originated from another organ, like cancer of the lung, breast, pancreas, colon, or stomach spreading to the liver. Most cancer found in the liver are metastatic from other organs.

What is the incidence?

In the United States, the incidence is between 1 and 5 cases per 100,000 population per year. About 70% of cases of hepatoma worldwide are due to chronic hepatitis B infection, compared to only 20% in the United States, where 60% to 80% are alcoholic cirrhosis-related. Among those not caused by hepatitis B virus, 50% to 70% were due to chronic hepatitis C infection. Mean age of hepatoma patients is 55-62 years, and with a male to female sex ratio of 3-4 :1

What causes hepatoma?

Those with chronic hepatitis B or C infection are prone to develop liver cancer. Other causal agents include alcoholism and chronic liver cirrhosis.

Will hepatitis lead to hepatoma?

While those who have hepatitis B or C have increased risk of developing hepatoma, not all persons with a history of hepatitis B or C infection will automatically develop hepatocellular carcinoma. For these persons, a healthy lifestyle could help boost the immune system and conceivably lessen the risk.

What are the other risk factors?

Chronic use of oral contraceptives, unsterile intravenous drug abuse, primary biliary cirrhosis, hemochromatosis, some metabolic disorders (Niemann-Pick), chlonorchiasis, gallstones, and choledochal cyst, chronic exposure to vinyl chloride polymers.

What are the symptoms?

Some cases have no symptoms at all till the hepatoma has progressed, and different individuals may experience symptoms in variable ways. Some of the most common symptoms and signs are abdominal pain, weight loss, fever, nausea, vomiting, swollen abdomen, fatigue, jaundice (yellow discoloration of the skin and eyes), large mass in the right upper quadrant of the abdomen.

How is hepatoma diagnosed?

A complete medical history and physical examination by a physician is essential. Some tests are liver function test, abdominal ultrasound, computed tomography or CT scan, magnetic resonance imaging or MRI, hepatic arteriography, liver biopsy with a needle for specific microscopic pathological diagnosis, laparoscopy, and, if needed, exploratory laparotomy.

What is the prognosis?

Unless the diagnosis is made very early, which is not the usual case, life expectancy after the diagnosis of hepatoma is established generally ranges between 6 and 8 months.

How can one prevent hepatoma?

Vaccination against hepatitis B virus to prevent getting hepatitis B infection is an effective way to significantly reduce the risk of developing hepatoma. Hepatitis B is transmitted sexually and through blood transfusion, like hepatitis C. So preventive measures in this regard is fundamental. On top of this, abstinence from, or moderation in intake of, alcoholic beverages will help.

Any sign that vaccination helps?

Yes, since universal immunization against hepatitis B was implemented among children, statistics show that the incidence of hepatoma has been reduced to 1/4 to 1/3, compared to the period before the use of the vaccine. Global immunization against hepatitis B among all infants will surely help in minimizing, if not eradicating hep-B-caused hepatoma.

What are the treatments available?

The attending physician, who has all the data available including the stage of the liver cancer, will determine and recommend the appropriate treatment strategy and options. The patient, as always, especially in cases of hepatoma, has the final say.

The management could include surgery to remove the entire liver (and liver transplant for specific candidates that qualify) or partial resection of the liver with cancer, depending on the extent of involvement, external beam radiation therapy to kill the cancer cells, or, in advanced cases, to shrink the size of the tumor for pain relief, chemotherapy intravenously, or intra-arterial chemo given directly thru a catheter in the liver artery, chemo-embolization to clog the artery and cut the blood supply to the liver and anticancer drugs delivered to the liver directly. Radio-frequency ablation, uses a special probe to kill the cancer cells with heat. Laser and microwave therapy also utilize heat to kill the cancer cells. For a few patients who qualify, liver transplantation may be an option, provided the cancer has not spread to other organs. The team of physicians and surgeon, led by the oncologist, will formulate a treatment plan for each individual patient.

We all look to the day when deadly diseases like hepatoma and all other cancers could be prevented with the use of vaccines or effectively treated with oral medications, like in the case of tuberculosis, which used to spread and ravage all the organs of the body like cancer, until French scientists Calmette and Guerin discovered the BCG vaccine against TB in 1906; and later, streptomycin was isolated on October 19, 1943, by Albert Schatz, a graduate student, and first randomized trial of the drug used against TB in 1947.

Herbal Warning

For thousands of years, China has been known to be the capital of herbal medicine. Other countries have their own version of treating diseases and health conditions using herbal products. Today, we still hear an abundance of anecdotal testimonials about the efficacy of these natural "medications" from indigenous foods, plants, minerals, some of them from regular food we eat every day.

Folk remedies are our earthly natural gifts, and traditional plant and herbs are still man's sources for about 85% of the world's developing nations. Some of the problems with herbals drugs include lack of quality control, contamination with adulterants, and bacteria.

There is no question that many plants, fungi, flowers, roots, leaves, and fruits have chemical substances in them that are beneficial to the human body, not only as a source of nutrition but as herbal items with medicinal values. Modern science has harnessed some of them, reconfigured their molecular structures and properties, and transformed them into medicine. Penicillin is one of the multitudes of drugs that have their origin from these natural elements.

Most herbal products today have not been scientifically investigated the same way all Western drugs on the market have been studied and tested. So we do not really know which are safe and efficacious and what side effects they may have. Not all herbal medicines are dangerous, but a few have been shown to cause kidney failure, liver failure, cancer, clot blockages in the kidney veins, seizures, etc. Some of them have caused deaths.

Some time ago, a Chinese herb known as Aristolochia fangchi or *A. fangchi* was linked to kidney failure and urinary cancer. This herb is used in Chinese medicine to treat asthma. *A. fangchi* is also an ingredient in a Belgian weight-loss formulation, where the linkage was discovered. This was not the first time where herbal medicines have caused severe, if not fatal, complications. Other herbals to stay away from, to mention a few, are pokeroot, comfrey, and liferoot, which have been reported to cause liver damage. Ginseng can affect hormonal balance and gingko biloba, excessive bleeding during surgery, among some people. A warning has been sounded by the United Nations health agency regarding the use/misuse/overuse of herbal medications.

It is one thing to take a substance and discover after days or months that it is not effective; it is another to find out months or years later that the substance is toxic, or causes cancer.

Alternative medicine could be a wonderful natural option; but with today's sophisticated medical science, it is most prudent for all of us to use only those herbal products and drugs that have been investigated by the US-FDA, studied, tested, and proven safe, effective, with minimal side effects and potential complications.

There are many fruits, vegetables, grains, nuts, spices, and herbs that we eat daily, which have medicinal values in them. These are the "herbals" that are good and safe. And much, much, less expensive too. For example: water, cleansing and detoxifying; apple, antiviral and lowers cholesterol; mustard, antifungal and antibacterial; salt, antibacterial and preservative; corn, induces urination; garlic, circulatory stimulant and lowers blood pressure; wheat, antiaging; cucumber, anti-inflammatory; onion, lowers blood pressure, cholesterol, and blood sugar; watercress is a tonic that detoxifies; potato, antiviral and anti-inflammatory; honey, antiseptic and expectorant; pepper, decongestant and immune-system enhancer; and green leafy vegetables, antioxidant like most of the above and also anticancer, etc.

One caveat: There is no one single drug on earth that is a cure-all for every illness known to man, and taking an untested drug or substance with unknown side effects and complications could be downright dangerous in the long term and potentially fatal.

High Blood Pressure:
The Silent Killer

What is High Blood Pressure?

High blood pressure, or hypertension, is a condition where the person's blood pressure is persistently elevated beyond what is medically considered normal level. Normal blood pressure has a wide range from person to person. When taking blood pressure, there are two sets of figures noted by the physician: the systolic and the diastolic pressure, expressed in millimeters of mercury as systolic pressure over the diastolic pressure, like 117/74.

What is systolic and diastolic blood pressure?

The systolic pressure is the force of the flow of blood as it travels inside and through the arterial pipe, while the diastolic pressure is the force exerted by the blood against (perpendicular to) the inner wall of the artery.

What is the normal blood pressure?

In medical school we were taught that the normal blood pressure was 120/80. However, new medical guidelines have set the normal blood pressure to be a systolic (upper figure) reading below 120 and a diastolic (lower figure) of less than 80 mm Hg, more like 115/75. Drug treatment is advised when the blood pressure is at or higher than 140/90. For BP below that level, but higher than what is now considered normal, dieting and exercise is the treatment recommended. If the systolic is higher than 120 and the diastolic pressure is higher than 75 on at least three separate office visits, then strictly speaking, the diagnosis of hypertension applies. So a blood pressure of 121/76 technically is higher than normal and is hypertension but mild. And this slight elevation is an indication that the person is prone to develop a more full-blown hypertension, unless dieting (plus low-salt intake) and exercise are implemented. The older the patient is, the higher the diastolic pressure; and the higher the diastolic is, the more severe the hypertension is. Medical guidelines state that a normal blood pressure for most adults is less than 120/80 mm Hg. Drug treatment is recommended if your blood pressure is at or above 140/90 mm Hg. For people with diabetes or chronic kidney disease, drug treatment is recommended for a blood pressure level of 130/80 mm Hg or higher.[1]

Lowering your blood pressure to less than 140/90 to 120/80 mm Hg or below will help prevent other serious health problems.

How does one know if he/she has high blood pressure?

Obviously by having the blood pressure taken, preferably by an experienced nurse or a physician. Other factors and conditions in the patient will be considered by the physician before making a diagnosis of hypertension.

Once a hypertensive always a hypertensive?

Basically, yes, once you are diagnosed to have high blood pressure, you are always a hypertensive, even if your pressure is "lowered to normal level" and well controlled by medication. Once a hypertensive always a hypertensive, the reason why high blood pressure requires medication for life to maintain a normal blood pressure.

What is "white-coat" hypertension?

"White-coat" hypertension is a condition where the patient's blood pressure goes up when he/she goes to visit the doctor. Somehow the white lab coat of the physician taking the blood pressure seems to jack up anxiety and the adrenalin level in the waiting patient, leading to a rise in the blood pressure of this patient, but only temporarily if the patient is really not a hypertensive. And when a nurse takes the blood pressure, it is back down to normal.

What are the signs or symptoms of hypertension?

Not all persons with high blood pressure have symptoms. As a matter of fact, many of them do not have symptoms, especially the mild to moderate hypertensives. This is why it is called the "silent killer." Some simply develop a stroke or a heart attack before learning they have hypertension. Classically, though, some of the symptoms might include headaches, feeling of "wanting to explode," being short-tempered, of being flushed, and nervousness, irritability, impatience, etc.

What is primary and secondary hypertension?

Primary hypertension, also called essential hypertension, is one where the cause is not known. Heredity is implicated in its etiology, but there are other probable causes that medical science still does not fully understand. To date, we still do not know what causes high blood pressure. Secondary hypertension is high blood pressure caused by certain conditions or diseases, like bilateral kidney disease, pheochromocytoma (tumor of adrenal gland), hyperthyroidism, etc., or ingestion of contraceptives or excessive alcohol intake. The most common high blood pressure condition is the primary or essential hypertension.

How common is high blood pressure?

About 20% or 50 million of the population of the United States have high blood pressure (systolic higher than 140 and diastolic higher than 90 mm. Hg). Hypertension occurs more in black than in white Americans. In a northern province of Japan, inhabitants consume the highest amount of salt per capita, and the incident of hypertension in that area is the highest in the country.

Does ingesting salty food really aggravate high blood pressure?

Yes, because when one eats salty food, water is retrained in the body, increasing the volume of total body fluids, which leads to elevation of blood pressure, especially among hypertensive persons. There is another mechanism, a chemical one, that goes into effect when the person with high blood pressure ingests salt or salty food, aggravating the high blood pressure. This is why physicians strongly recommend a low-salt diet as an essential part of the treatment strategy for patients with high blood pressure.

Are the so-called salt substitutes better?

Salt substitutes are potassium and not sodium. It is the sodium in the regular table salt that is harmful to hypertensives and to persons with heart disease. Potassium is medically acceptable for these patients. Potassium salt tastes a bit bitter.

What else is bad for a person with high blood pressure?

Smoking, lack of exercise, eating eggs and red meats (pork, beef, etc.), stress, and lack of rest and relaxation are some of the aggravating factors in a patient with hypertension.

Is hypertension curable?

No, there is no cure for high blood pressure. The only exception to this are conditions or tumors in the adrenal glands (located on top of the kidneys), where the high blood pressure ceases after surgery. The commonest high blood pressure condition—called essential hypertension or primary hypertension—is not curable. It is controllable with medications.

Can a person with high blood pressure live normally?

Yes, with current day treatment, a person with high blood pressure who is under effective management with pills, low-salt and low-fat diet, exercise, and no smoking can live a normal life. As long as the treatment is taken daily and as long as the blood pressure is controlled well, the person could even have a normal life span. With several medications available today in the physician's armamentarium against hypertension, persons with high blood pressure nowadays, who are compliant with the treatment, can be as "healthy" as the next person who does not have high blood pressure. However, there are some persons with the so-called malignant hypertension, who are resistant to the conventional treatment. These are the ones whose blood pressure is not well-controlled; and these individuals are prone to develop complications of hypertension.

How often should the blood pressure be checked?

It depends. If the blood pressure is erratic or hard to control, like when the patient is starting on a new medication for hypertension, the blood pressure should be taken once a day until the medication is adjusted and the blood pressure is basically controlled. If the blood pressure is within normal limits (as described above) as a response to treatment, the medications should be continued for life, and the blood pressure could be taken once a week. If it is really stable at the normal range, then it could be done once every two weeks or once a month. It is important to continue taking medications daily or regularly (as prescribed by the physician) for life, even if the blood pressure is well controlled and now normal. What is keeping it "normal" is the medication! So do not stop unless ordered by your physician.

A Bit of Medical History

Allow me to take you back in time to revisit some of the great moments in medical science, which made possible the great strides man has made in the treatment of cardiovascular diseases that benefit all of us today.

The management of heart diseases was still in the Dark Ages during my undergraduate years in the late '50s. Physicians then did not have the vital information we have today. Looking back, the physicians then did not even know that simple aspirin had any potential role in the prevention or treatment of heart attacks or cancer. Treatment was mainly symptomatic, using pain pills or pain shots. The most sophisticated pill was the nitrate pill, which is a vasodilator that "relaxes open" the coronary artery, since the "current" knowledge in physiology then said angina pectoris (chest pain) was due to spasm in the coronary arteries that supply the heart muscles with oxygen and nutrition.

The first milestone that started it all was in 1628 when an English physician first described blood circulation. Inspired by that, these historical events followed:

1706 Raymond de Vieussens, a French anatomy professor, first described the structure of the heart's chambers and vessels.

1733 Stephen Hales, an English clergyman and scientist first measured blood pressure.

1816 Rene T. H. Laennec, a French physician, invented the first stethoscope.

1903 Eillem Einthoven, a Dutch physician, developed the first electrocardiogram.

1912 James B. Herrick, an American physician, first described heart disease resulting from hardening of the arteries, a fundamental concept that led to the modern therapy of today.

1938 Robert E. Gross, an American surgeon, performed the first heart surgery (close-heart, not open-heart).

1951 Charles Hufnagel, an American surgeon, developed a plastic valve to repair the aortic valve.

1951 John Hopps, a Canadian, invented the external heart pacemaker. That same year, Willem Greatbatch introduced the concept of an implantable (internal) heart pacemaker.

1952 F. John Lewis, an American surgeon performed the first successful open heart surgery.

1953 John H. Gibbon, an American surgeon, introduced the heart lung machine (which he published as a concept in 1937) and first used this mechanical heart and "blood purifier" to do the first "real open heart surgery" utilizing the heart lung machine, precursor of the modern day cardiopulmonary bypass machine.

1960 The first self-contained implantable heart pacemaker made by Medtronic was inserted by W. C. Lillihei. Over the years, this has been improved, made more versatile, smaller, better, and longer lasting.

1960s Denton A. Cooley of Houston, Texas, rose to world fame for his extraordinary dexterity in performing thousands of congenital heart surgeries in infants, and for being the first to successfully remove pulmonary emboli (clots in the lungs).

1961 J. R. Jude, an American cardiologist, led a team in performing the first external cardiac massage to re-start the heart, the foundation for today's CPR.

1965 Michael De Bakey and Adrian Kantrowitz, American surgeons, implanted mechanical devise to help the diseased heart.

1967 Christiaan Barnard of South Africa, performed the first whole-heart transplant from one person to another.

1968 Denton Cooley performed the first heart transplant in the United States on a 47-year-old man, using a donor heart from a 15-year-old. The patient lived for 204 days. He had done 22 heart transplants over the next year, a record at the time.

1969 Denton A. Cooley implanted the first artificial (mechanical) heart on a man to "tide him over" and keep him alive while waiting for a donor heart.

1972 In the field of clinical application, Denton A. Cooley had, by this time, performed more than 10,000 open heart surgeries, more than any other surgeon in the world. That year, in his honor, the Denton A. Cooley Cardiovascular Surgical Society was founded. Its members are the more than 900 heart surgeons from 52 countries around the world whom he trained at the Texas Heart Institute (THI) in Houston. The THI has been doing more than 30 open-heart surgeries per day since then.

1970s Michel Mirowski, MD, and his associates, Morton Mower; Stephen Heilman, MD; Alois Langer, PhD; and a company called Medrad in Pittsburgh developed the automatic implantable cardiac defibrillator. In 1980, the prototype AICD was implanted at Johns Hopkins to prevent sudden cardiac death.

1982 Willem DeVries, an American surgeon, implanted a permanent artificial heart, designed by Robert Jarvic, also an American physician. O. H. Frazier and his team under Dr. Cooley at the Texas Heart Institute has performed more than 600 heart transplants and doing extensive works on artificial (mechanical) hearts. Someday, they will be available on the shelf, like pacemakers today, and heart bypass and cardiac valve surgeries would be a thing of the past.

A Crazy Idea

A most worthy pioneer was Werner Forssmann, who, as a surgical resident in Germany in 1929, experimented with himself by inserting a catheter through a vein in his arm and into his heart. He walked to the basement where the X-ray machine was and x-rayed himself to prove that the catheter was in his heart. In another experiment, he injected dye to his heart through that catheter and took X-ray film. Many of his fellow physicians were outraged by his "daring and insane" acts.

This, by the way, was the origin of what we know today as coronary or heart angiogram or cardiac catheterization that made possible lifesaving procedures, like angioplasties and heart bypass surgeries all over the world. Thanks to Forrsmann's "crazy idea." In 1956, Forrsmann was awarded a Nobel Prize, shared with Dickinson Richards and Andre Cournand, physicians in New York who studied heart function and physiology using catheters.

Against Conventional Wisdom

It was not until the early '70s that the full impact of Forrsmann discovery was realized when Marcus De Wood, MD, of Spokane, Washington, used coronary angiography to search for blockages in the coronary artery. As late as that time, the accepted concept was that heart attacks were "merely the last gasp of a dying heart," a gloomy and hopeless situation that could not be treated or altered or improved. His concept and research were ostracized and derided. In 1980, De Wood was able to prove by angiography his theory that virtually in every heart attack there was a clot blocking the artery. This was a revolutionary change in cardiology which has led to the modern clot-dissolving therapy to prevent a full-blown heart attack and save heart muscles and save lives. This has dramatically improved survival from heart attack.

In 1977, the first angioplasty was performed by Andreas Gruentzig, MD, of Zurich, Switzerland, to "open up" a tight blockage in a coronary artery. This was improved on by the invention of "stent" (a tiny mesh tube of coiled spring, like car shock absorbers) to keep the angioplastied artery from collapsing and reclosing. The stainless steel stents were then improved on with the introduction of drug-coated stents that keep the angioplastied artery patent (open) much longer.

The past half-century brought us lifesaving knowledge and discoveries in cardiovascular medicine. Since then the mortality rate from coronary heart disease has coasted down in a steep plunge from its record peak in the early 1960s.

No one discovery or invention could be awarded all the credit for improving the standard of care. Most of the new innovations have built upon, improved on, the ones before them. Each technology—from computer science to medical science—has made possible the development of better, safer, and more effective diagnostic procedures and/or therapies. Many of the great minds in medicine who dared to espouse new concepts or to alter the "status quo" had faced ridicule and contempt of their peers who thought their "ideas and concepts" were inspired by "misinformation," if not by "insanity and stupid audacity." However, as medical history shows, these pioneering physicians were vindicated, and humanity was better because of their vision and audacity.

HIV-AIDS: Global Trend

A person between the ages of 15 and 24 around the world is infected with the HIV every 14 seconds. Or about 4 cases every minute. More than thirteen million children today are orphans because of AIDS.

Globally, there are 42 million people living with HIV today, up from 40 million in year 2001, and mostly among young people (15-49). Majority of these live in the poorest countries around the globe. In Asia and the Pacific, 7.2 million have HIV infection (more than a million in China alone), a ten percent increase from 2001. Since the epidemic started in the late '70s, the total deaths from AIDS worldwide at the end of year 2000 was 21.8 million. Last year alone, 3 million died of AIDS worldwide, about 8000 a day! Roughly 50% of people with AIDS are women. In Indonesia, it is reported that 43,000 intravenous drug addicts were infected with HIV last year, predicted to double by the end of 2003. In Africa, 25.3 million people have HIV/AIDS. Seventy five percent of adults and 80% of children with HIV-AIDS live in Africa, and in year 2000 alone, there were 2.4 million Africans who died of AIDS and related causes. In Eastern Europe and Central Asia, 1.2 million; Latin America, 1.9 million (210,000 acquired in 2002); Japan, 83,000 got infected with HIV in 2002. In the Philippines, there were 1,921 cases of AIDS in 2003, 13 cases of these were acquired thru blood products (about 80% thru sexual intercourse). This covers the period from January 1984 to August 2003. Interestingly, the rate in this Asian country has remained low and slow, compared to other affected parts of the world.

Hodgkin's Lymphoma

What are lymphomas?

Lymphomas are cancers that develop in the lymphatic system. This system is composed of a network of thin lymphatic channels that branch into tissues all over the body, much like blood vessels. Circulating in this system is a colorless, watery fluid called lymph, which contains infection-fighting cells known as lymphocytes. Along this network are small organs called lymph nodes, clusters of which are found in our neck, armpit, chest, abdomen, groins. Other parts of this system are the spleen, tonsils, thymus, and bone marrow; and lymphatic tissues are also found in the skin, stomach and intestines.

What is Hodgkin's disease?

Hodgkin's disease is one of the lymphomas, an uncommon one, less than 1 percent of all cases of cancer in the United States. The other variety is called non-Hodgkin's lymphomas. Our body cells, under normal condition, grow and divide in an orderly and timely fashion to produce more cells when our body needs them. Carcinogens (cancer-causing agents) can cause the cells to grow in a disorderly, rapid, and uncontrolled fashion, forming a mass (tumor) of extra tissues. This could either be benign (not cancerous) or malignant (cancerous). Since lymphatic tissues are all over our body, Hodgkin's can start in almost any organ, affecting groups of lymph nodes, spreading to the next contiguous group of nodes.

What causes lymphomas?

The etiology of Hodgkin's or the other forms of lymphomas is still unknown, but it is an established fact that it is not caused by injury and that it is not contagious. Why some people get it and others don't, we still do not know.

What are the risk factors?

Persons who develop Hodgkin's disease are usually between 15 and 34 years old and among those older than 55. It is more common among males. It has some familial predisposition, since siblings have higher-than-average chance of getting the disease. Epstein-Barr virus is suspect in increasing the risk of Hodgkin's, but remains to be proven.

Are lymphomas linked to sexually transmitted diseases?

No, there is no known link between sexually transmitted diseases (syphilis, gonorrhea, AIDS, etc.) and the lymphomas, which cannot be transmitted by sexual contact.

Does having TB make one more prone to Hodgkin's?

Pulmonary tuberculosis in a person does not increase his/her chances of having Hodgkin's lymphoma. There is no scientific evidence that shows those afflicted with tuberculosis are more at risk of developing lymphomas of any type.

What are the symptoms of Hodgkin's?

The signs and symptoms may include unexplained fevers, night sweats, painless lymph nodes in the neck, armpit or groin, itchy skin, unexplained weight loss. Most often, though, patients with these symptoms have been found to have less serious medical conditions, like influenza. However, if these symptoms persist, medical consultation is strongly recommended.

How is the diagnosis made?

After the routine history and physical examination (especially for enlarged lymph nodes in the neck, armpit, or groin), the physician may order X-rays, CT (computerized tomography) scan, or even an MRI (magnetic resonance imaging). For definitive tissue diagnosis, a palpable lymph node may be biopsied for microscopic evaluation, in search of cancer cells (Reed-Sternberg cells, large abnormal cells found in Hodgkin's).

If it is Hodgkin's, then what?

If the biopsy confirms the diagnosis of Hodgkin's, the physician needs to know the staging (extent or location and severity of the spread, if any). Biopsy of lymph nodes and in some cases including those in the abdomen, liver, bone marrow, etc., is the gold standard in staging lymphomas.

Which specialists should be consulted?

The comprehensive treatment of Hodgkin's is best handled by a team of specialists, composed of the referring family physician, medical and surgical oncologists, oncology nurse, and/or radiation oncologist.

What is the treatment for Hodgkin's?

The usual treatment for Hodgkin's is either radiation or chemotherapy. Following the diagnosis and staging, the specialist develops a plan according to the patient's age, needs, general health, the size of the lymph nodes, the symptoms present, and very importantly, the stage of the disease.

Are there side effects of treatment?

Yes, just like radiation treatment or chemotherapy for other malignant tumors, the therapy for Hodgkin's also has side effects. These usually depends on the type, dose, and length of treatments. The oncologists will explain all the details of the treatment and the side effects of the therapy as a part of an informed consent for the patient.

What is the prognosis of Hodgkin's?

Today, most patients with Hodgkin's disease are curable, or at least the disease can be controlled for years. The research on cancers has progressed so much, especially with Hodgkin's, that most of these patients now have increased survival rates and improved quality of life. Majority of them can now be cured.

Can treated Hodgkin's patients live a normal life?

The main aim of treatment is to enable the patient to lead a normal life, especially among Hodgkin's patients, where therapy is very successful. Except for the expected lifestyle changes brought on by the illness, diagnosis, and treatment, patients are encouraged to live and be as active as normally possible, according to their condition and endurance. The general outlook for most of them is very good.

How about follow-up care?

Regular medical checkup is most essential in the treatment of Hodgkin's, and the follow-up will be for the rest of the life of the patient. One of the main reasons for this close monitoring is the observation that patients with Hodgkin's are more prone to develop leukemia and those with non-Hodgkin's, cancer of the colon, breast, lung, thyroid, and bone.

Where can one get more information on cancers?

Today, one of the best sources of information in general is the Internet. For medical information, www.webMD.com is a very popular site. There are, of course, at least half a dozen others. Most other websites (like Yahoo, MSN, etc.) have a health section or link. In the United States, publications and brochures on health and diseases are available from the National Cancer Institute (NCI), phone 1-800-4-CANCER.

Human Bar Code

Bar codes for commercial products and services are today a standard armamentarium of the business world. Its use has transformed daily transactions, inventory, record-keeping, accounting, auditing, budgeting, projections, etc., into simpler, more accurate, faster, more efficient, and time-saving endeavors.

A very impressive example on how the use of bar codes has made life a lot easier for all of us every day is grocery shopping or doing purchases in stores in general. Today, we zip through the counters a lot speedier compared to manual counterchecks of yesteryears.

However, "human bar coding" is totally another matter. The idea of implanting a microchip into a person, whose personal identity data and sensitive private information are on the chip (which could also pinpoint the exact real-time location of the wearer), is creating a lot of controversy. There is concern among various sectors of society that this "human bar coding" would curtail individual civil liberties and violate the person's constitutional freedom and right to privacy, confidentiality, security, and safety. There is also the fear that this technology could be used by unscrupulous people or criminals, by competing corporations, or even by some agencies in the government for illegal information gathering or surveillance or for some immoral objectives.

Is there such microchip today?

Yes, it is no longer science fiction. Available today, the implantable microchip radio frequency identification device (RFID) is inert (does not cause adverse reaction on contact with human tissues), encapsulated, the size of a grain of rice or the tip of a ballpoint pen (12 mm by 2.1 mm) that is powered and transmits information when activated by a chip reader. It is tamperproof, practically undetectable and indestructible, and is implanted under the skin.

What is it made of?

The microchip is a tiny (transmitter-computer) chip that has a special polyethylene sheath that encloses it, which makes the skin and subcutaneous tissue adhere to it, causing a tissue envelope around the chip and preventing the chip from migrating. It contains no chemical or battery. The chip is dormant until activated by a small radio frequency energy from a proprietary scanner. The chip never runs down and has a life expectancy of 20 years.

How is the chip implanted?

The chip is small enough to fit inside a special "intravenous needle" introducer. It is inserted using a syringe-type inserter, which comes with the chip preassembled and sterile. It is injected much like a regular injection into the area under the skin in the fleshy part of the inner aspect of the upper arm. A little sting is felt by the recipient during the insertion. No anesthetic agent is needed.

Any possible health complications?

The microchip acts like any foreign body when implanted under the skin, much like a large a sliver or splinter. It causes foreign body reaction and scar formation around (encapsulating) it, a natural body defense mechanism to isolate the foreign body. Unless the person is extremely allergic to the material and "rejects" it, which would be rare, the implant should not cause any complication.

What are the applications for the RFID?

There are various areas where the implantable microchip could be used, besides for personal universal identification and tracking down people. The extended applications include: financial, banking, and public transportation (airport, docks, railways, busses, automatically recording flight manifest log or passenger list, etc.) security, health data storage, access to residential and commercial buildings, access to sensitive government installations, national research laboratories, nuclear power plants, correctional facilities, and for tracking down parolees, ex-convicts, criminals. It could also be useful in homeland security and the fight against terrorism. At the present, the implantation is purely voluntary.

How about its practical use?

Microchips will someday come in various forms, features, specs, and capabilities, to suit the needs and objectives of the individuals or their employers. At the present, the memory of the implantable microchip is rather limited. The scenario could be as follows (depending on the type of chip and what data the person, or the requiring employer, wants on the chip): this implanted micro-chip shall contain a unique verification number, the wearer's identity, like name, sex, date of birth, social security number, Medicare Number, name of spouse and children, addresses (home, office, vacation home or hideaways, street and e-mail), phone numbers (landline, fax, and cell, etc.), attending physician and contact number, clinic or hospital), blood type, allergies, illnesses (including sexually transmitted diseases), medications and dosages, credit card numbers, banks and account numbers, various insurance policy numbers, etc. The chip could also contain confidential code for access to specific private, business, or governmental buildings. The receiver scanner records each entry and exit, with date and precise time. On top of this, the chip can be made a tracking device that could precisely pinpoint the location of the person (a child or a pet) with the implanted chip. This is most helpful in locating a missing person, alive or dead. Paramedics on an accident scene or physicians/nurses attending to an unconscious patient in the hospital can simply use a scanner to extract vital information from the injured. The features of, and the data on, the microchip can be tailored to the needs of the employer company and/or the individual. Right now, the VeriChip, for instance, includes a memory that holds 128 characters only. Larger microchips and highly specialized and more sophisticated ones are underway. With all these features and capabilities, it is easy to imagine how this device could be abused or used for evil purposes.

Is RFID compatible with other security devices?

Yes, as a matter of fact it could supplement advanced biometric devices, such as face recognition or thumbprint readers, retina scanners, and provide foolproof security.

Who makes these implantable microchips?

There are various companies manufacturing the implantable micro-chips, who also maintain a global chip subscriber registry for a fee of about $10 a month. The information on the chip could be updated through the Internet or by calling the registry office.

What's the future of implantable microchips?

In a perfect world, universal implantation of this radio frequency device on everybody (data and info adjusted for each age or professional group, personal, company or government needs, etc.) and used only for legitimate, legal, and noble purpose, this microchip could make life better for all of us, provide better security and peace of mind for us and our loved ones, and even save lives and tremendously benefit mankind as a whole. However, this is not a perfect world. That's why there are concerns and fears. But just like any offspring of the advances in science and technology, the actual and potential benefits of the RFID and its more sophisticated models will someday make implantable microchip a common "household" item. Who knows? Perhaps fashion might even jump in and create a "designer series" of microchips.

Boost Your Immunity

The integrity of our natural personal immune system confers upon our body a defense mechanism which determines our susceptibility to, or the degree of protection we have against, various diseases.

Besides a healthy diet, regular physical exercise, abstinence from tobacco and other harmful substances, moderation in alcohol intake, and taking daily multivitamins-mineral (from A to zinc) supplements, there are food items which can boost our immune system and provide us greater resistance to illnesses and daily stress.

The following foods do amazing job of boosting our immunity: low-fat yogurt, broccoli, wheat germ, sweet potato, garlic, tea, grapefruit, watermelon, cabbage, oyster, blueberries, acai berry, elderberry, button mushroom, spinach, almonds.

Watermelon, cabbage, and broccoli have the antioxidant gluthathione, which also has the side effect of whitening the skin in a natural way. (This should not be confused with the glutathione preparations being advertised as skin whitener, because the use of these commercial items still has some safety health issues. The final word on their long-term adverse health effects on the body as they are used as skin whiteners are still unknown).

Low-fat yogurt (live and active cultures are preferred) is good for the gastrointestinal system, digestion, lowering cholesterol, and boosting the immune system, even against common cold.

Broccoli has nutrients that minimize the damages of natural wear-and-tear to our body. Besides providing fiber, it also acts as "brushes to scrub and clean" the inner walls of the gastrointestinal tract, especially the colon (a protection against cancer).

Wheat germ has antioxidants, zinc, vitamins, and minerals and some good fats. This is a good substitute for regular flour in baked goods.

Sweet potatoes have beta-carotene, an antioxidant which neutralizes the cell-damaging free radicals in our body. They boosts vitamin A, which helps slow down the aging process and also reduces the risk of developing some forms of cancer.

Garlic contains several antioxidants that fight the enemies of our immune system and is an effective substance against the *h. pylori* bacterium that causes ulcers and stomach cancers. When using garlic, it is best to let it sit for about 15 minutes after peeling and chopping, to maximize its excretion of its immune-boosting enzymes.

Tea, black or green, contains a lot of flavanoids and polyphenols, which are antioxidants that ward off diseases by destroying free radicals that damage the cells. Both regular and decaffeinated teas are similarly effective.

Grapefruit has a load of vitamin C and is a booster of the immune system. If you are not too fond of grapefruit, you may try orange or tangerine. Caution: As we have stated in a previous column, grapefruit affects the absorption and potency of some medications.

Watermelon, a member of the cucurbitaceae family (squash, cantaloupe, pumpkin), is also an effective immune system booster with its antioxidant, gluthathione, which is in the red pulpy flesh near the rind. The other 3 members are also immune booster. Like tomatoes, watermelon also has lycopene, a substance protective against prostate cancer.

Cabbage also has gluthathione and vitamin C and provides high-fiber which is good for colonic health.

Oyster, the mythical aphrodisiac, contains a high level of zinc, a deficiency of which causes infertility. Zinc is known for its antiviral and wound-healing effects. Always remember that uncooked foods like raw oysters are possible harbinger of bacteria.

Berries in general have high levels of vitamin C and are rich in antioxidants, anthrocyanins, which have anti-inflammatory properties. Berries appear to fight flu viruses as well.

Button mushrooms are rich in selenium and antioxidants. They also have the B vitamins niacin and riboflavin, which are essential in metabolism. Studies in animals revealed button mushrooms to possess antibacterial, antiviral, and antitumor power.

Spinach, which some people dismiss as a vegetable good only for comic character Popeye, is actually a "superfood" rich in nutrients. Spinach contains folate, which is needed in the body's production of new cells and in the repair of our DNA. It is also rich in vitamin C and antioxidants. Spinach is best when eaten raw as a salad.

Almonds have niacin, riboflavin, vitamin E, fiber, anticholesterol properties, and are a booster of the immune system. Almond is one of the best nuts for our overall health, especially the cardiovascular system.

Green leafy vegetables, in general, are also boosters of the immune system, besides being good for our complexion, our gastrointestinal tract, bones, and joints and the cardiovascular system. These vegetables are also great aids in weight control and in warding off metabolic illnesses, like diabetes, arthritis, etc.

Impotence and ED

What is impotence?

With the advances in medical science, experts have replaced the word *impotence* with a less pejorative and less derogatory name. Today, impotence is referred to as erectile dysfunction (ED), the inability to attain and maintain an erection for a satisfactory sexual intercourse. While the word *impotence* is used to connote a hopeless and permanent condition, erectile dysfunction nowadays is synonymous with a disability that can be treated with great success in most cases.

How common is ED?

Erectile dysfunction affects an estimated 20 million men older than 18 years of age in the United States alone. The prevalence is 52% among men aged 40 to 70, and the incidence increases with age. Normally, men who are otherwise healthy can enjoy sex throughout life, even after age 70, albeit less frequently, with softer erection and the amount and force of the ejaculate somewhat diminished. With currently available medication, the quality of erection can be improved more than 95% in majority of cases.

What are the causes of erectile dysfunction?

The etiology of ED could be *primary* (the man *has* never been able to get and maintain erections at all); and this is almost always due to some psychologic reasons, like fear of intimacy, sexual guilt, severe anxiety, depression. Rarely, the primary factor is biogenic, usually associated with low levels of testosterone and associated with hypothalamic-pituitary-gonadal axis (brain-hormonal disorders). The other cause could be *secondary,* where the man previously was able to attain and sustain erections but presently could not. More than 90% of these are organic (caused by a medical disease), which can be treated.

What is the major cause of ED?

The major cause is usually vascular, where the arteries supplying the male genitals are blocked with arteriosclerosis (hardening of the arteries) due to cholesterol deposits, like those blockages found in the coronary arteries of the heart that cause heart attacks. Others include hormonal disorders (hypo or hyperthyrodism, etc.), drug use (those taking medications for high blood pressure, etc.), and neurologic disorders (stroke, multiple sclerosis, spinal cord injuries, etc.).

Can the penile arteries be blocked?

Yes, the tiny arteries to the male organ itself can be obstructed by cholesterol deposits; and as a result, not enough blood enters the male genital to fill it up to cause distension and erection. To attain and maintain erection, the penis must be fully filled with blood to keep it engorged and hard.

What causes cholesterol blockages in the arteries?

There are many factors. Among them are smoking cigarettes (a major culprit!); eating red meats (pork, beef, and any dish made of any of these two), eggs, butter, cheese, and other foods that are high in cholesterol; and lack of daily physical exercises. The healthier diet consists of fish, vegetables, fruits, high fiber oats, bran, and wheat and a daily multivitamin-mineral supplement. We do not have to eat red meats and eggs to stay healthy. As a matter of fact, it would be healthier for all of us if we stayed away from them. Diabetes also aggravates hardening of the arteries.

How does smoking cause harm?

Smoking has many bad effects on our health. It causes thickening of our blood that leads to blood clot formation on the walls of the arteries throughout our body. As a result of this, the clotted blood becomes so hard it blocks the arteries, like junk blocking our kitchen sink or sewer pipes. This blockages (arteriosclerosis) affect the coronary arteries of the heart, the cerebral arteries of the brain, arteries of the genitals, arteries to the legs and feet. The other harmful effect of smoking is from the poisonous smoke (the nicotine/tar/other chemical combination in the cigarettes) that constantly irritates the sensitive mucosal lining of our breathing pipes and the lungs. This causes not only emphysema ("burned" lung tissues) but cancer of the throat, breathing pipes, the lungs, breasts, and other organs in the body in both males and females. Erectile dysfunction is another side effect of smoking.

Does prostate surgery cause ED?

Yes, surgery of the prostate gland in men causes erectile dysfunction in most, if not all, patients. Those with TUR (transurethral resection for removal of BPH, benign prostatic hypertrophy: super-enlarged prostate gland that blocks urine flow) have 40% incidence of erectile dysfunction. But nowadays, this condition is no longer a hopeless situation like it was about five years ago. Today, we have a medication that takes care of this surgical complication.

What is this "wonder" drug?

The "magic" medication is a nitric oxide enhancer that causes penile venous engorgement and erection, which we have written about when it was first introduced in the United States in 1998. Two other similar drugs, Cialis and Levitra, have since been introduced. This oral tablet has revolutionized the management of impotence, which has since then been renamed erectile dysfunction, a much less ominous condition. The success rate in the treatment of ED is so high this condition does not pose much of a problem anymore in majority of cases.

What warning is there about these pills?

The vital warning relevant to the use of any of the pills for ED is that individuals taking medications with nitrates (as in some heart pills) should NEVER take the pills for erectile dysfunction, because the combination can lead to severe fall in blood pressure and shock. Before taking any of these pills, it is advisable to consult a physician.

Does alcohol cause ED?

One drink does not cause erectile dysfunction, but excessive alcohol ingestion (two or more drinks) could cause temporary ED. This condition can also be situational, involving time, place, damaged self-esteem, a particular partner, or some perceived competitive defeat. The psychological component is very strong. Hence, it is very important that a romantic ambiance and a happy rapport between lovers are a prelude to sexual intimacy in order for the partners to experience the fulfillment and true joy of sex.

When is penile prosthesis implanted?

Penile prosthesis is a device that is surgically inserted into the penis to keep it erect, but recommended only for impotence which does not respond to medication or other treatments. This prosthesis has been relegated to the background since the introduction of Viagra and vascular bypass surgery that redirects blood to the genitals, especially among diabetic patients.

How does one know which treatment is best?

After an interview, physical examination and some appropriate tests, the physician (usually a urologist) will determine and prescribe a treatment regimen for the patient. The management is tailored to the individual situation. It is for this reason why it is very important to seek medical help as promptly as possible, because the earlier it is diagnosed, the simpler it is to manage and the greater the success rate is.

Infertility

How prevalent is infertility?

Infertility is the inability of a couple to conceive after one year of unprotected intercourse. This condition affects about twenty percent (1 in 5) couples in the United States. Its escalating incidence reflects today's intentional delay in marriage and in having the first child.

What causes infertility?

The factors leading to infertility are sperm disorders (35%), ovulatory disorders (20%), female tubal dysfunction (30%), abnormal cervical mucus (5%), and unidentified factors (10%).

Is infertility more common among females?

It appears that is the case, in the approximate ratio of about 55 to 35, female to male.

Does fever affect sperm production?

Spermatogenesis (sperm production) is continuous and requires about 72 to 74 days for maturation. Production is most efficient at 34 degrees centigrade (93.2 degrees Fahrenheit), so exposure to excessive heat or prolonged fever within 2 to 3 months of sperm analysis can adversely affect sperm count, motility, and morphology (size, shape).

What are the sperm disorders?

The most common disorders are varicocele (abnormal dilatation of the veins of the testicles), which has about 25% incidence; azoospermia (no sperm in semen); retrograde (reverse) ejaculation into the bladder; and endocrine (hormonal) disorders.

Do mumps cause male infertility?

Only if the mumps are associated with orchitis (inflammation of the testicles). Fortunately, most cases of mumps are not associated with orchitis. Also, not all with mumps orchitis develop infertility. If orchitis develops, it leads to abnormal, poor, or absence of sperm production.

What is ovulatory dysfunction?

This is a condition where a woman is unable to ovulate (produce viable eggs for fertilization), as in polycystic ovary syndrome or chronic anovulation, luteal phase deficiency, and hypothalamic amenorrhea. The other causes of infertility in the females are tubal dysfunction (associated with past event of pelvic inflammatory diseases), abnormal cervical mucus (normal cervical mucus acts as a biologic filter to prevent influx of vaginal bacteria that could kill the sperm), and some are due to unknown causes.

What are the diagnostic tests for male infertility?

History and physical examination is essential to help the physician in deciding what tests to order. The usual diagnostic aids are semen analysis (the major test), performed after 2-3 days of sexual abstinence; immuno bead test for antisperm antibodies; hemizona assay; sperm penetration assay; and, rarely, testicular biopsy.

How about tests for female infertility?

Ovulation monitoring (daily measurements of basal body temperature), which is not very accurate. More reliable are: pelvic ultrasound monitoring of ovarian follicle diameter and endometrial biopsy. To detect ovulation, there are now predictor kits available that detect an increase in the urinary luteinizing hormone (LH) excretion 24 to 36 hours before ovulation. Other biochemical parameters can be used by the physician to determine if ovulation has taken place.

How successful are the current treatments for infertility?

More than ever before, the success rate today, especially among females, is better, depending on the underlying cause of the infertility. In general, the rate of success among males are much lower, depending on the underlying factor. For more detailed information, consult your family physician, urologist, or gynecologist.

What is assisted reproduction?

This is the science of helping women have a successful pregnancy. Onetechnique is in vitro fertilization, used among patients with tubal disease, endometriosis, husbands with oligospermia (low count) and/or sperm antibodies, and unexplained infertility. The procedure involves drug stimulation of the ovaries to produce oocytes (eggs), retrieval of the oocyte by ultrasound-guided needle biopsy of the follicle transvaginally, fertilization of the oocyte in the "test tube" with washed sperm, culturing the embryos for about 40 hours, after which 3 to 4 embryos are transferred to the uterine cavity (womb). The rest of the embryos may be frozen in liquid nitrogen for future transfer in subsequent natural cycle, if needed.

What is the success rate of this technique?

Although multiple embryos are transferred into the uterus, the average-term pregnancy with in vitro fertilization is only about one in five (20%) to one in four (25%) at best per attempt.

What are the other "surgical" assisted means?

GIFT or gamete intra fallopian tube transfer, where the in-vitro-fertilized embryos are transferred to the distal fallopian tubes laparoscopically or transvaginally guided by ultrasound. When other techniques have not succeeded, intracytoplasmic sperm injection is done, where the sperm is injected directly to the oocyte to ensure sperm penetration and attachment.

If all these and hormonal treatment fail, then what?

The procedures described above are obviously emotionally taxing, very expensive, and many times unsuccessful. The option left is not only a practical one but a very noble and very humane one: adoption. With millions and millions of unwanted babies and uncared for children and orphans in our own country (and in the whole world), adoption could satisfy the motherly and parental desires of childless couples at the same time doing a most admirable act. Adopting children is today considered all over the world as an honorable and dignified way of having and caring for children. After all, being parents in today's modern society no longer means "contributors of sperms and eggs," but rather being benefactors and providers of genuine love and family to children. It is good parenting, and not conceiving and giving birth to a child, that makes a couple real parents.

Insomnia

What is insomnia?

Insomnia is a condition where a person has difficulty falling asleep or in staying asleep, or has a disturbed sleep patterns causing inadequate sleep. The individual wakes up not rested and feeling tired.

How prevalent is insomnia?

Roughly 10% of the population suffers from insomnia, and 50% of these people have the severe form. This is indeed a common symptom.

What are the types of insomnia?

Primary type is long-standing and has not related to psychic events or somatic (body) ailment. Secondary insomnia is one that is due to some physical or emotional problems, pains, or the use of, or withdrawal from, certain drugs. Drinking heavily in the evening can impair sleep and cause some withdrawal symptoms in the morning.

What is initial insomnia?

Commonly associated with an emotional dilemma, like anxiety, fear or depression, stimulant drugs or beverage (coffee, coke, etc.), pain, withdrawal of sedatives or hypnotics, poor sleep schedule, and sleep disorders, initial insomnia means difficulty in falling asleep.

Is early morning awakening normal?

This may be normal for some, especially the elderly, as long as the person falls asleep normally and feels rested upon awakening. However, in many cases, the individual awakens early and cannot fall back to sleep, or drifts into a restless and unfulfilled sleep. Depression and some psychological dilemma could cause this. Early morning awakening is a common phenomenon of aging.

What is sleep rhythm reversal?

This is a circadian disorder, where the persons sleeps during the day and stays awake at night. Examples of this are jet lag, working irregular night shifts, sleep apnea (holding breath on and off while asleep, leading to poor oxygenation, restlessness, and impaired sleep), misusing sedatives, or damage to the hypothalamus of the brain following head injury. Rebound wakefulness is another condition. This results from withdrawal of hypnotics (sleeping pills) among persons who regularly take large doses of this drug.

Are hypnotics the answer?

No, they are not the answer to insomnia. The proper way to deal with the situation is to determine the cause of the impairment in sleep. Is the sleep schedule appropriate? Is the insomnia due to ingestion of stimulants like coffee, cola drinks, or to alcohol or nicotine? Is misuse or abuse of hypnotic or sedative a factor? Or is there a psychological problem or emotional stress or depression? If the insomnia is recurrent, persistent, and unexplained, we recommend clinical investigation in a sleep laboratory.

When are sleeping pills helpful?

Occasional use of sleeping pills, under the supervision of a physician, is safe, so long as there is no medical condition that would require further diagnostic tests. In many cases where psychological or emotional stress is present, discussion and reassurance may help alleviate the anxiety to the point that insomnia is minimized, if not controlled.

Do naps cause insomnia?

Taking afternoon naps can certainly lead to a sleepless night among majority of people. We see this a lot among postsurgical patients who take naps during the day and are awakened by the nurses at night for shots, etc., leading to a reversal in sleep pattern and in impaired sleep.

What is the role of exercise?

Physical exercise (scheduled in the afternoon but not close to bedtime) is one of the best ways to deal with insomnia. Exercise and relaxation can help in warding off insomnia. Some people induce sleep by drinking a glass of milk before bedtime.

Does melatonin help?

Melatonin and other herbal drugs have been advertised to help promote a restful sleep; but we caution the public because these are unregulated drugs, whose content, purity, efficacy and potential harmful side effects are fully unknown. Melatonin is a hormone secreted at night by the pineal gland (in the brain) to regulate the circadian system. Because it can reset the rhythm, it has been used in clinical studies in insomnia and jetlag. There are some reports melatonin could cause cardiac arrhythmia (heart irregularity), one reason why many physicians are reluctant to prescribe this drug.

What are some strategies to improve sleep?

1. Adopt a regular bedtime and wake-up time schedule each day, including weekends.

2. Make it a habit to have regular evening routine to set the mood for sleep, like washing or showering, brushing your teeth, moisturizing your face and hands, setting the alarm clock, etc.

3. The bedroom ambiance (dark and comfortably cool) should be conducive to, and used only, for sleep and sexual activities and not for eating, paying bills, watching the television, etc. Earplugs to reduce external noise can be helpful, where needed.

4. Pillows must be fluffy; and putting one between the knees or using a body pillow, could add comfort for a more restful sleep.

5. Do daily physical exercise earlier in the day, away from bedtime.

6. Avoid stimulants like coffee, caffeinated beverages, chocolate, alcohol, smoking, diet pills, diuretics (water pills) before bedtime.

7. Try to indulge in relaxation technique, like taking a warm shower or bath before bedtime, reading, listening to soft music, saying your night prayers, etc., all of which will help reduce the stress and anxiety of the day, and induce sleep.

8. Planning for a happy morning after, a day of sunshine, to look forward to, can also help.

Interesting Medical Trivia

How many cells do we have in our body?

The figures often quoted are between 50 and 75 trillion cells. The average life span of the cells is: red blood cells, 120 days; white blood cells, over a year; platelets, ten days; bone cells, 25-30 years; brain cells, lifetime; colon cells, 3-4 days; skin cells, 19-34 days; stomach cells, 2 days; and sperm cells, 2-3 days. Obviously, these cells regenerate under normal conditions.

What is the force of a human bite?

Tightly clenched teeth can generate a force as much as 55 pounds (25 kilos) on the incisors and 200 pounds (90.5 kilos) on the molars. For the molars, a greater force at 268 pounds (122 kilos) has been recorded.

Which is the largest organ in our body?

The skin is the heaviest and largest organ in the human body. The total surface area is 20 square feet or 1.98 square meters for an average individual and 25 square feet or 2.3 square meters for a larger person and a weight of about 5.6 pounds or 2.7 kilograms. The liver is the second largest organ (1.1 to 1.5 kilos) and serves about 500 functions as the main chemical factory of the human body.

How long is the human intestine?

Our small intestine is about seven meters (22 feet) long, and the large intestine (colon) is about 1.5 meters (5 feet) in length.

How much blood do we have?

A male weighing about 70 kilos (154 pounds) would have about 5.5 quarts or 5.2 liters of blood. A female of about 50 kilos (110 pounds) would have about 3.5 quarts or 3.3 liters. This blood is circulated through blood vessels that stretch to about 60,000 miles (95,500 kilometers), if placed end to end. The largest artery in the body is the aorta, the largest vein, the vena cava.

How fast does human hair grow?

On the average, human hair grows about nine inches each year. It grows faster in the summer because warm weather increases blood circulation to the hair follicles. The fingernails, on the other hand, grow about 0.8 inches (2 centimeters) every year. The middle fingernail grows the quickest. Fingernails grow four times faster than toenails.

How many muscles do we use to smile?

To produce a smile, we use seventeen (17) facial muscles. To frown, we use 40% more muscles, 43. So let's exert less effort, use less muscles, and smile more.

What does the term LASER stand for?

The acronym LASER stands for light amplification by stimulated emission of radiation. The applications of laser technology is far reaching and wide: micromatching of components and circuit boards for our computers; fiber-optic communications in long distance telephone networks; bar coding scanners; medical diagnostics and therapeutics; desktop printers, color scanners, etc; military target designators, etc.

Can human voice break glass?

Yes, this has been proven in several experiments. The amplified high-pitched singing voice of a soprano or a tenor standing about ten feet from a wine glass cracked the glass in less than half a minute. Without amplification, this could conceivably be done with the glass about two feet away. The sheer force of the vibration from the vocal cords does it.

Will a resected heart beat?

Yes, a human or animal heart cut out of the body will continue to beat on its own, until all the stored energy (glucose and derivative enzymes, etc.) in the cardiac muscle cells are used up. This is usually within five to eight minutes. The heart is the only organ in the body that has automaticity and rhythmcity, hence it beats automatically and with rhythm even after resection from the body (as in the preparation for heart transplant).

How does icy temperature cause frostbite?

Prolonged exposure to extremely low temperature, mostly during winter in parts of the world where subzero weather is the rule, causes the capillaries (most distal tiny blood vessels), arterioles and venules (small arteries and veins), and regular-sized blood vessels to constrict (go into spasm) and shut off the circulation to the toes, fingers, and ears, depriving these parts of the much-needed blood. Frostbites, and even gangrene, are very common. Holding your finger directly against ice for prolonged period can also cause frostbite.

Kidney Stones

What are kidney stones?

Renal calculi (kidney stones) are chemical crystals that form into a hard salt solid structure that looks like and feels like a common stone we find on the streets. They vary in size, shape, and consistency, according to their chemical composition. They could be calcium oxalate stone, cystine stone, uric acid stone, infection stone, or even a combination.

Where do these stones come from?

Our two bean-shaped kidneys are important blood filters which eliminate chemical waste from our body and excreted into the urine. Without our kidneys, the buildup of chemical waste in our body could reach a poisonous, even deadly, level within a few days. In people who have a high risk of forming stones, these chemical crystals solidify in the kidney calices (cup-shaped areas of the kidney). Some of these stones could travel down the ureter (a small muscular tube that connects each kidney to the bladder), causing severe colicky pains from ureteral irritation and spasm.

How large are these stones?

Renal stones vary in sizes, from the size of a grain of sand to as large as a golf ball. Many small stones (silent stones) are passed naturally. Medium stones are often crushed with ESWL (extracorporeal shock wave lithotripsy), popularly known as lithotripsy for short. Large stones may need percutaneous lithotripsy. Very large stones may need surgical removal, especially the staghorn calculus, which "staghorn" shape and large size lodge it in the kidney pelvis (main chamber) and prevent it from entering and passing down the small ureter. Some stones have round, smooth, surface and could pass down the ureter to the bladder with lesser pains. Others have sharp, jagged edges, causing more pains when they travel down, or get caught, in the ureter.

What factors increase the risk of kidney stone formation?

Not drinking enough fluids, dehydration, eating certain foods, urinary tract infection, living in hot climate, and family history of kidney stones are the more common factors that increase the risk of kidney stone formation. Metabolic or endocrine problems are rarer causes.

How much water should one drink a day?

In a normal average daily situation, it is advisable to drink about 8 glasses of fluids (water, juices, preferably not pop) a day, whether one had kidney stones before or not. Those who had kidney stones in the past are advised against cola drinks, tea, chocolate, spinach, and peanuts, which are high in oxalate, and dairy products which are high in calcium. Those with cystine stones are advised against eating foods high in methionine, like fish.

Is it true that renal colic is more painful than childbirth?

Yes, women who had kidney stone colics and had given birth say so. The pain is most excruciating, and in men, it could radiate down to the lower abdomen and to the scrotum of the affected side where the stone is. One thrashes around to find a more comfortable position, only to find none. Narcotic shots are given for the relief of the severe renal colic. Sometimes, renal colic could mimic, or be confused with, acute appendicitis. In some patients, there could be blood in the urine from the irritation of the ureter where the stone is lodged.

What are the diagnostic tests for kidney stones?

After a thorough history-taking and physical examination, your physician may order urinalysis, urine culture (for bacteria), blood count, blood chemistry, a KUB (plain X-ray of kidney, ureter, bladder), an IVP (intravenous pyelogram, X-ray with dye to see locate the stone), an ultrasound (a "3-Dimensional" picture of the kidney); and/or a CT Scan (computed tomography, an X-ray technique showing cross-sectional images of the abdominal area to locate and identify the stone). Twenty four-hour urine sample may also be taken to find out the levels of stone-related chemicals in the urine. Provocative tests may also be done to see how the kidneys handle chemicals. Stone analysis is essential to determine the chemical composition of the stone, which will help identify the cause of the stone formation and aid in the preventive treatment in the future.

Are some stones dissolved by medications?

Yes, bicarbonate can dissolve uric acid stones and cystine stones. This is why it is important strain the urine when one suspects kidney stones, to find out what the chemical composition of the stone is. Medications prescribed to dissolve kidney stones are taken for a lifetime. Unfortunately, not all stones are dissolved by medications. However, many kidney stones are passed naturally.

What are the preventive measures for the various stones?

Uric acid stones are found among those who overproduce uric acid (gout) and can be worsened by a high-meat diet (high in purines), especially pork and beef. Allupurinol is one drug that reduces uric acid. Cystine stones come from too much cystine (amino acids) in the body, caused by an inherited condition. Penicillamine or tiopronin reduces cystine. Prevention in this case includes diet low in methionine (a normal chemical found in fish). Infection stones, as the name suggests, is caused by a urinary tract infection. Antibiotics are given before the stones are removed. In all these three conditions, drinking lots of water helps a lot in preventing recurrent kidney stones.

What is ESWL?

If the stone or stones cannot be dissolved by medications or are too large to pass down the ureter, extracorporeal shock wave lithotripsy is an option. There are several types of ESWL, but the principle is the same for all. The patient lies down or sits up in a water bath, high-energy shock waves from the high-tech machine are precisely aimed at the stone (with pinpoint accuracy). The waves, passing through the water cushion, travel at a high speed, pass through the soft tissues of the body without harming them, and "shatter" the stone (only) into very fine sand. The procedure is done with mild sedation and may last about an hour and done as an outpatient or on an overnight stay.

What are the invasive treatments?

If all of the above therapies fail, invasive or surgical approach is the final option. This includes fishing out the stone in the ureter with a ureteroscope. Percutaneous lithotripsy is used for stones larger than one inch in diameter and where ESWL did not work. A small skin incision is made in the affected flank, and the stone is shattered by painless ultrasound. With the available modern technology today, open surgery is now reserved only for those with very large or oddly located kidney stones. #

Kissing Disease

What is kissing disease?

Kissing disease, medically known as infectious mononucleosis, or mono for short, is a viral illness that presents as fever, sore throat, enlarged neck lymph nodes, and fatigue (severe tiredness). Mono is very common, affecting children, adolescents, and adults. In the United States, about half of the children population have had the infection, usually mild, before age five. The incubation period (time from exposure to mono to appearance of symptoms) is from 30 to 50 days.

Is Mono caused by kissing?

No, kissing is not the cause of Mono. The illness is caused by a virus called Epstein-Barr virus (EPV), one of the herpes viruses, which can be transmitted by a person with mono to another person through mouth-to-mouth kissing or through intimate contacts. Persons who are not infected with the virus can kiss all they want, French kissing and all, and be as intimate as they want and not catch Mono.

Why is mono transmitted by kissing?

The Epstein-Barr virus abounds in the saliva of a person that is infected with infectious mononucleosis, and mouth-to-mouth kissing transfers the virus from the mouth of the infected person to the mouth of partner. The mucus membrane (inner lining of our mouth) absorbs the virus into the body.

Can the virus be transmitted by hand-holding or hugging?

No, physical skin-to-skin contact alone does not transmit the virus, unless the skin is contaminated by EPV-infected saliva. The virus is *not* very contagious. However, since mono could be very debilitating, it is best to be prudently careful when dealing with someone with this condition. Washing hands is a simple and yet very effective way of preventing many infectious illnesses.

How does the illness start?

Among children under five years old there are usually no symptoms. In other age groups, there may or may not be symptoms either. Those who present with symptoms, Mono usually starts as a feeling of malaise (being sick) that lasts for several days, followed by fever, sore throat, and enlarged lymph nodes, most notably in the neck. The fever could peak to 103°F in the afternoon or early evening, and there could be puslike material at the back of the throat. Fatigue is usually marked in the first 14 to 21 days. The acute phase is about 14 days, after which the individual can usually go back their daily routines. In some cases, fatigues could continue for several more weeks.

Is mono fatal?

No. While there are rare reports of deaths from mono (around 1%), usually these are caused by the complications like asphyxia (airway obstruction), encephalitis (inflammation of the brain), meningitis (inflammation of the lining of the brain), or rupture of the spleen. This is most seen among those with impaired immune system like transplant patients or persons with AIDS. In general, most mono patients recover fully.

Why the airway obstruction?

In a few cases, airway obstruction with dyspnea (difficulty breathing) and asphyxia in more severe situations, occurs as a result of the swelling of the lining of the throat and breathing pipe. In these cases, corticosteroids are prescribed by the attending physician.

Does mono cause cancer?

Infectious mononucleosis does not cause cancer. The EB virus is reportedly associated with Burkitt's lymphoma, a form of malignancy that is seen in Africa. In those patients with impaired immune system, it could cause B lymphocyte tumors and some cancers of the throat and nose. The role of the EBV in these conditions is not clear.

What can a partner of one who has mono do?

Both partners must totally abstain from mouth-to-mouth kissing and intimate contacts for at least 2 months from the onset of the acute phase. Since kissing mouth-to-mouth and sex are two of the most pleasurable romantic expressions among humans, especially among adolescents, the total prevention of mono may be difficult. But since prevention is the key, as with other human diseases, this is the only prudent option a concerned partner can take if this viral infection is to be avoided.

Is mono the same as chronic fatigue syndrome?

While chronic fatigue syndrome (CFS), which is twice more common in females and mainly happens to adults (20 to 40 years old), is an entity whose cause is unknown—hence, a syndrome—the EBV has been implicated before, but there is no scientific proof today that EBV is causally related to this syndrome. Severe and debilitating tiredness and lack of concentration are features of this condition. In some cases, there is a low-grade fever and swelling of lymph glands.

Any other similar conditions?

Other illnesses that can be confused with infectious mono are CMV (Cytomegalovirus disease), toxoplasmosis, and even some side effects from some drugs can mimic the symptoms of mono. A blood test can confirm the presence of infectious mono and rule out the other suspected illnesses. This is the reason why consultation with a physician is essential, if only to make sure the symptoms are not due to a more serious disease.

Is rest important in the treatment?

Yes, rest is very important because use the patient usually has severe fatigue and malaise for 2 to 3 weeks. Since the spleen in this individual is congested and enlarged, contact sports, heavy lifting, and other strenuous activities should be avoided for at least 2 months to prevent rupture and hemorrhage.

Does the drug acyclovir help?

While the drug Acyclovir minimizes the production of the Epstein-Barr virus in the body of the patient, this medication has insignificant effect on the clinical presentation of the patient with infectious mononucleosis.

Is aspirin used in mono?

In adults, acetylsalicylic acid (aspirin) may be used as antipyretic (to lower the fever) and as an analgesic (pain killer); but aspirin is no longer prescribed for children, because of the possibility of the occurrence of Reye's Syndrome, which can be fatal. Important warning: aspirin should never be given to children unless specifically prescribed by a pediatrician for a distinct medical reason.

Lactobacillus: Friendly Bacteria

What is *Lacobacillus acidophilus*?

L. acidophilus is the most popularly used probiotic or "friendly bacteria." They live in the intestines and vagina and prevent the entrance and proliferation of disease-causing organisms, thus protecting the individual.

Are there other friendly bacteria in the body?

Yes. Actually there are several trillion friendly bacteria (over 400 species) in the human gastrointestinal tract. Literally, we carry about four pounds (1.8 kilos) of microbacteria in our guts. A healthy predominance of the good bacteria over the bad bacteria spells well-being for the person. If the bad or pathogenic bacteria "outnumber" the friendly ones, ill health occurs.

How does *L. acidophilus* do it?

There are a variety of mechanisms through which L. acidophilus accomplishes its good job. Example: the breakdown of food by this probiotic results in the production of lactic acid, hydrogen peroxide and a few other by-products that create a hostile environment for the bad bacteria. Lactase, the enzyme that breaks down lactose (milk sugar) into simple sugars, for proper digestion and absorption, is produced by *L. acidophilus* too. Those with lactose intolerance or lactase deficiency may be helped by *L. acidophilus*.

Who develops lactase deficiency?

While it is possible that some people could be born with lactase deficiency state, most of those with lactose intolerance (lactase deficiency) develop the condition secondary to lifestyle. People who, during childhood, do not drink milk or do not eat dairy products regularly, acquire lactase deficiency. Lack of this enzyme prevents milk and dairy products (cheese, ice cream, even beans) from being digested and absorbed and properly. This leads to what is known as lactose intolerance, where the milk sugar (lactose) is not effectively broken down to simple sugars, a process needed for proper digestion.

How prevalent is lactase deficiency?

To some degree or another lactase deficiency is found in 75% of adults worldwide. Among Chinese, it is 100%. Twenty-five percent of the US population has some degree of lactose intolerance. About 90% of Asian-Americans, 80% of Afro-Americans, 53% of Mexican-Americans, about 80% of Native-Americans (American Indians), and 15% of Caucasians suffer from lactose intolerance of varying degrees. The incidence for southern Italians and Ashkenari Jews, 70%. A high prevalence is also reported among the majority of Mediterranean Arabs. Exception includes northwest Europeans, where the incidence is below said to be 20%. It has been postulated that those with lactose-intolerance also have a higher risk of stroke, colon cancer, hypertension, osteoporosis. Whether decreased calcium intake (as a result of lactase deficiency) is a predisposing factor in the development of these disease is still not known.

What are the symptoms of lactose intolerance?

Diarrhea and abdominal discomfort/distention, nausea, bloating, passing a lot of flatus, intestinal cramps following ingestion of lactose-containing food items, like ice cream, cheese, even salad or beans. Children who have lactase deficiency will fail to gain weight. The symptoms of lactose intolerance could be mild to severe, depending on the degree of lactase deficiency.

Are there pills for those with lactose intolerance?

Yes. One popular brand in the United States is Lactaid, an over-the-counter medication that has really been effective for those individuals with lactase deficiency. Taking this pill allows them to drink milk and eat dairy products in moderation. For children, pretreated milk (where commercially prepared lactase has been used to predigest the lactose) are available, labeled as lactose-free milk. For infants, strict glucose-galactose-free diet is a must and where fructose becomes the main carbohydrate. For those people on lactose-free diet because they have lactose intolerance, calcium supplementation is highly recommended. Some of the nondairy sources of calcium include green leafy vegetables, fish (especially salmon, tuna, and sardines, where the bones are soft and edible), brussels sprouts, tofu, and broccoli.

What are the claims about *Lactobacillus*?

The major claims include the assertions that *L. acidophilus* lowers cholesterol, boosts the immune system, maintains a healthy flora in the digestive tract, and that it prevents cancer. While there are some probably positive preliminary studies on the first three claims, the last one has yet to be proven. Currently there is no scientific support for the claim that L. acidophilus prevents cancer or that it is safe to take this substance regularly.

Is it effective for bacterial vaginal infection, diarrhea?

L. acidophilus, when taken by mouth (like yogurt) or as a vaginal douche, tablet, or suppository has been proven effective in treating vaginal infections caused by bacteria. For chronic or recurrent diarrhea, this "friendly bacteria" may be of some help but further clinical studies are needed to determine the safe and effective dosage.

How about for other illnesses?

L. acidophilus has also been tried in dozens of other conditions, like acne, AIDS, cancer, canker sores, constipation, cardiovascular illnesses, Cohn's disease, heartburn, hives, indigestion, infections, stomach ulcers, ulcerative colitis, urinary tract infection, thrush, asthma, and many others. The studies done on some of them were flawed and scientifically not significant and worthless. There is no medically validated study to date that proves *L. acidophilus* is effective in any of those conditions listed above, or any other illnesses, except for the bacterial vaginal infection and some form of diarrheas.

Is *L. acidophilus* safe?

As aptly reported by Natural Standard in cooperation with Harvard Medical School, "there is *limited* scientific evidence about the safety and effectiveness of L. acidophilus in humans." Interactions with other drugs or herbs have not been adequately studied. Some people with weak immune system may be at risk of acquiring serious infections when taking *L. acidophilus*. The naturally occurring lactobacillus acidophilus in our intestines is a friendly bacteria, but the commercially manufactured and sold preparations are the ones that need further clinical evaluation in humans before it is approved by the US Food and Drug Administration. Before taking any lactobacillus preparation, consult with your physician.

Is eating yogurt safe?

Yes, safer and healthier than taking *L. acidophilus* or eating ice cream, cakes, or drinking pop beverages (the cola and noncola drinks) that are full of sugars, loaded with carbohydrate that leads to weight gain fast. Yogurt, also spelled yogourt or yoghurt, is a semisolid fermented milk product which originated in Bulgaria centuries ago. In the United States, the starter culture for the production of most yogurt is a symbiotic blend of *Streptococcus salivaris* subsp. *thermophilus* (ST) and *Lactobacillus delbrueckii* subsp. *Bulgaricus* (LB). This produces the best, most stable, and safest combination. Eating yogurt daily has been proven for centuries to be safe and healthy. Since yogurt contains the enzyme lactase, it is easily tolerated by lactose-intolerant people. Other food items easier to tolerate are cheeses (swiss, cheddar, Colby). However, with the commercially prepared lactobacillus "potions for a host of diseases," more scientific studies need to be done to prove its effectiveness; the proper dosage; interaction with other medications; side effects on the brain, liver, kidneys, and other organs; complications; and, most especially, the safety of the therapeutic use of the available preparations of *L. acidophilus*. For use in some forms of diarrhea and urinary tract or vaginal infections *L. acidophilus* appears to be effective and harmless as an occasional beverage, but let's wait for the final verdict from the scientific community.

Wouldn't eating yogurt confer the same benefits?

Yes, eating yogurt, which is a health food acclaimed the world over, provides no less benefits, and perhaps more, than taking the commercially marketed lactobacillus preparations. Moreover, yogurt has been tested for centuries to be safe and healthy. Dieters around the globe consume yogurt with passion. It also comes in various flavors today.

Lead Poisoning

What is plumbism?

Plumbism is the medical term for lead poisoning. The Center for Disease Control and Prevention (CDC) in the United States considers childhood plumbism present when the PbB (lead blood level) is equal or greater than 10 microgram per deciliter, at which level cognitive deficits may start to manifest.

What are the common sources of lead poisoning?

The high-dose exposure includes swallowing pain chips among infants, young children, and mental patients; using lead glasses or kitchen wares; inhalation of leaded gasoline fumes; metallic lead objects (fishing weights, pellets, shots, curtain eights, etc.) in the stomach or joint spaces; burning lead-painted wood and inhaling the smoke; taking folk medicines containing lead; eating acidic foods and drinks stored in improperly lead-glazed ceramic wares; ingestion of lead-contaminated wine or whiskey; and exposure to lead without protection in the workplace. The low-dose source is from lead-contaminated dust and soil on items at home like miniblinds.

What are the signs and symptoms of plumbism?

Depending on the degree of exposure to lead, plumbism may take a while to occur. This could be associated with recurrent episodes of acute symptoms, which may have detrimental effects on the patient, like cognitive deficits in children and damage to the brain and kidneys in adults. When the blood concentration of lead is greater than 50 to 100 microgram/deciliter, the danger of symptomatic lead poisoning goes up. If the level is 100 mcg/dL or more, the risk of brain damage is greatly increased.

How does the condition present itself?

The onset of symptoms among young children is usually abrupt, within one to five days, ushered in by continuous and forceful vomiting, seizures, changes in consciousness, unstable gait, which could end in coma. These are all due to cerebral edema (swelling of the brain). Several weeks before these symptoms, the child may show reduced play activity and irritability. Sometimes, the condition may be mistaken for meningitis, acute encephalitis, brain tumor, or brain abscess (infection with a pocket of pus in the brain).

How about in older children?

In older children, it could present as mental retardation, seizure disorders, aggression, and developmental regression. Anemia in plumbism cases at any age group may be present due to the lead and also to iron deficiency. Psychosis may also be present if tetraethyl or tetramethyl lead is involved.

And among adults?

Among adults, the typical sequence of signs occur over several weeks, with headaches, changes in personality, poor appetite, abdominal cramps and colic, metallic taste in the mouth, constipation, and vomiting. Encephalopathy is uncommon.

Who could be exposed to lead?

The following environmental situations contribute to lead exposure: those who live in houses built before 1960, with peeling paint, and those who visit these houses often. This could be day-care centers, preschool buildings, or the home of a babysitter. Adults whose work or hobby involves lead and people close to them; those in houses built before 1960 which are being renovated; those who live close to battery recycling plants, active lead smelter, and other industry that release lead fumes to the environment; those who have family members or playmates who are being treated for lead poisoning; and those who eat fish and other item from waters contaminated with lead, discharged as waste products of some irresponsible industrial companies.

Do bullets lodged in the body caused plumbism?

Lead bullets in the body do not cause lead poisoning. The body encapsulates all foreign bodies with scar-like tissues, as a natural protective mechanism, which would prevent any significant amount of lead from getting into the blood.

Can biting on pencils and crayons cause lead poisoning?

Yes, if there was lead in the paint or coloring material used in them. This used to be a great and common sources of lead exposure for children, until the government enacted laws that prohibit the use of leaded paints and other coloring materials. Today, you hardly see any leaded paints anymore. There is also a move to phase out leaded gasoline in most countries to protect the global environment.

Are canned goods a source of lead?

The cans used for foods and beverages are made of aluminum. In spite of this, however, it is prudent to empty canned goods into a glassware and not store them in cans for more than a couple of hours.

How about water through lead pipes?

Yes, this is a possible source of lead, especially when the water that goes through them is warm or hot. Lead pipes have also been replaced by copper, galvanized iron, or polyethylene aluminum, and other materials.

What is the treatment for plumbism?

The treatment for lead poisoning is called chelation therapy. While some unscrupulous medical practitioners still claim and administer chelation therapy (for $4000-$5,000) "to wash away and get rid of cholesterol deposits and dissolve hardening of the arteries as a treatment for coronary heart disease" (which are unfounded claims and the use of which for that purpose is totally useless and is criminal), this therapy is most effective for metal poisoning, like plumbism.

When is chelation therapy started?

This treatment is initiated only after the source of the lead exposure has been removed. Among acute symptomatic patients, with presumptive diagnosis made, the chelation is given even before the blood and urine test results are in, to avoid unnecessary delay.

What are the contraindications of chelation?

Those patients who do not have symptoms and those with concurrent kidney or liver disease should not receive chelation treatment.

Any adjuvant therapy?

Yes, for those severe lead poisoning (class 4 and 5), chelation is combined with dimecaprol (BAL) and CaNa2EDTA treatment, as long as good urine flow is present. The maximum duration of treatment is 5 days to avoid depleting the body of other essential metals, like zinc.

Can these be used to prevent lead poisoning?

No, none of these drugs are recommended for prophylaxis against lead poisoning. Besides their potential adverse side effects, it does not make medical sense to use them while being continually exposed to lead. The best way to prevent plumbism is to avoid exposure to lead.

Leprosy

What is leprosy?

Leprosy, or Hansen's disease, is an ancient chronic bacterial infection of the nervous system and the skin, first reported in 600 BC, and is caused by *Mycobacterium leprae*. This microbe is very slow in replicating, taking two weeks to reproduce itself, unlike *E. coli*, for instance, which takes only 20 minutes to replicate itself. This explains why it takes two to 20 years for leprosy to manifest its symptoms and signs from the time the person acquires the infection.

Is leprosy infectious?

Yes, but contrary to myths, leprosy is one of the least contagious of the infectious diseases. The disease is not easily transmissible. It requires extremely prolonged close contact before it is transmitted to another person. Casual daily contact (including handshakes and hugs) does not cause transmission of the disease. The spread is by droplet of nasal mucus during sneezing, but this occurs only in the early stage of leprosy.

Is leprosy a sexually transmitted disease?

No, leprosy is not a sexually transmitted illness. One does not catch the disease by having sex with someone with leprosy.

How prevalent is leprosy?

It is estimated that there are about 20 million people around the world still with leprosy today. The current prevalence is 1 case per 10,000 population, which is statistically low, but the goal is still to eliminate leprosy totally from earth. If left untreated, leprosy can cause severe body tissue damage, like losing fingers and toes, blindness, and other forms of disfigurement. The overall goal set by the World Health Organization Hanoi Declaration in 1991 (a 90% decrease of leprosy as an initial objective for the ultimate global eradication of the disease) has been met. A lot still has to be done by the world community to totally rid our planet of leprosy.

What are the symptoms and signs of leprosy?

Since Hansen's disease affects the skin and nerves, the first sign may be the discovery that the fingers holding a lighted cigarettes have been burned, without the individual knowing or feeling it. This is because of the numbness, absence of sensation or feeling, that results from the damage to the nerves caused by leprosy. More obvious are the nodules, lumps, skin ulcers, blindness, and the disfigurement following damages to the tissues of the body, among others.

Does leprosy lead to cancer?

There is no medical evidence to show that persons afflicted with leprosy have an increased risk of developing cancer.

In which countries is leprosy still out of control?

Leprosy is still "endemic in sixteen countries in the world, representing 92% of the global dilemma where there is insufficient coverage of the network for control measures covering disease in the field, inadequate information and lack of education for patients and communities," says the *Journal of the World Medical Association*. Full control of Hansen's disease has eluded the following countries: Brazil, India, Madagascar, Mozambique, Myanmar, and Nepal. The key force in leprosy global elimination strategy is the Global Alliance for the Elimination of Leprosy chaired currently by India. While great strides have been made in lowering the incidence of this disease the past 15 years, there were still 800,000 new cases reported in 1998.

What were leper colonies all about?

Before science knew the truth about leprosy, its nature, transmission, etc., myths abound, spreading wrong reputation about the disease and its victims, making most people, including close relatives of those afflicted, ostracize and mercilessly drive these poor patients away, putting them in leper colonies, which were remote areas where lepers were camped and "cared for," but generally abandoned. Today, we know better and treat these persons with understanding and compassion. People now live safely with persons with leprosy, knowing it is hard to catch the disease and that the disease is curable with modern-day triple-drug therapy. Among educated people who have current knowledge, the stigma of leprosy is practically gone.

What is the proper message to spread out there?

For leprosy to be totally eradicated from the face of the earth, like what science has done to the historical killer disease, smallpox, we, the medical community and the lay people in general, must echo what the Nippon Foundation stated as it reaffirms its commitment to help eradicate leprosy once and for all: "We must take every possible opportunity to raise our voices and spread the message: leprosy is curable, treatment is free, discrimination must end." Information is indeed fundamental, especially in high-risk regions of the world, so that patients and their families, who were historically ostracized from their communities, are encouraged to come forward and receive treatment, according to the editorial of the *Journal of the World Medical Association.*

What was that reported breakthrough on leprosy?

A major breakthrough has recently been accomplished with the mapping of the genome of the bacillus *Mycobacterium leprae,* which has given the medical community new venues for the development of diagnostic tests for leprosy and possibly for potential discovery of future vaccine and cure for the disease.

Is there hope for persons with leprosy?

Yes, most definitely, now, more than ever before. Cure is now possible. Permanent complication, like blindness, will not recover, but many of the tissue damage that is present could be helped with plastic surgery and prosthetic devices and aids.

What is the current therapy for leprosy?

Chemotherapy with dapsone has been the regimen used with great success, but resistance to this is rapidly increasing. Now triple therapy with rifampicin, clofazimine, and ethionamide is in the forefront of treatment and has been found to be very effective. No vaccine has been developed as yet for prophylaxis. A vaccine would be ideal for the final eradication of the disease.

What are the types of leprosy?

The two forms of leprosy are lepromatous and tuberculoid. In the lepromatous form, there is no body immunity so the bacteria are present in enormous amount in the macrophages of the in the skin and nerves. This leads to large nodules and bumps, which can break down to form ulcers, causing extensive body tissue damage. The tuberculoid form happens when the body immune system is strong and is therefore milder and probably noninfectious.

Let's Be Health Nuts!

Are nuts good for the heart?

Yes, they are, according to clinical investigations upon which the US-FDA based its approval in 1997 for nuts and whole-oat foods to carry the labels "touting possible heart benefits." While animal fats are bad for us, the fats in nuts are the healthy unsaturated fats, which reduce the risk of heart attack. Food items like oatmeal and those whole grains made from wheat, bran, etc., besides providing high fiber in our diet (which reduces the risk for colon cancer) also helps lower the cholesterol in our blood, which protects the cardiovascular system. The study on 31,208 Adventists showed that those who ate nuts 1 to 4 times a week had 27% lower risk of dying from heart ailment compared to those who had nuts once a week. Those who consumed nuts 5 or more times a week had almost half (48%) reduction in the risk. This study considered and adjusted for standard risk factors such as gender, age, blood pressure, smoking, exercise, and other foods like fruits, cheese, legumes, and meats. This clinical investigation also revealed on this same subjects (years later) that those who ate nuts every day lived almost 4 years longer than those who rarely ate nuts. Two other similar researches, the Nurse's Health Study, involving 86,016 women followed for 14 years, and the Iowa Women's Health Study, showed similar results.

Those subjects in the study who consumed five or more ounces of nuts a week showed a reduction in their risk of death from heart attack by 35%, even after considering (adjusting or) others factors such as smoking, alcohol, obesity, blood pressure, dietary fats, fiber, vegetables, vitamin E intake. A more significant reduction of 52% was noted among those who did not drink alcoholic beverages and those who did not smoke. A 57% reduction in their risk of a fatal heart disease was seen among those who ingest nuts frequently compared to those who did not.

Why are nuts good for our body?

Some of the reasons why nuts are healthy for us are: (1) Nuts contain a protein which is high in arginine, a precursor of nitric oxide, which is a vasodilator that relaxes and opens arteries that improves blood circulation to organs, like the heart, brain, kidneys, liver, etc. (2) The fats in nuts are unsaturated fats, the good fats. (3) Almonds and walnuts help lower serum cholesterol level. (4) Walnuts have high alpha-linoleic acid (essential n-3 or omega) fatty acid that is cardioprotective by reducing heart disease and deadly arrhythmias (irregular heart rhythms). And (5) a good source of dietary fibers, nuts contain vegetable proteins, potassium, vitamin E, folic acid, magnesium, and copper.

Do nuts cause obesity?

One of the reasons why some people do not eat nuts regularly is the mistaken notion that the fats in nuts are like the saturated fats in red meat and egg yolk. The fats in nuts are the unsaturated kind that is healthier for our body. Nuts have been found to speed up satiety during a meal, making us feel fuller and satisfied sooner, thus helping control our calorie intake. The recommended amount is one to two ounces a day.

How about peanut butter?

Modern peanut butter contains hydrogenated fats which makes it less ideal and only weakly beneficial to our cardiovascular system. The old-fashioned peanut butter did not contain hydrogenated fats and are as good as the nuts themselves. Peanuts, unlike the other nuts, are really a legume.

Which nuts and seeds are good?

The variety of nuts and seeds commercially available are all good. They are peanuts, cashews, brazil nuts, almonds, walnuts, filberts, hazelnuts, pecan, macademia, sunflower seeds, sesame, and flaxseeds, either raw or roasted, alone or as topping for desserts, in salad or in a recipe. Peanut butter, almond butter, and tahini, as long as they are not hydrogenated, are also healthy for us.

Liposuction Deaths Alarming

Liposuction is the most common cosmetic procedure performed in the United States today. Medically termed lipoplasty, it is a surgical procedure for removal of fats under the skin using a suction equipment through small incisions. This is a short procedure performed usually in the office by a plastic surgeon and was first introduced about 30 years ago.

Like most plastic surgeries, liposuction is a purely elective procedure, one performed not to save lives or treat diseases, but "to achieve beauty."

The accepted medical standard mortality rate (risk of dying) in elective surgeries is 1 death in 100,000 cases. However, in liposuction, the mortality rate has been found to be around 19 deaths in 100,000, or 19 times riskier than what is acceptable. This was reported by the American Society of Aesthetic and Plastic Surgeons (ASAPS) and published in the *Plastic and Reconstructive Surgery* journal. This is even higher than the death rate for motor vehicle accidents in the United States.

This death rate is, indeed, too high a price to pay for vanity' sake, and for an effect that is not permanent or lasting and a condition that is expected to, or could, recur even within months among individuals not disciplined enough to diet properly and exercise daily after the liposuction.

The standard acceptable surgical mortality rate in major operations is usually around 1-3%. While even coronary (heart) bypass surgeries today can attain a 1% post-op rate, or 99% death-free result, well within the set acceptable standard post-op death rate, and in some series, the death rate was even zero in 100 consecutive bypass cases done, liposuction is, to this date, still unable to achieve the industry acceptable mortality rate of 1 out of 100,000 patients for this elective procedure.

The risk in major surgeries cases naturally varies according to accompanying co-morbidities (other diseases present), such as high blood pressure, diabetes, pulmonary disease, thyroid disease, etc., if any. Patients for liposuction, on the other hand, are usually healthy individuals only seeking for aesthetic improvement in their physical appearance.

Is liposuction a cure for obesity?

No, liposuction is not a treatment, much less a cure, for obesity. Most, if not all, plastic surgeons consider obesity as a contraindication for liposuction. The treatment for obesity is mainly reduction diet and daily exercises under a programmed regimen.

So what is liposuction for?

Liposuction is being used to contour the chin, neck, cheeks, breasts, upper arms, abdomen, buttocks, hips, thighs, knees, calves, and ankles. Because of patient expectation, some have been disappointed in spite of good surgical results. Plastic surgeons report that most patients like how they look afterward.

Will liposuction remove cellulite?

No, liposuction will not remove cellulite (dimpled skin). Daily exercises could help improve the looks of the areas involved by firming the muscles underneath.

What are the patient criteria for liposuction?

Liposuction candidates must meet the following minimum criteria: good physical and medical health, normal weight, psychologically healthy, bothered by pockets of fats that remain after dieting and exercise program. And of course, they must have enough money to pay for the procedure, which may need to be done repeatedly as time passes by.

What are the risks and possible complications?

Reaction to medications, problem breathing during the procedure, bleeding, infection, thrombus (blood clots), pulmonary embolus (clots to the lungs), fat embolus (pieces of fats go to the bloodstream and then to other vital organs), which could be fatal. The higher risk appears to be associated with the use of general anesthesia.

What are we willing to pay for "better looks"?

Cosmetic surgery has mesmerized our bulging-sagging-wrinkling-aging population as a crutch while we search for the elusive fountain of youth. And plastic surgeons today can really do amazing feats with one's looks, in the area of noselifts, facelifts, etc. How risky and temporary the good effects of liposuction is another story. I have read and heard of fatalities among young women following liposuction. These are useless and preventable deaths. Not to mention the prohibitive cost of this plastic surgery.

To me, the procedure is unphysiologic, useless in the long run, and not safe enough, to say the least. It is against our body physiology, because it is natural to develop more fats when we eat more calories than we expend with our physical activities. Common sense dictates for us to go on a diet and do daily exercises when we start to gain weight and fatty bulges develop in our face, neck, abdomen or arms or legs. Or even better yet, to diet and exercise before these bulges occur, instead of allowing them to form and then resort to a surgical procedure to remove them. Living a healthy lifestyle is much less expensive, more physiologic, safer, and wiser, and more effective for health and maximal longevity.

Suctioning the fatty tissues under our skin is not the solution, because if, after liposuction, we resume eating more calories than we burn, the fatty bulges will recur to deform us again within weeks or months. Shall we then have liposuction every two months or so? And more seriously, are we willing to risk, or even lose, our life with liposuction just to look a little less fat and prettier temporarily? Are we really that obsessed in dying to look good?

"Liquid Candy"—Unhealthy

In a previous column, we wrote that soft drinks ("liquid candy"), cola or uncola, diet or regular, are, by and large, unhealthy, especially for children. Not only because the regular ones are loaded with sugar (high carbo, super calories), but because of the other adverse effects all these soft drinks (without exception!) have on people's health.

Ravi Dhingra, MD, clinical instructor in medicine, Harvard Medical School, Boston, Massachusetts, reported that "both diet and regular soft drinks have brutally high acid levels."

"Drinking more than one soda a day—regular or diet—appears to increase the risk factors for heart disease," the Framingham Heart Study researchers emphasized.

The following findings of the Harvard research, which we are quoting in full, are a most convincing confirmation and reaffirmation of the other clinical studies in the past:

Risk Rises with Soda Consumption

Harvard Medical School researcher Ravi Dhingra, MD, and study colleagues looked at nearly 6,000 middle-aged men and women who had exams every four years. At the outset, all were free of heart disease and metabolic syndrome. Four years later, in comparison to people who drank less than one soft drink a day, researchers found that those who consumed one or more sodas a day experienced:

- A 25% increased risk of impaired (or higher than normal) fasting glucose and high triglyceride levels.
- A 31% greater likelihood of becoming obese.

- A 32% higher chance of lower HDL levels.
- A 44% increased risk of metabolic syndrome.
- These results were published in the July 31, 2007, issue of *Circulation: Journal of the American Heart Association.*

Study Results Were a Surprise

Dr. Dhingra and his colleagues were surprised that regular and diet soft drinks posed similar risks for metabolic syndrome—which remained the case even when the study was adjusted for dietary factors such as saturated and trans fats, calorie and fiber consumption, and levels of—physical activity. There are several theories as to why this might be—perhaps the extreme sweetness of soft drinks makes people more apt to eat sweet foods, or the caramel content may promote insulin resistance and inflammation. But these are theories, and no one knows for sure. To others though it is now obvious that high acidic levels will help cause these symptoms.

Adverse Health Effects

Drinking soft drinks of any kind has been linked to the development of obesity, type 2 diabetes mellitus, osteoporosis, lowered calcium and potassium level, heart disease, high blood pressure, metabolic syndrome, dental cavities, and nutritional depletion. There is also a claim that it may have an adverse effect on conception. These liquid candies also contain caffeine which could disrupt sleep and lead to anxiety and DNA damage and hyperactivity, especially among children.

The prevalence of obesity among Americans doubled between 1977 and 2001, and this trend was paralleled by a doubling of the consumption of soft drinks. An increase in the body mass index (BMI) of 0.24 kg/meter square was found among children for each (*one!*) soft drink they consumed. Studies on adults (50,000 female nurses on one study) revealed that drinkers of even one can of soft drink led to weight gain, and increased blood sugar among diabetics.

One study reported this interesting finding: "One four-week experiment compared a 450 calorie/day supplement of sugar-sweetened soft drinks to a 450 calorie/day supplement of jelly beans. The jelly bean supplement did not lead to weight gain, but the soft drink supplement did. The likely reason for the difference in weight gain is that people who consumed the jelly beans lowered their caloric intake at subsequent meals while people who consumed soft drinks did not. Thus, the low levels of satiety provided by sugar-sweetened soft drinks may explain their association with obesity. That is, people may who consume calories in sugar-sweetened beverages may fail to adequately reduce their intake of calories from other sources. Indeed, people consume more total calories in meals and on days when they are given sugar-sweetened beverages than when they are given artificially-sweetened beverage or water."

One alarming report: "In 2003, the Delhi non-profit Centre for Science and Environment published a disputed report finding pesticide levels in Coke and Pepsi soft drinks sold in India at levels 30 times that considered safe by the European Economic Commission."

Another study showed that those subjects who consumed soft drinks had lower bone mineral density, placing them at increased risk of suffering, not only osteoporosis but bone fractures. More scary is the increased risk for the development of metabolic syndrome (a group of conditions that include type 2 diabetes, coronary heart disease, stroke, high blood pressure, obesity, high blood fat, low level of good cholesterol).

It is our government's role and responsibility to protect our children by not allowing our schools, public or private, to have vending machines that sell soft drinks and other unhealthy products, much like outlawing the vending machines that used to sell cigarettes.

The Departments of Health and Education and other agencies concerned must also ensure the public that all schools require a course in nutrition for all students and offer only healthy menus in their cafeteria. After all, a healthy citizenry translates into a healthy nation.

Maximizing Longevity

Only about a century ago, the average lifespan of American men was 46; and today it is 73, an added bonus of 27 years, according to statistics from the US Centers for Disease Control and Prevention.

Biologists have estimated that the human body has the potential to last 120 years, if not abused, and properly cared for. The "fountain of youth" appears to be a healthy lifestyle. How we live will forecast 75% of how far we can get.

There are a few "strategies" proven by scientific researches which can maximize longevity. The studies also "calculated" how many "added years" each regimen will confer upon the person who uses any of them.

While the benefits are not cumulative, the more strategies one uses, the greater the chance of enjoying a longer life.

For instance, cutting down on the use of cell phone while driving adds 45 seconds to your life for each call you do not make. According to Dr. Donald A. Redelmeier of the University of Toronto, every day, 99 years of life are lost because of driving accidents while one driver is on the phone.

Have sex often, if possible, and live longer. Studies revealed that there is an inversely proportional "dose-response" relationship between orgasms and heart problems. The more sex, the lesser the risk of suffering a heart malady. One study of 918 men showed that those who had sex the most often had 50% less risk of death from heart ailment.

Cutting down on calorie intake (amount of food you eat) by one-third of what you now eat can lower cholesterol and increase your life by 2 to 3 years. Leaving the dining table less than full is a healthy practice.

While this next one may sound funny, this observation is based on a study made by the University of California at San Diego: Individuals with positive initials, like J.O.Y. or W.O.W., lived almost 4.5 years longer that those with "neutral" initials. Those with D.U.D. and A.S.S. as their initials lived 3 years fewer, and some initials are associated with shortened life span, such as I.L.L. or D.E.D.

A UCLA School of Public Health study shows that men who took 300 mg vitamin C or more a day lived 5.5 year longer than those whose intake was less than 50 mg. Getting enough vitamin C from vegetables and fruits is the best way of doing it.

Helping your spouse take care of your children has been found to increase longevity.

Lowering the cholesterol from 239 to 200 adds 6 months to one lifespan, and dropping a high level of 300 down to 200 gives an additional 4 years to life. This can be achieved by diet, exercise, and if needed, by cholesterol-lowering drugs.

Go to church twice a week and extend your life to 7-14 years longer, as reported in *Demography*. Besides, learning abstinence from tobacco and alcohol, religion in this case also provides strong social and psychological ties and other good practices conducive to a healthier lifestyle.

A research has shown that an active social life can add nearly 10 years to life. Those with practically no friends, minimal social contacts, live 4.5 years shorter.

Among 10,000 men studied, those who have the highest level of aerobic fitness lived 8.7 years longer than those least-fit individuals.

Having regular medical checkup increases longevity by 2 to 3 years by preventing diseases and detecting diseases in their early, curable stages.

Eating less red meat extends life up to 9 years. A diet of fish, soy, legumes and beans and other vegetables increases life expectancy by 13%. Limiting red meat to 3 ounces twice a week, if not eliminating it totally, in exchange for chicken meat, will do the trick.

Get a dog and walking him every day will add 5 years to your life. The studies at the Cooper Institute reported that men who walked briskly for 30 minutes a day, five times a week, prolong their lifespan by five years.

Those who smoke and won't quit, but who do moderately physical exercises daily, are able to delay life-threatening disability by one year, compared to those who just sit around. But naturally, the best is to abstain from tobacco and live five years longer, compared to a smoker.

A normal or medically controlled blood pressure increases your longevity by five to 5.3 years. The standard normal blood pressure level, which used to be 120/80, has been lowered to about 115/70.

You can cut your risk of dying by 13% in the next two decades by ignoring fast-food fries/hamburger chains, as borne out by a study on 3,000 men.

Controlling body weight to normal confers between 8 and 20 added months to longevity.

Believe it or not, a study on 7,841 men showed that those who ate 3 candy bars (dark chocolates, especially) per month, regularly, lived one year longer than those who did not. But those who ate 3 or more sweets a week had 30% increased risk of premature death.

While curiosity kills the proverbial cat, inquisitiveness among seniors has been found to increase their lifespan by five years. "Higher curiosity levels may mean better adaptation to changes, stress, or challenges," said Dr. David Larson of the National Institute of Healthcare Research.

People who have stomach aches and who availed themselves of prompt medical care to cure their ulcer add 2.3 years to their life.

A study conducted by a Scottish neuropsychologist on 1,000 eccentrics found that those "unencumbered by the usual stupid worries that so-called normal people obsess over, live 5 to 10 years longer."

Professional men live 2.6 years longer than average, and unskilled workers live about 4.6 shorter life than average.

Studies from Harvard found that "men who had two to six drinks per week had a 21 to 28 percent lower risk of death from all causes compared to abstainers."

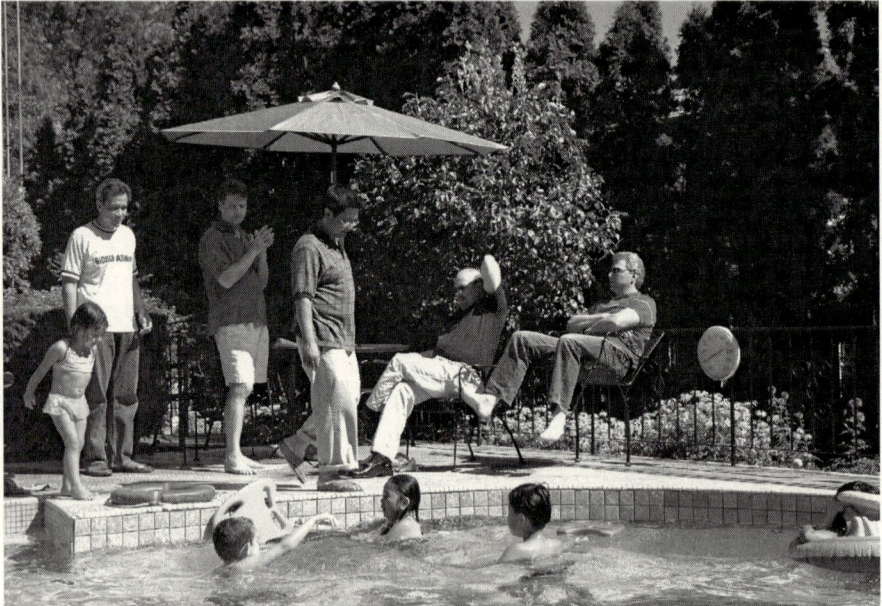

Studies have universally shown that having a family promotes health, stability, inner peace, and longevity. A regular family get-together is a wholesome activity that stimulates the secretion of happy hormones that are beneficial for the body.

Lovemaking and Health

Why is lovemaking good for us?

Scientific evidences suggest that clean sex is good for us in more ways than one. Here are some of the dozen reasons why it is so.

1. Sex is a beauty treatment. Medical tests show that when women make love they produce amounts of the hormone estrogen, which makes their hair shine and skin smooth.

2. Gentle, relaxed lovemaking reduces your chances of suffering dermatitis, skin rashes, and blemishes. The sweat produced cleanses the skin pores and makes your skin glow.

3. Lovemaking can burn up some of those calories you piled on during that romantic dinner, albeit only about 90 calories (22.5 calories after 15 minutes of foreplay and about 67.5 calories during actual intercourse for 15 minutes).

4. Sex is one of the safest sports you can take up. It stretches and tones up just about every muscle in the body. It's more enjoyable than swimming 20 laps, jogging a couple of miles, and you don't even need special sneakers! But this is not enough exercise and not a substitute for daily brisk walking, dancing, aerobics, etc.

5. Sex is an instant cure for mild depression. It releases endorphins into the bloodstream, producing a sense of euphoria and leaving you with a feeling of well-being.

6. The sexually active body gives off greater quantities of chemicals called pheromones. These subtle sex perfumes drive the opposite sex crazy!

7. Sex is the safest tranquilizer in the world. It is 10 times more effective than Valium and other sedatives when it comes to providing the individual the sense of relief, satisfaction, fulfillment, and tranquility.

8. Kissing each day will also keep the dentist away. Kissing encourages saliva to wash food from the teeth and lowers the level of the acid that causes decay, preventing plaque buildup.

9. Sex actually relieves headaches. A lovemaking session can release the tension that restricts blood vessels on the surface of the brain.

10. Lovemaking can unblock a stuffy nose. Sex is a natural antihistamine by producing adrenalin in the bloodstream. In many cases it can help prevent asthma, hay fever, or mild allergies.

Individuals who have special concerns on this matter should consult with their physician for appropriate medical advice.

However, lovemaking is only a small part of true love and caring between husband and wife or lovers. As long as you are able to feel and give love to that special person in your life, the actual physical and sexual expression of this sentiment is secondary. And as couples grow older together, the physical affection is gradually transformed into a longer-lasting, sacred, and spiritual love for each other. A love that truly binds two soul mates into one for the rest of their lives.

Low Back Pain

How common is low back pain?

Low back pain (LBP) is extremely common, is the second most frequent reason for patients to seek medical help, and the number one cause of disability for persons 45 years old and younger. LBP accounts for about 15% of all sick leaves. Lifetime prevalence (chances of getting it during one's lifetime) is about 60-90%. Only 1% of these develop pinching of the nerve, leg pain and numbness, and only 1-3% have herniated (slipped) disc.

What causes low back pain?

The most common form (about 85%) of LBP is called musculoskeletal back pain (MBP), which results from sprain, spasm, or strain of the paraspinal muscles and/or ligaments on either side of the spine and irritation of facet joints. MBP results from lack of exercise; obesity; chronic poor posture while sitting, standing, or walking; and/or wrong lifting technique. After years of abuse, the back succumbs to LBP.

What is slipped disk?

Slipped disk occurs when the disk (filled with jellylike material for cushion) between the vertebrae (spine bones) bulges out and presses on the adjacent nerves. This commonly happens when one twists while lifting. When the herniation (bulging) of the disk is severe and the pains and numbness from the resultant pinching of the nerves are medically intractable, surgery is recommended.

What is the classification of low back problems?

The three clinical categories are: (1) potentially serious spinal condition, which is a rare cause of back pains, includes spinal tumor, infection, fracture, cauda equina syndrome (compression resulting from massive ruptured discs causing urinary and fecal incontinence, unilateral or bilateral leg weakness or pain; (2) sciatica, nerve root compression causing pain along the course of the sciatic nerve from the hip area to the legs and feet; and (3) nonspecific back symptoms, low back pains that suggest neither of the two classification described above.

Does smoking increase the prevalence?

Yes, studies have shown that the incidence of low back pains, sciatica, and spinal degenerative disease is higher among smokers compared to nonsmokers. Smoking also delays bone healing, not to mention it is the major cause of lung cancer and cardiovascular diseases, like stroke and heart attack.

Can cancer elsewhere cause back pains?

Yes, cancer in another organ in the body, like of the prostate, breast, kidney, thyroid or lung cancer, can metastasize (spread) to the spine and cause back pains.

How common is spontaneous relief?

About 90% of patients with LBP will improve within one month even without treatment, and among those with sciatica, 80% will eventually recover with or without surgery. Therefore, conservative management is the initial treatment of choice.

What is the treatment strategy for LBP?

Bed rest is usually not necessary but is an option if the pain is severe. Even so, 2 to 4 days should be max in order not to lose the benefit of physical activity. Greater part of the treatment regimen is good education about low back pains; modification of behavior and activities to tolerable level; temporary limit to lifting and using the correct technique when lifting, no matter how light the object might be; avoidance of prolonged sitting, bending and twisting; gradual return to exercise (those who resume physical activities fare better than those who do not do exercises). Those with cauda equina syndrome and those with persistent, medically intractable pain are candidates for surgery.

What are not effective for low back pains?

The following have been tried in the management of low back pains but scientific studies have shown that they do *not* provide the benefits they claim to have for patients with LBP: muscle relaxants, spinal manipulation therapy (SMT); traction; epidural injection with steroids; transcutaneous electrical nerve stimulation (TENS); lumbar corset and support belt; biofeedback; acupuncture; and herbal medications. Unfortunately none of the above have been found to be an effective treatment for low back pains, but the public is continuously bombarded with infomercials and marketing scams, and unwittingly many have fallen victims to them.

When is support belt useful?

Lumbar support belts when lifting something are of value as a prophylactic measure to prevent the development of low back pains, but they do not relieve back pains when the person already has them.

What is the proper lifting technique?

The correct way to lift an object from the floor is for the individual to sit (not bend his back) and grab the object with both hands and slowly and evenly get up, using the knees and leg muscles, instead of the back muscles, to lifting. The back must be straight, holding the object as close to the body as possible, and avoidance of twisting the body. When picking up something from a table, or walking while carrying anything, it is also best to keep the object as close to the body as possible, to minimize strain on the muscles of the back. Push rather than pull heavy objects. Again, avoid twisting and bending.

Do lifting light objects need the same technique?

Yes, it has been shown that lifting or carrying anything, no matter how light (a glass of water or a book, etc.) causes some strain on the muscles of the back, especially when the carrying arm is extended or away from the body.

What is the best position to minimize LBP?

Good posture is essential. Take frequent breaks when you have to sit for a long period of time, and move around and stretch. Wear flat shoes with low heels. If you must stand for a long time, rest one foot on a low stool, and switch foot every 5 to 15 minutes. Turn by moving your whole body rather than twisting at your waist. The best way to sit is to use chairs with low back support, maintaining a good posture, keeping the knees a little higher than the hips, with feet on a low stool. Use a swivel chair to avoid twisting. When driving a vehicle, sit straight and move seat forward for a comfortable position. Use back support. To reduce pressure on the back, the best way to sleep is on your side, with a pillow between your knees, on a firm mattress.

What exercise can strengthen the back?

Gently stretch your back muscles. Lie on your back with knees bent, and slowly raise the left knee to your chest. Press the lower back against the floor. Hold for about 5 seconds, then relax. Repeat the same exercise using the right knee. Do about 10 of these exercises for each leg. Staying active and living a healthy lifestyle are fundamental. Other exercises, like swimming, walking, etc., unless medically contraindicated, are good regimen for cardiovascular and musculoskeletal fitness.

Lung Cancer

What is lung cancer?

Pulmonary (lung) cancer is a malignancy where the normal lung tissues are replaced by wild, aggressive, viciously invasive, rapidly multiplying abnormal cells, resulting in a tumor mass and loss of the aeration function of the lungs. As the tumor grows, it crowds out and invades the remaining normal lungs adjacent to it, transforming them into a large useless mass. This uncontrolled growth of malignant cells tend to metastasize (spread) to other organs around it, like the lymph channels and glands, blood vessels, nerves, the heart and its covering, and also to distant organs like the bones, adrenals, brain, etc.

What causes lung cancer?

Smoking is the cause of 90% of pulmonary cancers. It is also the culprit in most cardiovascular diseases, like stroke, heart attack, and implicated as contributing risk in the development of type 2 diabetes. Smokers are 13 times more prone to develop malignancy of the lungs, besides other forms of cancers in the body, compared to nonsmokers. The risk is doubled among pipe and cigar smokers. One cigarette is one too many. Tobacco is a vicious killer. Other causes are radon, asbestos, uranium, vinyl chloride, mustard gas, arsenic, coal products, nickel chromates, gasoline, chloromethyl ethers, diesel exhaust, and high levels of talc dust.

Is secondhand smoking as bad?

Secondhand smoke, also known as passive smoking, is even worse and a more deadly cause of lung cancers. Tobacco smoke contains about 4,000 (yes, four thousand) chemicals, 200 of them known poisons. Each year, between 5,000 and 10,000 people in the United States develop cancer from secondhand smoke.

What are the other risks?

Polluted air, industrial chemicals (like nickel, chromium, asbestos, arsenic, etc.) and radiation increases the risk of lung cancer. Chronic exposure to asbestos alone brings the risk to 4 times as high. Combining asbestos exposure and cigarette smoking makes one 90 times more prone to develop lung cancer.

What is the most common lung cancers?

The most common (cell) type of pulmonary cancer among smokers is adenocarcinoma of the lung. It is also the most frequent type of lung malignancy among nonsmokers, among women, and among those who are younger than 45. Compared to the other types (small-cell carcinoma, squamous-cell and large-cell carcinoma), adenocarcinoma spreads less aggressively; and it responds better to treatment, especially if caught early. About 17% of these patients survive 5 years. Breast cancer was the leading cause of death among women for four decades, until 1987, when it was replaced by lung cancer, because of cigarette smoking.

What are the symptoms?

The classical symptoms are cough, weight loss, wheezing, discomfort breathing, recurrent cold or pneumonia, chest pains, hoarseness, and symptoms referable to metastases (spread to distant organs, like bone pains, etc.). Many patients are already far advanced (stage 4) by the time any symptom appears.

How is the diagnosis made?

The medical interview, physical examination, chest X-ray, and CT scan are the most commonly used tools to make a diagnosis. To check for spread, any of the following may be performed: bronchoscopy (looking into the breathing pipe with a lighted scope), biopsy of the lymph nodes in the neck or behind the breastbone, fine-needle lung biopsy, CT abdominal, bone and brain scan.

What is the treatment for lung cancer?

If caught early (or incidentally on a routine or executive chest X-ray), the best treatment is surgical resection. This is the best scenario. If spread to any other organs (bone, brain, liver, adrenals, etc.) is present, X-ray and or chemotherapy may be resorted to, depending on the cell type and other medical considerations.

How is this deadly disease prevented?

Avoidance of exposure to tobacco (active or passive smoking) and the other chemical agents or air pollution listed above is the primary step. Moderation in alcohol intake, living a healthy lifestyle (eating low-fat, high-fiber, high-grain diet of fish, vegetables, nuts, and fruits), and daily exercises are overall strategies to maintain a fortified immune system to ward off diseases, including cancer.

Lyme Disease

What is Lyme disease?

Lyme disease, also known as Lyme borreliosis, is an inflammatory disorder that is transmitted by minute ticks of the *Ixodes ricinus* complex, and the infection is caused by a spirochete, *Borrelia burgdorferi*. The primary reservoir (carrier) for *B. burgdorferi* in the United States is the white-footed mouse, and the preferred host for the adult tick is the deer, but in Europe it is the sheep.

How common is Lyme disease?

First recognized in 1975 in a cluster of cases in Lyme, Connecticut, this tick-borne illness has been reported in 49 states in the United States, with 17,730 cases in year 2000 alone. Majority (more than 90%) of these were in Massachusetts, Maryland, Wisconsin, Minnesota, California, and Oregon. This disease is also found in Europe, across the former Soviet Union, in Japan, and in China.

Who are the usual victims?

The incidence is highest in young children (5-10) and in adults (50-59) living in heavily wooded areas. The onset is usually summer and early fall. Very few of these patients recall the tick bite. The infection rate following the tick bite is about 1.4%. Although this rate is not high, it is obviously important that one prevents tick bites because the complications can be serious.

How is the disease transmitted?

Deer ticks are very small and hard to see. When the ticks in their nymphal stage attack humans, they attach themselves to the skin and engorge on blood for days. *B. burgdorferi* becomes infective only after it has been in place for 36-48 hours, the reason why screening for ticks after exposure and removing them can aid in avoiding Lyme disease. When the *B. burgorferi* enters the skin at the site of the tick bite, it spreads to the lymph glands and also circulates with the blood to various organs.

What are the signs and symptoms?

The best clinical indicator (obvious sign) of Lyme disease is erythema migrans, which begins as a red macule or papule on the skin of the proximal (nearest the body) portion of the arm or leg, especially the thigh, buttocks, and axilla (armpit), between 3 and 32 days after a tick bite. This usually lasts for a few weeks. A flulike muscle and bone syndrome frequently accompanies erythema migrans, manifesting as fatigue, chills, fever, malaise, headache, bone aches, muscle pains, and stiff neck. The symptoms are usually changing and intermittent. Fatigue and malaise may linger for a month or longer.

What are the possible complications?

About 15% of cases develop neurologic (brain and nerve) abnormalities, which last for months but which recover completely. Cardiac findings, like heart block leading to very slow heartbeat and inflammation of the heart muscles occur in 8% of patients within weeks of the erythema migrans, most of which usually recover. Arthritis happens in 60% of cases, with painful and swollen joints, especially the knees, which could last up to more than 6 months in 10% of patients.

How is the diagnosis made?

When the patient is in an endemic area and the classical erythema migrans is noted, no laboratory confirmation is needed. The clinical acumen (knowledge and experience) of the attending physician is enough to make the diagnosis and start the appropriate treatment. ELISA serum test has a sensitivity of 98% and specificity of 72% and reserved for those cases where the index of suspicion is high. Identification of *B. burgdorferi* takes weeks and difficult. Although testing the fluids from the joints of untreated patients for spirochetal DNA could be useful, the test is not generally available yet. Examination of the synovial fluids/

membrane, and other blood and immune system indicators could also be helpful in ruling out other diseases that could mimic Lyme disease and arrive at the correct diagnosis.

What diseases may be confused with Lyme disease?

Illnesses that can present like Lyme disease include juvenile rheumatoid arthritis in children, Reiter's syndrome and atypical rheumatoid arthritis in adults, ehrlichiosis (an emerging infection transmitted by the same tick), idiopathic (cause unknown) Bell's palsy, as well as lymphocytic meningitis, chronic fatigue syndrome, peripheral neuropathies, and other central nervous system disorders.

How can Lyme disease be prevented?

Those who live in endemic areas or persons high at risk must be educated about tick habitat, the disease in particular, and about tick-borne illnesses in general. Those with occupational exposure can be protected by insect repellant spray on their clothing and appropriate repellant for the exposed skin. After being in the wooded areas, individuals must routinely examine themselves for ticks, using a magnifying lens is necessary. Arbitrarily taking antibiotics "to prevent Lyme disease" is not recommended because of potential adverse side effects.

Is there a vaccine for Lyme disease?

New vaccines, based on recombinant outer surface protein specific to *B. burgdorferi*, are being clinically tested. Thus far, they have been found effective and safe among adults in the study.

What is the treatment for Lyme disease?

Appropriate antibiotic regimen is the treatment of choice for Lyme disease. The attendant symptoms are managed accordingly. Complications like heart block may require a cardiac pacemaker and effusion in the knees may need to be tapped, etc. Each stage of the illness is treated respectively, and the prognosis is generally good for most patients. The standard of care is outlined in the guidelines drafted by the Infectious Diseases Society of America. As we have stated earlier, routinely treating all persons exposed to, or bitten by, the tick with antiobiotics is not recommended, because only less than 1% of the totally asymptomatic (symptoms-free) patients eventually develop the disease. Persons with tick bites should be closely monitored for skin rash and fever for one whole month following exposure. Each patient must be individually evaluated, because a shotgun approach will cause more harm than good.

Mad Cow Disease

What is mad cow disease?

Mad cow disease (MCD) is a degenerative central nervous system disease in cattle also known as bovine spongiform encephalopathy or BSE. It was first diagnosed in cows in Great Britain in 1986. The name "mad" was used because the animal afflicted acted crazy, dementia, with mood swings, nervousness, agitation, and instability when standing. The picture is similar to that of Alzheimer's disease but on a greatly accelerated course. The cattle with MCD die within 14 days to six months. There is no cure for this illness.

Does MCD affect humans?

No. However, there is a human version of the illness known as new variant Creutzfeldt-Jakob disease (nvCJD), caused by ingestion of infected beef. The theory is that prions from animals infected with MCD are the sources of nvCJD. The "old" form of CJD is a rare brain malady affecting 2 out of one million people, caused by a viruslike organism and is also found in the United States. The nvCJD is a similar brain disease but different in many respects. It is the human version of mad cow disease and is caused by ingesting food (any food) contaminated with the organism that causes MCD. The malady is fatal. Various USA governmental agencies reported that there have been no cases of MCD or nvCJD in the United States, where import restrictions on cattle from the United Kingdom have been strictly adhered to since 1989.

What does nvCJD do?

The disease attacks the brain, punching tiny holes in vital nerve tissues in it, causing irreparable and widespread damage, eventually resulting in dementia and death.

Have there been cases of nvCJD reported?

Yes. More than 80 people in England, 12 cases in Ireland and three in France have fallen fatal victims to the new variant CJD. Mad cow disease, on the other hand, has also been found in cattle in France, Portugal, Ireland, the Netherlands, Switzerland, Liechtenstein, and Belgium. The epidemic is spreading across Western Europe. No cases of nvCJD among humans and no MCD affecting animals have been reported in the Philippines. But we cannot be complacent and let our guard down. Our government and the public must be ever-vigilant in preventing these diseases coming to our shores and into the country.

How many cases of MCD have there been?

There have been more than 178,000 cases of mad cow disease in cattle worldwide since it was first reported in the United Kingdom in 1986. As a result of MCD, about 5 million suspect cattle have been destroyed prophylactically in England and about the same number in other European countries to prevent further spread of the disease.

Are animal parts used as cattle feed?

In the United States, it is illegal to feed livestock with feeds containing animal parts, precisely to obviate potential risk and prevent the possible contamination, onset, and spread of the disease, although no cases have been reported in the USA. Health authorities put on notice hundreds of animal feed manufacturers that they could be shut down or prosecuted if they violate a 1997 law enacted to protect the people from MCD. Even one contaminated cow can result in an epidemic of catastrophic proportion.

Can MCD or CJD be transmitted by blood?

It is still not known if MCD or CJD can be transmitted by blood transfusion. The US-FDA has been investigating all other possible pathways. An advisory committee to the FDA has recently suggested expanding the ban on blood donations from long-term residents of Ireland, UK, Portugal, France, to ensure uncontaminated blood supply in the United States. Persons who lived in any of these countries for 10 years or longer from 1980, including US citizens, would not be allowed to donate blood. Last August, the FDA approved to ban blood donations from persons who had stayed at least 6 months in the UK from 1980-1996, for concerns that they might have eaten British beef contaminated with MCD. This ban cuts the risk of CJD from transfusion by 90% but also reduced by about 2.2% the amount of blood donation in the United States where there is already a blood shortage. The authorities would rather err on the side of caution to protect its entire national blood supply.

How about contaminated vaccines or supplements?

Since vaccines and dietary supplements that utilize or contain animal proteins or glandular extracts (from brains, tonsils, testicles, and other organs of cattle) may have the potential risk of contamination, the FDA has been vigorously monitoring the situation and has issued stern warnings to pharmaceutical and food supplement manufacturing companies. Let the public beware!

What is foot-and-mouth disease?

Popularly called FMD, foot-and-mouth disease is a highly contagious illness that can spread like wildfire among cloven-hoofed animals like cattle, sheep, pigs, goats, and deer. This disease can easily devastate any country's wildlife and livestock industry and would take billions of dollars to contain and eradicate. The United States has been free of FMD since 1929, but there is an increasing number of outbreaks worldwide.

Does FMD affect humans?

In general, no, foot-and-mouth disease does not pose any health hazard to humans. Humans are not susceptible to FMD, but humans can carry the FMD virus in their body (throat and nose), clothing, shoes, and personal items. Once a carrier contaminates even a single cloven-hoofed animal, a horrible epidemic could rapidly ignite throughout the country.

What precautions can travelers take?

For MCD or CJD and its new variant, the prudent prophylactic measure to take is not to eat beef, in suspect countries, or in countries where these diseases have been reported. For FMD, avoid visiting farms, stockyards, sale barns, animal laboratories, fairs, zoos, and other animal facilities for at least 5 days prior to travel back to your home country. Do not bring in any agricultural or animal products. If you visited one of those animal places, launder or dry-clean all clothing. Dirty shoes may be cleaned with cloth soaked in chlorine solution (using a solution of 5 teaspoon of household bleach in one gallon of water), and so with all personal items if they are soiled. Upon arrival, avoid contact with livestock or wildlife for at least 5 days. This will help minimize, if not prevent, the introduction and subsequent spread of foot-and-mouth disease. Remember, it only takes one stupid mistake by a careless person to cause a national disaster that could devastate our country's wildlife and livestock industry.

Mammogram Controversy

There is public uproar and protests from the medical community against the US Health and Human Services Department about the recent guidelines issued by the US Preventive Services Task Force (USPSTF), an outside consultant "group of experts who make health recommendations based on best available evidence," which call for women "to start mammogram every-other-year screening for breast cancer at age 50 unless they are more comfortable with starting earlier."

This was a change from the annual screening starting at age 40 recommended by the previous guidelines. If the new guidelines are officially adopted, women who are younger than 50 opting to have a screening mammogram will not be covered by their health insurance.

The change is "ill-advised and dangerous . . . and a step backward and represents a significant harm to women's health," according to the American College of Radiology and the Society of Breast Imaging. The two associations claim that the new guidelines will lead to "countless unnecessary breast cancer deaths each year." They advocate the return to the former guidelines: annual screening starting at age 40 and starting at age 30 (or earlier) for higher-risk women.

The USPSTF countered that "to extend the life of just one woman, 1,904 women ages 40-49 and 1,339 women ages 50-59, must be screened." While statistics show that breast cancer risk rises sharply at age 40, the USPSTF "calculates that breast cancer risk gets large enough by age 50 to justify the 'potential harms' of screening," referring to anxiety over false positive results and painful unnecessary biopsies." The radiology societies argued that "the risk at age 40 already justifies such harms," and that "at least 40% of the patient years of life saved by mammographic screening are of women ages 40-49."

The American Cancer Society "still stands by its recommendation of routine mammogram and breast cancer screening for all women at the age of 40 and above . . . and performed every two years."

What is mammography?

A mammogram is a low-dose X-ray examination to detect any abnormality in the breasts which may not be noticeable with the naked eye or by palpation (manual feel). A 20-minute radiological test, a mammogram usually takes about 20 minutes. Since this is a low-dose radiation exam, the exposure is not even part of the debate. There are two types of mammography: screening and diagnostic.

How do they differ?

Screening mammogram is done as a routine exam, a preventive measure, to check for any abnormalities in women without symptoms. Diagnostic mammogram is performed when symptoms of breast cancer are suspected. This test takes longer, and the patient is exposed to more radiation since more films are taken to check more views of the breasts for more accurate evaluation.

What are some signs of breast cancer?

One should be suspicious of any change in the shape or size of the breasts, or the consistency of the skin, when it feels thicker than before, or the presence of pain or discharge from the nipple. This is where familiarity with your own breasts is important, the reason why awareness and or a weekly self—breast exam is of great value.

When should awareness begin?

Starting at the age 20 or even sooner, women should be aware and familiar with how their breasts look and feel, whether they are symmetrical or not, of same size or not, how their nipple and areola (circumferential surrounding area around each nipple) look like. These are then the normal baseline from which any changes may be detected. Not all changes mean they are abnormal. The best thing to do when a woman suspects any abnormality in her breast is to seek medical consultation. As a matter of fact, even without symptoms, it is recommended that women have breast exam every 3 years as a part of a periodic health exam.

What is the incidence of breast cancer?

The incidence of breast cancer in the United States is about 13%, or one in 8 women. In 2009, about 192,370 cases of invasive (wild and deadly) breast cancer and 62,280 new cases of non-invasive (in situ, or localized) have been detected. In men, 1,990 new case of invasive breast cancer were found. Less than 1% of breast cancer occurs in men.

What are the risk factors in breast cancer?

Only about 10% of breast cancers are due to heredity, and 90% are due to genetic abnormalities that occur with aging and environmental factors or lifestyle. Some of the risk factors are regular alcoholic intake, smoking, trauma to the breast, and, very importantly, lack of awareness and familiarity with one's own breasts and carelessness and neglect about medical checkup. The heredity-related breast cancers are due to gene mutation from one's father or mother. The most common are mutations of the BRCA1 and BRCA2 genes. Those with these genes have up to 80% risk of having breast cancer even before they are 50 years of age and also at risk of developing ovarian cancer. Men with BRCA1 gene have 1% risk by the age 70, and those with BRCA2, 6%.

How deadly is breast cancer?

The estimated US cancer deaths from all types of cancer in 2009 in women was 269,800, and in men, 292,540. Fifteen percent, or 40,470, of these deaths in women was due to breast cancer, and 26%, or 70,148, from lung cancer. For men, 9%, or 24,282, from prostate cancer, and 30%, or 80,940, from lung cancer. The death rates from breast cancer have been decreasing since 1990 due to awareness, early detection from screening, and advance treatment modalities for cancer. In 2008, 2.5 million women in the United States survived breast cancer.

Measles Can Be Serious

What is measles?

Measles is a highly contagious airborne disease caused by paramyxovirus and transmitted by virus-loaded droplets circulating in the air coming from an infected patient. One patient can potentially infect as many as 18 or more unvaccinated persons breathing in the contaminated air. Places that are congested and over-crowded spread the disease more readily.

What are the signs and symptoms of measles?

About 14 days after exposure to a patient with measles, the following start to show: flulike symptoms, fever (about 39C or 102.2F), general weakness and occasionally conjunctivitis (red eyes), sensitivity to light, barking cough, sore throat, and Koplik's spots (grayish spots, the size of sand, appear in the mouth) just around the molar teeth, seen a day or two before the skin rash appears. The rash (clear red color) usually starts as small (2 mm) spots that double in size fast and joined together, initially around the ears and then in the body and legs. When the rash appears, the fever may shoot up to 40C (104F) for a couple of days and normalizes when the rash disappears (leaving some brown spots). After 7 days, the child will feel well again. Children can return to school/childcare facilities *only* after they have recovered and the temperature is normal.

When is measles contagious?

The patient with measles is contagious for about 9 days (starting 4 days before the rash appears and five days thereafter).

Is measles dangerous?

While measles is a viral infection that is self-limiting (generally leads to spontaneous full recovery), it can be serious, especially among those with weak immune system, where complications are prone to develop. Among these complications are diarrhea, corneal ulceration causing corneal scarring and blurred vision, otitis media (ear infection) pneumonia and encephalitis (inflammation of the brain), meningitis (inflammation of the tent-like covering of the brain); the last three account for most of the deaths among patients with measles. Fortunately, the last two complications are not that common.

Can adults catch measles?

Yes, unvaccinated persons, who had never had measles, can get infected when exposed to a patient with measles. Measles is usually more dangerous to adults who catch the disease. One of my professors in medical school caught measles and died from its complication (pneumonia). Children usually breeze through measles, but it is wise and prudent for all children to have the MMR vaccination, which includes measles-mumps-rubella (German measles). Chicken pox vaccine is likewise essential for all children to have.

When should the MMR be given?

For children, the first dose is given on or after the first birthday, and the second dose at age 4 to 6, before the child enters kindergarten or primary school, or anytime after 28 days from the first dose. For adults, at least one dose for those who never had MMR or the measles vaccine; and a second dose is recommended for those who are at higher risk of exposure to, and catching, measles. The vaccine confers up to 90% immunity against the virus. Children under one year of age who are exposed to measles must be given an immunity injection *within* 5 days to ward of the disease

How can measles be prevented?

Vaccination is the best way to prevent measles, on top of a healthy lifestyle for the children to maximize their immunity and resistance to illnesses in general. The other is to avoid exposure to patients with measles. Children who had measles will never catch the disease again ever, because infection with measles confers a lifelong immunity to it.

Can measles occur during pregnancy?

Yes, measles can infect women during their pregnancy, if they had never had measles before or never had been vaccinated against measles in the past. While measles during pregnancy does not cause any congenital anomaly, it can infect and kill the unborn. It is best for pregnant women to have measles vaccination unless they already had measles as children. If unsure, consult your physician for possible MMR vaccination.

What's the home treatment for measles?

Basically, this is limited to the management of the symptoms, tiredness with bed rest, fever with acetaminophen (like paracetamol or Tylenol) and cough syrup prescribed by your physician, and a lot of fluids to prevent dehydration. Aspirin is not recommended for children as they can be dangerous for them. Children usually tolerate measles well, but if the fever persists for more than 4 days, or if the child has shortness of breath or if there is any doubt at all, urgent medical consultation is recommended.

Caution on Med Combo

Combining a popular blood pressure medication and either of two commonly used antibiotics may lead to dangerously low blood pressure, or even shock, in elderly individuals.

This was revealed in a 15-year study led by senior author Dr. David Juurlink of the Sunnybrook Research Institute and the Institute for Clinical Evaluative Sciences in Toronto, Ontario, Canada, published in the January 2011 issue of the *Canadian Medical Association Journal.*

The medication is calcium-channel blockers (CCB), a class of pills used for treating high blood pressure, and the two anti-infection pills are macrolide antibiotics called erythromycin or clarithromycin. When a CCB pill is taken by an elderly person in combination with either of the two macrolide antibiotics, the blood pressure of the individual could drop to an unsafe low level. Some may even go into shock.

However, azithromycin, also a macrolide antibiotic, when taken with a CCB did not have such an adverse reaction. Dr. Juurlink recommended that "when clinically appropriate, it (azithromcin) should be used preferentially in patients receiving a calcium channel blocker."

Menopause

What is menopause?

Menopause, also called climacteric, means "change of life," when the woman's ovaries stop producing ova (eggs) and her menstrual bleeding decreases and eventually ceases, all of which are a result of her body's marked decrease in the production of the female hormones called estrogens and progesterone. The diagnosis is established when amenorrhea (bleeding cessation) persists for one year. This natural event in a woman's life usually begins between the ages of 40 and 55, but the average age is about 51. During this stage, the woman can no longer get pregnant because her ovaries no longer "manufacture" eggs.

What do estrogens do?

Estrogens are a group of female hormones necessary for the reproduction and for the development of the breasts, uterus, external genitalia, and the bodily changes associated with puberty. Estrogen also prevents heart disease and osteoporosis (loss of calcium within the bones, causing the bones to be thin, weak, brittle, and fragile and susceptible to fractures). This hormone also helps preserve normal sexual libido and maintain normal vaginal lining and lubrication.

Do all women get premenopausal symptoms?

Not all women have the same premenopausal symptoms. Some do not have symptoms at all, while the others have moderate to severe debilitation symptoms. Others go "crazy" with their violent mood swings and personality changes and drive their husband and children crazy.

Do men undergo menopause?

Yes, men also undergo the change of life at about the same age as women, but usually preceded by minimal or subtle symptoms. Many of them experience this middle-age crisis and start acting a bit weird, like in dressing and behaving like twenty-some-year-olds, or developing sudden interest in text messaging, motorcycles, or buying a sports car, etc. Some become a bit moody or a little depressed, but majority have indiscernible changes. Others undergo male menopause without even knowing it.

What are the symptoms of pre-menopause?

In women, the symptoms are more pronounced and could include hot flashes, skin flushing, and profuse sweating, which affect 75% of women. Most have hot flashes for about a year and 25% to 50%, for more than 5 years. Some of the other symptoms include chills following the hot flashes, irritability, vaginal dryness, decreased sexual drive or interest, fatigue, insomnia, depression, headache, anxiety, nervousness, constipation or diarrhea, muscles aches, palpitation, irregular menstrual, depression, insecurity (with self-pity), mood swings which may extend to "borderline insanity" as a woman once described it to me. Some get upset and hot tempered, impatient, supersensitive to noise and loud music, and simply "hard to get along with," according to children, husbands, friends of premenopausal women. If this happens to men to the same degree, we, too, will be hard to live with.

Can these women control themselves?

No, because their behavior is caused and controlled by the hormonal chemicals (or lack thereof) in their body. The drop in the level of female hormones during premenopause makes some women feel like their being deprived of a drug they used to take, causing severe withdrawal symptoms. We, husbands and children of these premenopausal women must recognize the "pain and torture" our wives or mothers are subjected to during this premenopausal period and should be very understanding, patient, forgiving, and fully supportive of them during this agonizing and trying phase in their life. They are the victims of this "change in life," and we are the natural casualties. Since this phase is only temporary, these women return to their normal selves after their body has adjusted to the change, which time varies in different women from one to three years. Luckily, many women only have mild premenopausal symptoms.

What is the treatment for premenopausal symptoms?

Women should accept menopause as a normal and natural part of their life and that premenopausal symptoms, if present, are temporary and that natural menopause in most women does not need any treatment. Discussing with a physician the physiology of menopause, the concerns, fears, and stresses related to this phase of every woman's life helps a lot in alleviating or somewhat minimizing the symptoms. If severe psychological problem occurs, psychotherapy, antidepressants, and mild sedatives might be indicated. Fortunately, most women do not have severe symptoms.

Estrogen replacement therapy (ERT), also called hormone replacement therapy (HRT), relieves hot flashes, profuse sweating, vaginal dryness and irritation, and other symptoms and also reduces the risk of osteoporosis and heart disease. Fosamax (iandronate sodium) once-a-week tablet is used as a part of a regimen for the prevention and treatment of osteoporosis. Preliminary clinical data seem to suggest that ERT may also help prevent Alzheimer's disease and decrease the risk of cancer of the colon. Estrogen, when given alone, increases the risk of cancer of the uterus, hence in ERT estrogen is combined with progesterone or testosterone to decrease the risk. On the other hand, ERT has been suspected to increase the incidence of liver tumors, gall bladder diseases, blood clot formation, and uterine cancer. Estrogen use has also been linked to cancer of the breast, but experts say the medical evidence is still inconclusive. Some of the side effects of ERT include vaginal bleeding, nausea, vomiting, abdominal bloating, breast tenderness, and uterine cramps. Every woman should, therefore, confer at length with her gynecologist to fully discuss and understand the individual merit, risks, and benefits of estrogen replacement therapy. Self-medication, for convenience and/or to save money, is not only very dangerous, but could be a lot more expensive and more inconvenient in the long run.

Any alternative to ERT?

Yes, a healthier lifestyle is a good alternative or even in conjunction with ERT. This includes diet rich in fish, vegetables, fruits, whole grain, high fiber, and avoiding those foods high in saturated fats (pork, beef, eggs, dairy products) and those high in trans-fatty acids (hard margarines, shortening, commercial baked goods). Abstinence from smoking, caffeine (regular coffee and cola drinks), reducing salt and excessive alcohol intake, and daily physical exercises are vital part of a healthy lifestyle. A glass or two of red wine with dinner; green tea; daily multivitamin with added vitamin B and C; some plant estrogens (phytoestrogens) found in soy beans; flaxseeds; whole wheat; berries; cimicifuga racemosa or block cohosh; isoflavones from tofu; and acupuncture have been used to minimize the symptoms of premenopause. Success with acupuncture varies. Meditation, yoga, and other relaxation techniques as a part of stress management have likewise been found to be of great benefit, not only for premenopausal women, but for all of us in general.

Migraine Headache

What is migraine?

Migraine is a form of throbbing, debilitating headache, the worst a person could have. It may last from four to 72 hours, affecting one (usually) or sometimes both sides of the head, moderate to severe in intensity, associated with nausea or vomiting, and with increased sensitivity to smell, light, loud music or noise, and aggravated by exertion. While migraine affect both genders, even during infancy, it is more common in adult women and most frequently starts between 5 and 35.

What causes migraine?

The cause is not known. What seems clear is that there are blood-flow changes in the brain cortex during an attack of migraine: vasodilation (opening up) of tiny blood vessels in the brain, followed by inflammation and irritation of the tiny nerves around the small blood vessels. Some theorize the opposite: vasoconstriction (clamping down) of the vessels in the brain leading to reduced blood flow and diminished oxygen supply to the cortex of the brain. A cascade of events then ensue in either scenario that ignite the severely disabling headache into a full-blown migraine.

What triggers migraine?

The mechanism in the development of migraine is not clear, but there are triggers known to the clinician. Cycling estrogen is one, and this probably explains why women are affected 3 times greater than men and why estrogen replacement therapy for postmenopausal women usually makes migraine worse. The other triggers are smoking, barometric pressure (altitude) changes, hypoglycemia (hunger), insomnia, stress, fatigue, flickering or glaring light, certain foods, or the weather.

What foods can trigger an attack?

This depends on individual reaction to certain foods. Some people develop migraine after yogurt, lima beans, nuts, dishes with MSG (taste enhancer); others sufferers do not. Some scientists postulate that migraine could be precipitated by foods that contain tyramine and by some cold medications, both of which can constrict arteries, or it could be an allergic reaction to these foods and medications.

What are the symptoms of migraine?

There are two types of migraine: classic and common. The classic form is the one preceded by a prodrome or an "aura" ten to 30 minutes before it strikes. The prodromal symptoms may include temporary blindness, vision of flashing lights or zigzag lines, weakness of an arm or a leg, tingling in the hands or face, speech difficulty, and confusion. The pain is intense, pounding or throbbing, affecting the forehead, temple, around the eye, ear, or jaw and starting on one side but may spread to the other side, lasting for 1 to 2 days. The common migraine is labeled as such because it occurs more commonly in the general population. It has no "aura," although some people have vague symptoms before it sets in, like mood changes, mental fuzziness, fatigue, and even fluid retention and swelling. Nausea and vomiting, diarrhea, and increased urination may be present during the actual headache phase. Common migraine may last 3 to 4 days.

Can migraine cause paralysis?

Yes, among patients who have what is termed as hemiplegic migraine, where a temporary form of paralysis of one side of the body occurs during the attack. Some may have vertigo and or double vision. In the status migrainosus type, which is rare, the very intense headache can last up to 72 hours or longer, requiring hospitalization. Many of these patients were depressed and anxious before the event occurs. The headache-free migraine does not cause any pain, but patients have dizziness, nausea, vomiting, fever, constipation, or diarrhea.

How is migraine diagnosed?

The history, clinical presentation (symptom pattern), and the absence of any evidence of intra cranial pathology (diseases in the brain) are the most important information needed to make the diagnosis of migraine, especially when a family history of migraine is present. No tests will clinch the diagnosis, except exclusion of other causes of headaches. This is why consultation with a physician is important. In the United States there are now headache clinics and headache specialists who treat nothing but headaches.

Why do bright lights or noise aggravate migraine?

The oversensitivity of the patient to external stimuli brought on by migraine makes bright lights, noise, loud music (or even some odor or aroma of food) irritating to persons having an attack of migraine. The perception of all these are so magnified out of proportion that they make the sufferer hurt more.

Is it true some migraine patients have committed suicide?

Yes, there are reports to this effect. The very severe excruciating and intolerable pain in the head has led some patients to bang their head against concrete walls, leading to serious, even fatal, head injuries. And some people have committed suicide because they could no longer take the torture from the recurrent exquisite migrainous headaches. Luckily, nowadays there are more effective treatment regimen to help migraine patients.

What is the modern regimen?

One of the drastic forms of therapy for migraine during the Stone Age was cutting with flint instruments pieces of the skull of the patient for relief of pains. In the 19th century in the British Isles, the patients were given a vinegar cocktail of cow's brain, juice of elder seed, and goat's dung (manure). Compared to those, suicide might seem to be a more pleasant alternative.

Fortunately today we have drug therapy, stress management, biofeedback training, and activity/diet control (keeping a migraine diary to keep track of what activity or food to avoid to prevent migraine attacks). Prevention of hypoglycemia (low blood sugar from hunger) among migraine patients helps control the occurrence of an attack. Abstinence from cigarettes also minimizes migraine attacks. Regular exercises (ballroom dancing, vigorous walking, swimming, and aerobics) can also minimize the severity and frequency of attacks.

Once the migraine sets in, those same activities will aggravate the pains. Yoga or whirlpool baths and other relaxing activities also help prevent attacks. During the attack, the patient should be alone in a dim-lit and quiet room, with just the right temperature. Cold compress over the painful throbbing part of the head or pressure on the pulsating artery by the temple helps. There are two strategies in the use of drug therapy for migraine: one set for prevention and the other for relief. The drugs to prevent attacks should be taken at the first sign of a headache. Even simple aspirin or acetaminophen may help at the onset (as a first step) to minimize the pain, and antidepressants have been prescribed for prevention.

Personal discipline plays a major role in preventing or minimizing the attacks of migraine. For the actual relief, a variety of medications are now available also, starting from the different formulations of ergotamine tartrate. Since treatment has to be individualized, migraine sufferers should consult with their physician for a personalized and comprehensive management. Outlook for migraine victims today is much more hopeful, much better and more pleasant than it was decades ago.

Caution on Mineral Oil

One of the most versatile oils known to man is mineral oil. Commonly called liquid petroleum, mineral oil is a by-product of the crude oil that results from distillation of petroleum in producing gasoline and other petroleum-based products. It is colorless, tasteless, and odorless and is insoluble water and alcohol. It is abundantly available and is inexpensive.

Mineral oil is a common ingredient in baby oil or lotion, ointments to reduce or prevent diaper rash, alleviate mild eczema, as cold creams and cosmetics such as eyelashes strengthener, make-up and temporary tattoo remover. Mineral oil is present in more than 450 skin moisturizers in the market.

Mineral oil is also used in protecting alkali metals like lithium, which are submerged in mineral oil for storage and transport. It is also used to protect and prevent oxidation in weapons, metal tools, guitar strings, poker chips, leather goods, preserve wood products, and as lubricant and coolant for machines, as transformer oil and hydraulic fluid. In some custom-built projects, computers are immersed in mineral oil to absorb the heat and cool down the system. This petrochemical is also the basis for most engine oils.

Mineral oil has also been used on cooking utensils or to grease cook wares and bake wares to prevent food from sticking. It is also used to remove adhesives and sticky gums. It is also used as pesticide for edible plants. It is a dust suppresant on furniture surfaces and useful in cleaning stains from heavy oils.

Medically, mineral oil is used as laxatives for people with constipation and/or hemorrhoids, to soften stool and help ease bowel movement.

Since it coats the gastrointestinal tract, mineral oil use can prevent the absorption of certain vitamins and important nutrients. Chronic use of mineral oil as laxative can be harmful.

Mineral oil has also been found effective in cleaning ear canals of ear wax, except for those with perforated eardrums, where mineral oil can cause infection of the middle ear. It is also used to lubricate the birth canal for delivery. It is not to be used with latex condom as lubricant as it will impair its integrity. It is not safe to use mineral oil in combination with other stool softeners. If applied to hair, it will cause dandruff. Inhalation of mineral oil can damage the lungs.

The US Food and Drug Administration has approved mineral oil "in personal care and cosmetic products, as well as for an additive for food to 10 mg/kg of daily consumption." Also as a laxative, under a physician's supervision.

Minimally Invasive Surgery

The trend in surgery today is toward minimally invasive techniques, all geared for patient comfort, lesser blood loss, lesser pain, lesser morbidity, shorter hospital stay, faster recovery, less obvious scars. These procedures are performed by surgeons specially trained in robotic surgery and/or minimally invasive surgery.

For example: while standard open cholescystectomy (surgical removal of the gall bladder) requires a 5-8 inch incision in the right upper quadrant of the abdomen, all laparoscopic cholecystectomy needs are four small one-inch ports (thumb-size incisional holes), which postoperatively are smaller and much lesser painful compared to the large incision in the open technique.

The Access and Monitoring

The abdominal cavity (or the chest, for heart, lung, and esophageal surgery) is accessed thru small ports and the cavity is inflated with carbon dioxide (safe and harmless for this purpose) to provide a large and unobstructed view of the organ being operated on as the rest of the other organs are pushed away from the operative site.

Trocars (5-10 mm tube cylinders) are inserted through the thumb-size ports, and through one of these trocars is inserted a flexible fiberoptic scope with a lens (lighted magnifying video camera) at the tip, which will send real time and live images to a TV monitor for everyone in the operating room to view as the surgeon manipulates the various instruments to perform the surgery. Thru the other ports are inserted the long-stem needle (suture) holder, scissors, grasping/dissecting instrument, endoknife, suction tip, etc. The images on the monitor are magnified to about 5 the normal size of the structures for easier surgery.

The Surgical Procedures

Minimally invasive procedures are now performed for almost all surgeries: neuro (brain and nerves), cardiovascular (heart and blood vessels), gastrointestinal (food pipe, stomach, intestines, pancreas, liver, gall bladder), orthopedic (bones), and gynecological (womb, tubes, ovary).

The "Nonsurgical" Procedures

The following are the minimally invasive medical procedures: endoscopy (scoping the food pipe, stomach, or colon), subdermal implants (pacemaker and IV access ports), arthroscopoy (scoping the knee), endovascular surgery (intra-arterial surgery), spinal and brain electrode implants, coronary angiogram and angioplasty/stenting, interventional radiology, etc.

Complications

Just like in conventional surgery, there are possible complications that could occur with minimally invasive procedures. Reaction to medications or anesthesia, a bit of hypothermia, internal organ injury, bleeding, infection, blood vessel tear, blood clots in the lungs, breathing problem, and rarely, death.

While the minimally invasive surgery benefits the patient a lot, it is harder technically for the surgeon, because of the space and mobility restriction inherent in minimally invasive procedures.

Conversion to Open

When uncontrolled bleeding, organ damage, or lack of clarity as to the anatomy is encountered, or when the patient does not tolerate the procedure, with unstable vital signs, a conversion to the conventional open technique, with the standard full incision, is done in a timely fashion, usually "ASAP," within minutes, to enter the chest or abdomen, whichever the surgical site is.

Robotic Surgery

In 1985, with CT scan guidance, a robot, the PUMA 560, was used to place a needle thru the skull for brain biopsy. Three years later, the PROBOT, built by Imperial College London, was utilized to do prostate surgery. Four years thereafter, in 1992 Integrated Surgical System's ROBODOC milled "out precise fittings in the femur for hip replacement." The robotic systems was refined and Intuitive Surgical came out with the da Vinci Surgical System.

Like playing most of the computer games at home or in game parlors today, where the players use joysticks to control the desired moves, the da Vinci robotic machine requires the even more precise hand-eye coordination in a new spatial dimension the surgeon has to get used to. With training and more frequent application, the operator gets to be adept at it.

Remote or Telesurgery

Telesurgery, also known as remote surgery, a form of telepresence, is an operation performed on a patient in a hospital by a surgeon who is at another location. This new technique in surgery has been used in the battlefield army makeshift hospital where the patient's trauma required a surgical specialist not available on site.

This cutting-edge science combines the elements of robotic system and today's lightning speed communication technology, like high-speed data connection and management information system. Telesurgery is "an advanced telecommuting for surgeons, where the distance between the surgeon and the patient is immaterial." This makes available the expertise of a superspecialized surgeon to any patient anywhere in the world and allows such surgeon to do surgery with neither of them traveling.

The Lindberg Surgery

On September 7, 2001, a remote surgery was performed across the Atlantic Ocean by Dr. Jaques Marescaux in New York. One of the earliest such telesurgery done, it was a gallbladder operation on a patient 6,330 kilometers away, in Strasbourg, France. The surgery was called Project Lindberg, honoring Charles Lindberg's transatlantic flight from New York to Paris.

Unmanned What?

If the Lindberg was mind-boggling, here's one that will surely bring back the memory of R2D2 in the 1977 Star Wars classic: unmanned robotic surgery.

The first unmanned robotic surgery was performed in Italy in May 2006.

As a cardiac surgeon, I wonder if human physicians will someday be replaced by RoboDocs ?

Mitral Valve Prolapse

What is mitral valve prolapse?

Mitral valve prolapse is a condition where the mitral valve is prolapsing (bulging) into the left atrium during systole and does not close competently as it should normally do. As a result, it allows some blood to leak from the left ventricle back up into the left atrium.

What causes mitral valve prolapse?

Mitral Valve prolapse, or mitral prolapse for short, is also known as MVP, floppy valve syndrome, click-murmur syndrome, balloon mitral valve, Barlow's syndrome, and click chick/straight back syndrome. The exact cause is not known and usually no other heart disease coexists with it. Microscopically, there are myxomatous tissue degeneration of the valve resulting in thin, flimsy, and redundant valve leaflets and elongated chordae. Occasionally, MVP may be associated with disorders causing inflammation of the heart, coronary heart disease, atrial septal defect (congenital hole between the two atria, the upper chambers of the heart).

How common is MVP?

Mitral valve prolapse varies in prevalence between 1 and 6% in otherwise normal population, predominantly among females. The prevalence is higher among persons with Graves' (thyroid) disease, Marfan's syndrome, atrial septal defect, rheumatic heart disease, Duchenne muscular dystrophy, sickle-cell disease, and myotonic dystrophy. About 25 out of a hundred of these patients with MVP have high-arched palate, laxity of the joints, funnel chest, scoliosis, and other skeletal abnormalities.

What are the symptoms of MVP?

Most people with MVP are active and healthy, without symptoms whatsoever. Many of them may not even know they have MVP. Among those few who may have, the symptom(s) could be one or a combination of the following: palpitation (skipped beats) and other heart rhythm irregularity, fatigue, dizziness, shortness of breath, chest pains, migraine, orthostatic hypotension (pressure falls when suddenly getting up from a sitting or lying position). In general, people with asymptomatic (symptom-free) MVP do not have to be overly conscious and anxious after diagnosis is made by a physician. It is rare for this condition to be serious or life-threatening. However, those with symptoms should seek medical consultation because the treatment could be as simple and as minimal as taking pills daily to ward off the symptoms.

Can stroke occur among MVP patients?

The probability of stroke or sudden death to take place in persons with mitral valve prolapse is very rare, less than 1%, and usually happens among those with the complete click-murmur syndrome (prolonged QT interval and low or negative T waves in II, III, AVF and the left precordial leads on EKG). This is more of an exception than the rule among MVP patients. The chances of a heart attack or cancer developing among chronic cigarette smokers are much higher than the probability of stroke or death among persons with mitral valve prolapse.

How is MVP diagnosed?

Auscultation (listening to the heart sounds with a stethoscope) is the primary method of diagnosing mitral valve prolapse. The anatomical deformities of the valve leaflets and chorda tendinae described above create abnormal heart sounds (an opening snap or click, a systolic honk, or a whoop). Two-dimensional echocardiography confirms the diagnosis in 95% of cases and only in 75% of patients when using M-mode echocardiogram. The positive yield is slightly more if the echo is done with the patient on standing position.

Is valve infection a worry?

MVP in itself does not make the mitral valve more susceptible to endocarditis (infection). It is when there is mitral regurgitation (leaky valve) that the mitral valve is more prone to endocarditis, in which case prophylactic (preventive) antibiotic is recommended, especially for those undergoing dental procedures or other surgery, or those with infection elsewhere in the body, including skin infection. Unless absolutely sure that there is no mitral valve leak, all patients with MVP, symptomatic or not, are prescribed prophylactic antibiotic under those circumstances.

Can MVP patients engage in sports?

This issue is still controversial. Some cardiologists advise MVP patients with definite click and murmurs to avoid competitive sports to prevent the occasional rupture of chorda tendinae that will lead to severe mitral regurgitation and serious heart failure. Others do not restrict their patients from sports activities, even those that require maximum effort. A scientific consensus has not been developed yet. The patient's tolerance (or lack of it) to strenuous physical activities (as evidenced by any symptom present) is one best guide to use in making the final decision. The vast majority of MVP patients enjoy full and active lives with no restrictions

What is the treatment for MVP?

As alluded to earlier, the overwhelming majority of patients with mitral valve prolapse do not have symptoms at all, will have no problem, and do not require any treatment whatsoever. MVP patients with leaky mitral valve may need antibiotics during dental or surgical procedures to prevent endocarditis as mentioned earlier. Those with symptoms listed above may obtain relief and benefit from beta blockers, which oral medications also raise the fibrillation (heart quivering) threshold, minimizing the occurrence of fibrillation among patients with dangerous tachycardias (excessively rapid and potentially fatal heart rhythm problem). This is the reason why patients with symptomatic MVP, or who are in doubt that they may have MVP, are advised to seek medical evaluation and care.

When is surgery indicated?

Surgery is seldom indicated for mitral valve prolapse. The operation is reserved for the rare case where the prolapse is so marked that severe chest pains and/or hemodynamically significant heart rhythm disturbances are medically intractable, and/or mitral regurgitation (valve leak) becomes excessively debilitating because of the resultant congestive heart failure.

Multiple Sclerosis

Multiple Sclerosis, or MS as it is popularly known, is an autoimmune demyelinating (nerve sheath destroying) inflammatory disease of the central nervous system (CNS) whose specific cause is still unknown. The pathology characteristically involves the optic (eye) nerve, periventricular white matter of the cerebellum, brain stem, basal ganglia, and spinal cord.

What are the presenting signs and symptoms of MS?

The patient afflicted with MS usually presents with an individual mix of neruopsychological dysfunction, which get worse over years and decades. The classic presentation includes optic neuritis (swelling of the nerve to the eyes), ophthalmoplegia (paralysis of the eye muscles), paresthesias (abnormal skin sensations), and a variety of other neurologic aberrations noted from the patient's history and physical examination, like bladder dysfunction, impaired swallowing or cough reflex, spasticity, gait instability, paralysis, and other CNS dysfunction.

What test can help establish the diagnosis?

The typical tell-tale findings on MRI (magnetic resonance Imaging), together with the above-listed findings, help confirm the diagnosis of multiple sclerosis. Persons suspected to have MS, but who have atypical signs and symptoms and/or atypical or normal MRI findings, may need evoked potential studies to reveal subclinical (subtle) neurologic abnormalities or a spinal tab for cerebrospinal fluid for analysis to rule out other neurologic conditions.

What does the spinal tap show?

Also known as lumbar puncture, spinal tap entails collecting samples of CSF (cerebrospinal fluid), blood serum, and ordinary blood specimen for analysis (by electrophoresis) and comparing them. This test does not clinch the diagnosis but the findings can be indicative of MS and help support a clinical diagnosis. The finding, a phenomenon termed IgG oligoclonal banding, if often corollary to MS. In 90% of MS, the immunoglobulin-G (IgG) is elevated to 0.7, which results in IgGo banding shown on electrophoresis. Viral infection and tumors may also exhibit this phenomenon, so clinical correlation and confirmatory tests by the attending physician is essential. In about 35% of MS, CSF helper T-cells is also increased; and in 80% of acute relapsing MS, myelin basic protein (MBP) levels are also elevated.

How prevalent is MS?

In the United States, multiple sclerosis is the most common debilitating disease in young adult, with an incidence of about 0.5 to 1 per 1000 people. An individual, in the general population, has a 0.2% lifetime risk of developing MS. Each year, about 25,000 new cases are diagnosed. Globally, about 1 per million acquires MS, which appears to be twice as common among the Caucasians than among Native American Indians and Asians, where it is rare, and unknown among Eskimos and Bantus. MS is also 5 times more in temperate climates than in the tropics. The risk of having MS is greater among those who have lived in temperate climate before age 15, but not among those to be moved to temperate regions after that age. It is also twice as common among females, and seldom happens before age 20 and after 50.

Does MS kill?

No, the disease itself does not. MS generally causes disabilities that adversely affect the quality of life of the individual. It is the worsening disability which leads to other problems that cause mortality. The fulminant type of MS, which is rare, can cause death; but usually the mortality in MS is secondary to pneumonia, pulmonary embolism (blood clots in the lungs), and infected decubiti (bedsores) and suicide precipitated by depression.

How is MS managed?

Approximately 70% of MS is the more favorable type called relapsing-remitting (RR), who typically have acute episodes with complete or partial remissions. The acute fulminant MS often results in death or morbidity within days, while the forme fruste or benign MS has a very slow progression over decades, if any at all. The management of MS is a multidisciplinary approach, including careful monitoring, medications to modify the disease, drugs to treat symptoms, such as antiviral meds, steroids, muscle relaxants, pills to reduce fatigue, physical and occupational therapy, and counseling.

For RR-MS, the US-FDA has approved for chronic use the use of beta-interferons and glatiramer acetate (a synthetic form of myelin basic protein (MBP), which has fewer side effects than interferon. This therapy has reduced about 33% the clinical activity and progression of the MS. For the chronic form of MS, the results are not as good, even with beta-inteferons, though modest response is noted with methotrexate. The management includes individualization of medical care according to the type of MS and the various complications that may develop. But research on the optimal form of treatment for each type of MS is still ongoing.

Multivitamins and Nutriment

What is nutriment?

The substance in the food we eat that nourishes the body is called nutriment, consisting of micronutrients and macronutrients. Micronutrients include vitamins (A, B, C, D, E, etc.) and elements (calcium, phosphorus, potassium, iron, zinc, iodine, etc.). Macronutrients are the carbohydrates, fats, and proteins.

Are vitamins important for our health?

Yes. The body is like a complex and sophisticated chemical factory synthesizing, producing, transforming, modifying, degrading, destroying, and eliminating countless chemicals in us to make our vital organs, our body, in a balance state (homeostasis) to function properly. In order to be able to do all these biological chemistries, the body needs all necessary ingredients to accomplish the proper chemical reactions, and vitamins are some of the essential components in the formula for a normal and healthy physiology.

Does our body contain silver and gold?

Yes, there are traces of silver and gold in our body, but they do not have any known metabolic role in our health.

Are vitamins safe?

Yes, vitamins, manufactured by a reputable drug company, are safe, so long as the user is not allergic to them, and that they are taken in the normal prescribed dose.

What is the recommended dose for vitamins and minerals?

For adults, taking one tablet of a one-a-day multivitamins and minerals (they come combined in one pill) is sufficient and safe. For children, there are specially formulated multivitamins and minerals designed for them. Anywhere in the world, some manufacturers may produce substandard quality drugs, including vitamins and minerals. So be careful. Read the labels well and use drugs and vitamins that are manufactured by established companies with a good record and reputation. Your physician can guide you accordingly.

Do vitamins have toxicity?

Yes, some do. Vitamins A, D, E, K, and B6 could produce toxicity if taken in excess. Vitamin C and most of the other Vitamin Bs are water soluble and, if taken in excess of not more than twice, are eliminated by the body, thus averting toxicity. In contrast, Vitamins A, D, E, and K are fat soluble and are not as easily eliminated by the body when taken in excess and therefore cause toxicity.

Who should take vitamins and minerals?

In this age of hurried life, stress, and fast foods, practically everyone could benefit from taking multivitamins and minerals. Since these come in one pill to be taken one a day, it is so convenient there is practically no excuse for not taken them. And even if one eats "well," multivitamins and minerals could still supply what the body needs, which we may not even know are lacking in the food we consume daily.

What happens if a person takes a double dose?

Unless the person is allergic to any components in the pill, chances are no ill effects will happen if this is done only once or twice. If done repeatedly, toxicity could occur. But there is no reason at all for a person to take more than one. The recommended dose of one pill a day gives the maximum benefit to a normal person. Taking double dose will not give any added benefit. It will only be more expensive.

What time should vitamins and minerals be taken?

Unlike some medications, multivitamins and minerals may be taken any time at the person's convenience. However, most people take them with breakfast in order not to forget taking them.

Should all children take multivitamins?

Yes, especially in this part of the world. Even pediatricians and the surgeon general in the United States officially recommend that normal babies and children be given daily multivitamins and minerals especially formulated for them. Parents should discuss this with their physician for advice.

Does taking multivitamins and minerals slow down aging?

There is no concrete evidence in the medical literature that proves taking multivitamins and minerals slow down the aging process in man. However, vitamin/mineral deficiency in us, which is not easy to detect, is a condition that could make the tissue aging process faster than "normal." Some lay publications claim that taking multivitamins/ minerals and antioxidants (which substance we shall discuss as a separate topic in the future) helps slow down the aging process to a certain extent.

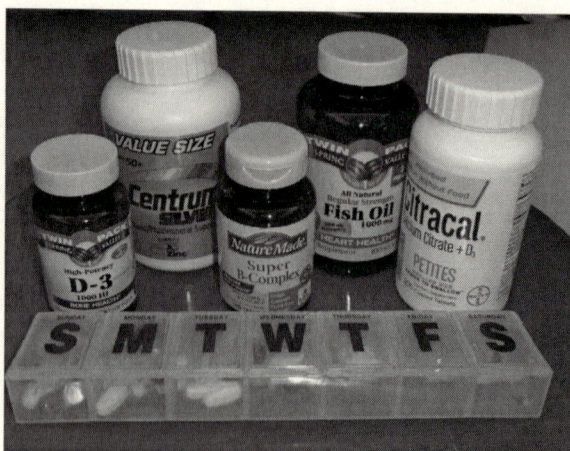

Strict compliance with prescribed medications and supplements is important to keep the effective blood level on an even keel.

Multivitamins and Prostate Cancer

Men taking multivitamins more than once daily, more than 7 days a week, have 30% higher risk of developing advanced prostate cancer and doubling the risk of death from this malignancy, reported a new study.

Taking too many multivitamins and/or mega-doses of "food supplements" is hazardous to health. Overdosing on anything is abuse and, therefore, unhealthy and unsafe.

The new findings from the National Cancer Institute (NCI) noted that regular multivitamin intake, once a day, was not associated with increase cancer risk. The research included more than 295,000 men who were enrolled in a diet and health study for five years.

What is interesting is that even excessive use of vitamins did not increase the risk of early or localized prostate cancer; abuse was linked to the increase risk of the development of advanced type of prostate cancer. The study found that the association "was strongest among men with a family history of prostate cancer and men who also took selenium, beta-carotene, or zinc supplements."

The study did not have any data as to which individual vitamin in a multivitamin preparation was responsible for the increased risk.

Scientifically, there is no evidence to date that taking multivitamins at any frequency help prevent cancer of the prostate. But taking one multivitamin once daily is safe and a general medical recommendation, especially for those who "eat and run," who may not be eating an adequate nourishing diet, for children and the elderly.

"Based on our findings, we would recommend that men adhere to recommendations for dietary supplements and consult with their physician before taking supplements in excessive doses," NCI researcher Michael F. Leitzmann, MD, PhD, tells WebMD.

In spite of warnings like this, we still know of individuals, some of them physicians and nurses, no less, who take megadoses of vitamins and "food supplements," thinking that these are antioxidants that will boost their immune system and that megadose will prevent cancer. This is simply not true.

The facts are (1) the most effective and safest sources of antioxidants are found in nature—like in fish, fruits, vegetables, and nuts—and not manufactured or synthetic food supplements; (2) taking megadoses of medications, including vitamins, is dangerous; (3) except for fish oil and multivitamins (which already contain vitamin D3 and vitamin B complex, etc.), most of the so-called food supplements (pills or potions or juices widely advertised in the market today) are medically useless for the consumers and only beneficial to the manufacturers and vendors in this billion-dollar food supplement industry; and (4) if one eats properly, all the individual needs is a daily dose of complete multivitamins with minerals (in one pill), perhaps an added vitamin D3 for cancer prevention and fish oil for cardiovascular health.

The analysis of 47 studies "assessing antioxidant supplementation, published earlier this year, found a slight increase in deaths among people who took beta-carotene, vitamin E, or vitamin A supplements."

As far as antioxidants being aggressively market on all media are concerned, Dr. Christian Gluud, coauthor of the investigation, reported "that there is little evidence of a benefit for antioxidant supplementation and mounting evidence of potential harm."

These clinicians and some others hypothesize that the notorious and dreaded "bad free radicals" being targeted by antioxidants, may, in fact, be "doing some good by targeting and killing harmful cells, such as those that cause cancers to grow." This is a theory that is being extensively studied in centers around the world.

The investigators stated that "our diets typically contain safe levels of vitamins, but high-level antioxidant supplements could potentially upset an important physiologic balance."

Health is exactly the maintenance of physiologic balance in our body. When that critical balance is upset, our body goes into "dis-ease," hence the word *disease*, whether the signs symptoms are obvious or not, overt or subtle, acute or chronic. Examples are hypertension (high blood pressure), hypercholesterolemia (high blood cholesterol), diabetes, etc., which usually starts without the person even knowing. This is why a medical check up, even as early as age 20, albeit symptom free, is important, if only to get a baseline data on these health parameters for reference or for detection of the disease.

Calcium and Vitamin D3

As we reported in this column on December 6, 2010, the science on calcium's role in bone health shows that 700 milligrams per day meets the needs of almost all children ages 1 through 3; and 1,000 milligrams daily is appropriate for almost all children ages 4 through 8. Adolescents ages 9 through 18 require no more than 1,300 milligrams per day. For practically all adults ages 19 through 50 and for men until age 71, 1,000 milligrams covers daily calcium needs. Women starting at age 51 and both men and women age 71 and older need no more than 1,200 milligrams per day.

As for vitamin D, 400-1000 IUs daily meet the needs of almost everyone in the United States and Canada, although people 71 and older may require as much as 1000 IUs per day because of potential physical and behavioral changes related to aging. Vitamin D3 is the preferred form of D for supplement.

Overdosing is Abuse

Overdosing on anything is unsafe. Multivitamins, calcium, D3, fish oil, cholesterol-lowering statins are among the great scientific discoveries of our time and are beneficial to our body when used properly as recommended by the prescribing physician. Abusing any of them is unwise and unsafe.

Cliché or trite, these are nonetheless words of wisdom: too much of even a good thing is bad. And this goes true with all medications, activities, food, and drinks.

Nicotine Addiction

Is nicotine addicting?

Yes, nicotine, which is a prime drug in cigarettes, is highly addicting. Cigarette smokes contains, believe it or not, thousands of substances, and one of them is nicotine, which is found only in tobacco leaf. Smokers who crave it find it hard to go without a cigarette. Those who are under stress or feel nervous are the ones at a higher risk of becoming addicted to nicotine.

Why do people smoke?

It almost always starts as an adventure among teenagers, peer pressure, rebellion against society and the nonsmoking elders who forbid smoking. Smokers also get hooked on the smell, taste, and feel of cigarettes. Also, smokers "link" smoking with certain activities, like after eating, or while on the phone, or while on coffee break, or when confronted with a stress situation, or when with friends or simply relaxing at home. This "linkage" makes the habit harder to break and addiction stronger.

How does nicotine work?

Just like many "central-acting" drugs, nicotine works on the brain and the "nerve" system. When one smokes a cigarette, nicotine is absorbed rapidly through the buccal mucosa (lining of the mouth) into the blood circulation, faster than heroin given intravenously in the arm. And when the smoker inhales the smokes, nicotine is drawn into the lungs and into the blood circulation also. This nicotine-filled blood is pumped by the heart to the brain and all over the body. It takes only seven (7) seconds for the nicotine to reach the brain, and this sudden burst of nicotine gives an instant "high." If the smoker is a pregnant woman, the nicotine also gets to the fetus through the connecting arteries.

How does nicotine provide "relaxation"?

Nicotine acts in a dual role. In the early part of the day, it acts like an "upper," speeding up many body reactions like a stimulant. Late in the day, it acts like a "downer" it seems to act like a sedative and help people relax. How nicotine affects the body depends on the amount of nicotine, time elapsed from the last cigarette, stress level, the personality of the smoker, and even the time of the day.

What are the effects of nicotine?

In large amount, nicotine, like other addictive drugs (heroin and cocaine), is a poison. Nicotine has been used to kill insects. Nicotine causes tachycardia (fast heartbeat), which causes tachypnea (fast breathing), resulting in increased oxygen consumption of the body. Nicotine also causes spasm in the arteries, narrowing its caliber and thus slowing the flow of blood. It also causes increased in the blood pressure as the arteries constrict to smaller caliber. Nicotine also thickens the blood, resulting in tendency of the smoker's body to form blood clots. It also increases the speed of hardening of the arteries, making the cholesterol (fats) adhere to the walls of the arteries at a faster rate. This can cause heart attacks, stroke, or blockage of arteries in the carotid (neck) arteries, renal (kidney) arteries, or leg arteries.

Why can't smokers use only one stick a day?

Most smokers are not satisfied with only one or two sticks of cigarettes a day. Just like drug addicts, they crave for more. Many who smoke for the first time feel nauseated and dizzy. As they continue, these unpleasant feelings and replaced with a "high" or an "upper" effect. As their system gets used to the level of nicotine in their blood, and soon, they are hooked and would need a higher nicotine level to achieve the same "high" they used to get with one or two sticks a day. Pretty soon, they would need a pack or two a day to be satisfied as their body tolerance and "nicotine need" increases. At this point, they are so addicted they only feel "good" or "comfortable" when the "necessary" level of nicotine is in their bloodstream. This is nothing but drug addiction.

Why should smokers quit?

Cigarette smoking kills. This has been scientifically proven beyond any doubt, time and again. One out of four smokers dies prematurely because of smoking. One person dies every minute (five persons have died since you started reading this article the past five minutes) of heart attack, a cigarette-related illness, not to mention those from cancer or the lungs and emphysema. In ths past it was "cool" to smoke; but today, it is considered a dirty habit, a deadly habit. The trend now is to have a smoke-free society, smoke-free public places, like airports, airlines, libraries, restaurants, etc. The air pollution from cigarette smokes also causes illnesses among nonsmokers exposed to secondhand smoke.

What other illnesses can cigarette smoking cause?

Emphysema of the lungs, stroke, cancer of the lungs, cancer of the urinary bladder, cancer of the breasts and other female organs, and cancer of the throat and the mouth are a few of them. These should be enough to scare us all. Among pregnant women who smoke, their fetuses are also adversely affected, making the children more prone to respiratory diseases, bronchitis, asthma, pneumonia, etc. Smoking is not only an act of "attempting suicide" but also an act that could cause harm to family members and other people, not to mention the expenses for this dangerous habit and its effect on our home, to the public, and to our environment.

What are the helpful hints and strategy to quit smoking?

First and foremost is making a firm decision to quit. Your mind must be convinced that smoking can bring you premature death, not to mention the illnesses, pain, suffering (physical, emotional, and financial), and other hardships you and your family will go through. Once you are convinced and resolved, plan a strategy:

1. Pick a good time to quit. Do not try to quit when you are under a lot of stress from certain incidents or situation in your life or during the holidays. Quitting "cold turkey" has been found to

be more effective by many who have successfully quit the habit than doing it "gradually."

2. Understand and accept that when you start to quit, you might feel strange, anxious, sleepy or excited, lightheaded, irritable, nervous, or nauseated, have abdominal cramps, improved appetite, develop headaches and, of course, you will have a craving for tobacco. You have to understand and accept these temporary side effects of quitting.

3. Start an exercise regimen, like walking so many miles a day or around your block, or in a gym, or do ballroom dancing regularly. Exercise is a big boost to the feeling of well-being as it increases the secretion of adrenalin and endomorphins circulating in our bloodstream. Exercise also improves our spirit and emotional stability.

4. Get plenty of sleep, have a balanced diet, and drink a lot of water. Instead of a cigarette in your mouth, chew gum or suck on candies as a temporary substitute.

5. Talk to your friends and family members, telling them your decision to quit, and ask for their patience and understanding while you go through the process of quitting from this addiction, when you are irritable, etc.

6. If you do not succeed, try quitting again and again until you succeed. Many quitters have been successful after two or three attempts. The stronger the personality and the more disciplined the person is, the easier he/she can quit. So do not give up. Keep on trying.

7. If there are two or more of you (husband and wife, couples who are friends, or two or more friends), quitting as a group has been found to be easier and more successful. You could even have meetings to hear about the progress of your "group project."

8. Talk to your physicians about nicotine "patches" or pills, which have helped thousands quit smoking.

Noise Pollution "Quietly" Kills

A reader was asking how deleterious noise was to health. She complained that blasting karaoke revelry from a restaurant 5 houses down from her home, even beyond midnight, was causing her whole family and the neighborhood from getting a good night's sleep, night after night. It's bad enough to have blaring car engines and tooting horns, inconsiderate people on the street shouting and laughing or even partying past ten, she added.

This is not an isolated incident or complaint. Noise pollution is a pandemic.

In the United States and in many countries, it is socially unacceptable to make telephone calls after 10 at night and before 8:00 a.m., except for emergencies or urgent matters, or when prearranged, with mutual consent.

A World Health Organization study reported that "noise has been such an important environmental problem that even in ancient Rome rules existed to regulate the noise caused by iron wagon wheels turning on stone pavements, which disrupted sleep and annoyed people . . . In Medieval Europe, certain cities banned horse carriages and horseback riding at night to ensure that inhabitants would get a good night's sleep."

We must indeed respect other people's privacy and personal rights to have peace and domestic tranquility, at the very least, during those ten hours, as stipulated by our laws. Besides, noise pollution is unhealthy and sleep is very important to health.

During other hours, noise pollution, which means sound level beyond the comfortable level, is obviously, bad for our body. This is why construction workers wear earplugs, noise screen, or headsets. Reasonable noise from construction or home repairs and other public noise is allowed only between before 8:00 a.m. and 10:00 p.m. to allow people to rest.

While we have been accustomed to street noise in our daily life, chronic noise pollution leads to increase secretion of adrenalin in the body, causing higher blood pressure, general stress to our body, especially to the immune system. All these lower our body resistance to many forms of illnesses in subtle ways, beyond our awareness, realization, or suspicion. We take all this noise as normal and harmless, but they are actually unhealthy.

A study released by the World Health Organization on August 2007 "suggest that thousands of people around the world may be dying prematurely or succumbing to disease due to the insidious effects of chronic noise exposure." There is no question that constant exposure to noise or any unwanted sound, even loud human voice, is hazardous to health.

Several studies revealed that noise "kills in much the same way as chronic stress by causing an accumulation of stress hormones, inflammation, and changes in body chemistry that eventually lead to problems such as impaired blood circulation and heart attacks." The adverse effects on the body and its immune system take place even if we are not consciously aware of the noise or even when we are asleep, because our body reacts physiologically even while we are not awake.

Clinical research in Europe also showed that "chronic and excessive traffic noise, for instance, accounted for three percent of deaths from chronic heart disease, which kills about seven million people in the world each year," which translates to mean that "210,000 of these deaths may actually be due to unwanted noise." Much like air pollution, noise, beyond the comfortable decibels, leads to slow death, whether we realize it or not. It is so subtle and generally accepted by default, most of us do not even recognize that noise is unhealthy and dangerous. It "quietly" takes a toll on our health and well-being gradually as time goes by. Chronic noise pollution also harms wildlife, not only humans, and disturbs normal ecological activities in general.

The Noise Abatement Act

Noise control in public in the United States dramatically became more effective when it passed the National Environmental Policy Act (NEPA) in 1969 and the Noise Pollution and Abatement Act, more commonly known as the Noise Control Act (NCA), in 1972.

The city of Portland, Oregon, has the most strict ordinance, instituted to aggressively protect its citizens, which fines offenders $5,000 per infraction, with provision that allows the authority to cite a responsible noise code violators multiple times in a single day.

Most countries have their own laws to control noise. Japan was pioneer in this regard, a few years ahead of the United States, but its anti—noise pollution laws are not as comprehensive as those in the United States.

If you think about it, what our society needs more than laws is our individual sense of responsibility, consideration, and respect for our neighbor.

Obesity and Dieting

What is obesity?

Obesity is the excessive accumulation of body fat, where a person has a weight 20% over that in standard height-weight tables. It may be mild (20 to 40% overweight), moderate (41-100% overweight), or severe (greater than 100% overweight). Body mass index is a more accurate gauge of obesity but more complex. The prevalence of obesity in the United States is 24% of men and 27% of women. In the United Kingdom, about 14.5% are obese, and in France only 7% of people are obese. Unfortunately, with the Western influence on lifestyle and behavior, there seems to be a trend among Asians toward these same statistics.

What causes obesity?

The specific cause of obesity is unknown but the mechanism is clear: taking in more calories than expended. There are at least 7 factors that contribute to obesity. They are genetic, social, endocrine, psychological, developmental, physical, and brain damage. Obesity could be exogenous (eating too much and too little physical activity: intake of calories more than output of calories) or endogenous (caused by internal medical condition, such as endocrine problem, etc.)

How does heredity play a role in obesity?

Heredity provides the genetic predisposition to obesity. However, children of an obese parent or obese parents do not necessarily become overweight, since there are environmental factors (health consciousness and social pressure) that could lead to lifestyle changes that prevent obesity. In cases where all children of obese parents are also obese, this could be due to perpetuation of parental lifestyle and behavior, or there could be some underlying endocrine or metabolic causes.

Why is it hard for some people to lose weight?

Body weight is controlled by a "physiologic regulator" in our body. The fact that in some people (genetically) this regulatory "set point" is higher, the "weight threshold level" is also increased. The bodies of those persons "follow the regulator" to attain that "set point" of weight for their bodies. Because each person has a different "set point," it is harder for some of us to lose weight or maintain a certain weight level compared to others. Proper medical workup and intervention and self-discipline can help majority of persons with obesity problem.

Are obese persons more prone to heart attacks and stroke?

In general, yes. People who are overweight have a greater tendency to have abnormally high cholesterol level in their blood and organs. The cholesterol is deposited in the walls of their coronary (heart) arteries, the carotid arteries (supplying the brain), and other arteries. These people are also more prone to develop high blood pressure. These cholesterol plaques (deposits) gradually build up and clog the inner arterial channels, depriving vital organs (heart, brain, kidneys, legs, etc.) of their blood supply, leading to a heart attack and/or stroke, etc. Overweight people are also more prone to develop diabetes and other illnesses. Normal weight confers not only a more attractive physical appearance but a healthier body.

Why do obese people have some difficulty breathing?

Obese persons have excess fats all over, including in their chest, around the heart and other organs, inside their abdomen, and the pressure from excess fat on the chest and on the diaphragm (the tentlike dome that separates the chest from the abdomen) makes the normal lung expansion more difficult. Air exchange is less efficient. Besides all these, the obese person has a lot more body surface, and therefore the heart and lungs and all other organs have to work much harder. Hence, there is more overall oxygen demand and consumption.

Is snoring really more common in obese persons?

Yes, somehow snoring is more common among persons who are obese. While many people with normal weights snore, this condition appears to be more common among those who are obese. In many of these "snorers" sleep apnea (breath holding while asleep) occurs, leading to poor oxygenation of the blood. This makes these people prone to have high blood pressure; and if the sleep apnea is prolonged, it could lead to hypoxia (insufficient oxygen for the body), heart attack or even death in some persons. This poor oxygenation is the reason why the "snorers" do not get a restful sleep and feel so tired and fatigued when they wake up.

Are diet pills, food, and drinks safe?

We do not recommend them. Diet pills are appetite suppressants. Most of them have side effects that could cause heart irregularity and could be dangerous. Some deaths have been reported among people taking diet pills. The diet food and diet drinks in the market are basically low fat, high protein, and loaded with vitamins and minerals. Depending on the formula, some of these could also have adverse side effects, like diarrhea and electrolyte imbalance. Without self-discipline and determination, even these diet pills and diet food products will not work, and most of these people gain back their weight much too soon. Dieting with these aids should be under the supervision of a physician.

What is the safest way to attain a normal weight?

Since most overweight problem is exogenous (eating too much and burning too little calories), the obvious initial strategy is to eat less and/ or exercise and lose more calories. The common sense approach is to cut down the food intake to half, take one-a-day multivitamin and minerals for supplement, and start a regular daily exercise regimen. Weigh once a week, naked or in underwear only, and record weight. If after one week of (honest and disciplined) reduction in the total food intake and the weight does not start to come down, it means either there is a need to cut down on the intake some more, or there is a need to increase the physical exercise. Too rapid weight reduction is not healthy, so adjust the food intake accordingly, but maintain the exercise regimen. If it works and the weight starts to come down (about 2-5 pounds a week, depending on the starting weight) simply continue this program. If no success is achieved after a month of this initial strategy, then it is time to consult a physician

Are special diet preparations more effective?

These commercial preparations are more expensive, yes, but not necessarily more effective. Besides, as we alluded to earlier, there could be adverse side effects from taking them. Eating regular food (obviously low fat, like fish, vegetables, and fruits) that is properly portioned in reduced quantity, is as effective, lesser expensive, and definitely safer than any special preparations in the market today. There is absolutely no medical or scientific reason to eat these special diet food preparation and spend more money when controlled intake of regular healthy table food will suffice to achieve weight reduction.

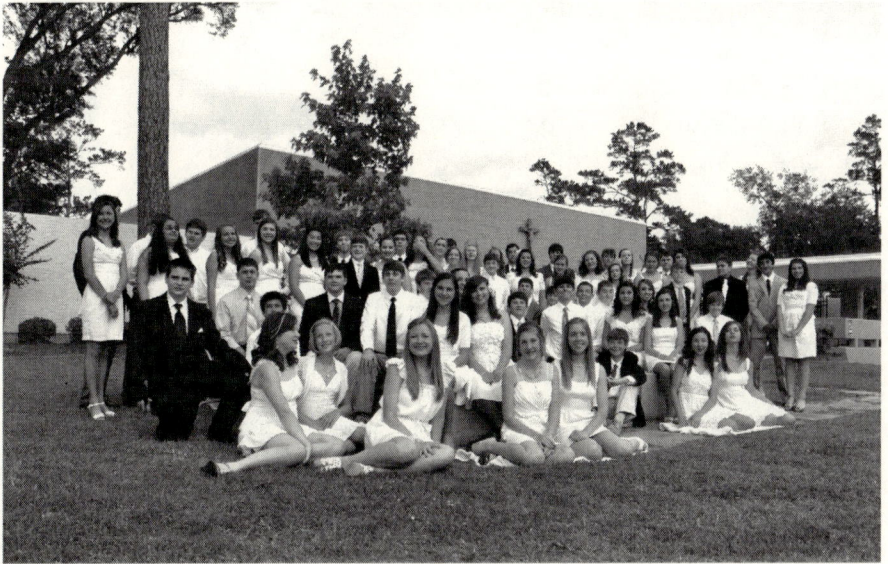

The future leaders and pillars of society, our children are for us, parents, to guide, inspire, nurture, and protect to assure generations of healthier, better-educated, more responsible, and more productive citizenry. Anything less on our part is an abdication of our responsibility and obligation as parents and role models.

Organic is Healthier

Most of the produce and products in the market today are "contaminated" with some type of chemical used in fertilizing them, protecting them, making them more appealing, preserving them, or enriching them. Our farmers and manufacturers all over the world have been so programmed and enslaved by modern automation that without much thought, they use environmentally destructive chemicals and substances just to maximize their bottom line, with the customer's health and safety lowest in the list of their priorities and obligations to society.

Versatile plasticware abound in the world, many of them releasing vinyl chloride and other toxic gases, or contain phthalates, which are cancer-causing and birth-defect-causing agents and which are also harmful to the lungs and liver. Surprisingly, unbeknownst to most of us, some plastics are also used in chewing gum, cosmetics, carpeting, mattresses, toilet paper, sanitary napkins, polyester clothing, and tissue paper. The use of glass containers, natural fiber clothing, personal care and cosmetic products made with natural ingredients, wooden toys for kids, and staying away from aluminum cookware to prevent aluminum poisoning are the healthier ways to go.

All white paper products are bleached with chemicals which leave behind residues of cancer-causing dioxin, which are likewise found in lunch bags, coffee filters, diapers, paper towels, napkins, tissue and toilet paper. Dioxin, like other harmful chemicals, enters the soil and eventually contaminates groundwater.

The use of organic household cleaners, "Green Your Clean Routine," is the safer and healthier alternative. An effective and safer cleanser, for instance, is diluted vinegar, for use in the kitchen and bathroom tiles, mirrors, and even in carpets, to inhibit mildew and bacteria.

Equally, if not more important, we must avoid processed food and opt for organic food such as fish and poultry products, and fruits that are organically raised and produced without pesticides, herbicides, hormones, antibiotics, preservatives, and artificial coloring. These are obviously safer and healthier alternatives. The current significant drawback is the prohibitive cost of organic food. Hopefully, as more consumers go organic, the price of these items will be more reasonable. We also hope that the manufacturers and purveyors will subjugate their material priority to the health and safety of the public and the world as a whole.

The basic principle in all this is for us, the inhabitants of planet Earth, to be responsible and good to our environment by not contaminating our natural habitat with poisons and to allow Mother Nature to flourish at her best. The purer and healthier the air we breathe in, the water we drink, the food we eat, the healthier the ozone layer is; and the healthier lifestyle we live, the healthier our world will be for humankind as a whole and for the future generations to come.

Our Dangerous Diet

We need to change our dietary protein sources, if we are to significantly reduce our risk of heart disease, stroke, and arterial blockages and damages all over our body, all of which make cardiovascular illnesses the number one killer in the affluent societies around the globe.

This most convincing confirmation of the deadly effects of saturated fats and high cholesterol foods (mostly from red meat like pork and beef) came from more than a quarter of century studies on 84,000 nurses, who were studied, tested, and followed up for 26 years.

Other studies have shown that consumption of saturated fats (red meats and products with red meat) also increases cancer risk, besides metabolic diseases, like diabetes and arthritis, etc.

The comprehensive investigation (Nurses' Health Study) was conducted by Dr. Adam Bernstein of Brigham and Women's Hospital in Boston, Massachusetts) and his colleagues, and was published in the August 16, 2010, issue of *Circulation*. The data from this systematic and meta-analysis on 84,136 nurses, between 30 and 55 years of age, who were all healthy at year one, reported 2210 incidents of nonfatal heart attack and 952 deaths from heart attack, involving those who ate red meat regularly.

The multivariable analysis revealed that consumption of red meat and high-fat dairy (eggs, cheese, regular milk, etc.) resulted in elevated risk for coronary heart disease, while greater intake of fish, poultry, and nuts significantly lowered the risk. One serving per day of nuts led to 30% lower risk of heart disease compared to one serving of red meat. The risk is 24% lower with fish and 19% with poultry.

Another study by Dr. Renata Micha at Harvard School of Public Health in Boston showed that processed red meat (bacon, hamburger, hot dogs, etc.) was worse: 42% increased risk for coronary heart disease and 19% risk for diabetes. Dietary iron from red meat, called heme iron, and compounds resulting from cooking red meat (heterocyclic amines and advanced glycation end-products) were positively linked to increased risk of heart attack and fatality, not to mention cancer in general.

"Replacing saturated fats with polyunsaturated fats significantly reduced the risk of coronary heart disease . . . When major sources of protein, such as nuts and fish, are used to replace red meat, saturated fat, heme iron, and sodium decrease, whereas intake of polyunsaturated (good) fat increases," concluded the study.

Our red-meat eating culture is obviously unhealthy. With all the scientific data we now know, it behooves all of us, men and women and especially children, to reevaluate our diet and seriously consider eliminating or drastically cutting down on red meat and choosing the healthier options of fish, poultry, beans, nuts, and vegetable protein sources.

Nuts, the Super Snack

Nuts, in general, are super food items, which provide the body protein, fiber, minerals, antioxidants, cholesterol-lowering monosaturated fats, immune—and brain-boosting nutrition. Each nut confers different benefits, so it is best to indulge in a variety of them within the week. But don't go overly nuts on them. Moderation is a key to almost everything. In alphabetical order, they include the following, their serving size and calories:

Almonds—serving size: 23 nuts, calories: 163. Contains the greatest natural calcium, vitamin E, and fiber among all nuts; they also lowers cholesterol.

Brazil Nuts-6 nuts, 186 calories. Larger in size than cashew nuts and looks partially peeled, contains selenium, good for the thyroid. Three to 6 nuts a day is good enough.

Cashews-18 nuts, 163 calories. Provides 10% of your iron daily requirement, a good source of folate and vitamin K, for strong bones and normal blood clotting.

Macademia-10 to 12, 204 calories. Contains monosaturated, heart-healthy, fats, good source of thiamine (vitamin B1). And its taste is superb, almost addicting.

Peanuts—a handful, 181 calories. Peanuts are, strictly speaking, not nuts. They do not grow underground, not on trees. They belong to the legume family (beans, peas, lentils), provide monosaturated fats, folate, vitamin B, E, and fiber.

Pecans-19 halves, 196 calories. Contains beta-sitosterol, plant sterol that lowers cholesterol and good for prostate health.

Pine Nuts-167 nuts, 191 calories. Shaped like rice, pine nuts is an excellent source of manganese, which helps in the metabolism of carbohydrate (sugar) and protein. There is a suggestion that pine nuts may actually boost the satiety hormone that curbs the appetite, for better weight control.

Pistachios-49 nuts, 162 calories. One serving provides about the same amount of potassium from one small banana, has antioxidant lutein, like the one in vegetables.

Walnuts-14 halves, 185 calories. Great source of magnesium, protein, fiber, has high level of brain boosting omega-3 fatty acid called alpha-linolenic acid.

Calcium and Heart Attack

Taking plain calcium supplement (without coadministered vitamin D) has been found to be linked to increase risk of heart attack, according to an article in the July 29, 2010, issue of the *British Medical Journal,* which reported on 15 randomized trials on 11,921 individuals.

This study justifies the reassessment of calcium supplement for prevention or treatment of osteoporosis, whose efficacy has been called to question anyway. Since vitamin D3 is cardio-protective, besides lowering the risk for colon cancer, the calcium supplement, if taken at all, is safer when it comes with, or taken with, vitamin D3.

The role of calcium in osteoporosis is marginal at best, and there are options today that are effective, sans the risk reported linked to calcium supplements. Of course, there are conditions causing hypocalcemia that justifies its continued used as a supplement, together with vitamin D3.

Dr. John Schindler of the University of Pittsburgh Medical Center, Pennsylvania, stated that the safest thing is "to get your dietary calcium from good dietary sources, such as yogurt, sardines, and skim milk that potentially might be all you need to ward off the risk of osteoporosis. Then we don't have to deal with this increased cardiovascular risk."

If you think about it, practically all things in the environment Mother Nature has given us, in their original pristine, unprocessed, unadulterated, uncontaminated form, are the healthiest, including the human mind.

Parkinson's Disease

What is the shaking palsy?

Parkinson's Disease, first described in 1817 by British physician James Parkinson, who called it "the shaking palsy," is a slowly progressive, degenerative brain disorder that leads to slow and reduced movement, rigidity of the muscles, tremors at rest and gait (walking and postural) instability.

How prevalent is Parkinson's disease?

It is the fourth most common brain deterioration disorder in the elderly. About 1% of those 65 and older, and about 0.4% of those older than 40 are affected. However, Parkinson's disease could also begin in childhood or adolescence. Ten percent occur under age 40. Generally, the onset of symptoms occur after the age of 40, and the incidence goes up among older people.

Who are some well-known personalities afflicted?

Pope John Paul II, US Attorney General Janet Reno, Rev. Billy Graham, actress Kathryn Hepburn, sitcom actor Michael J. Fox, former heavyweight boxing champion Muhammad Ali, country singer Johnny Cash.

What causes Parkinson's disease?

The cause of the primary form of Parkinson's is not known, hence it is called idiopathic. Secondary Parkinsonism could be due to other forms of degenerative disease of unknown cause or due to drugs or external toxins. The most common is ingestion of antipsychotic drugs or reserpine, which blocks dopamine receptors in the brain, causing

Parkinsonism. The less common causes are carbon monoxide or manganese poisoning, encephalitis, tumors, bleeding in the brain, and use of illegal IV drug called N-MPTP, a drug synthesized from meperidine.

Exactly what happens in the brain?

The brain is the most sophisticated, elaborate, and complex communications system there is in the world. Not even the fastest computer available today can match, much less equal, the human brain. Parts of the brain called substantia nigra, locus caeruleus, and brain stem have dopaminergic neurons (cells that produce dopamine, a neurotransmitter that helps direct muscle activity). In Parkinson's, there is loss of these neurons that produce dopamine, and the resultant depletion of dopamine characterizes Parkinson's disease. Without enough neurotransmitters, it is obvious that vital normal "connections" are impaired, which explains why these patients act and behave a certain way, presenting typical signs and symptoms of the disease.

How does the disease start?

In 50 to 80 of Parkinson patients, the condition starts insidiously with the so-called "pill-rolling" tremor of one hand. This is very typical. The uncontrollable coarse tremor looks like the fingers are rolling a pill or a marble continuously. This is severe at rest and decreases during movement and is not present when the patient is asleep. Emotional stress, tension, or fatigue aggravate it. The hands, arms, and legs are commonly affected in that order. In some patients, tremor is absent, and rigidity of the muscles is present. The face becomes masklike, expressionless, with diminished blinking and with mouth open.

How is walking affected?

The patient initially has difficulty starting ambulation. The gait becomes shuffling with short steps, with the hands flexed to the waist and do not swing with walking. The steps may gradually quicken beyond the patient's control, and the patient may find himself running to prevent falling because of instability of his gait. Sometimes, he could only stop when he hits an object. His center of gravity is displaced forward (or backward) due to loss of postural reflexes.

What are the other symptoms?

The speech among Parkinson patients becomes hypophonic (monotonous) and stuttering. The legs have lead-pipe rigidity when the physician examines and moves them. The sensation and muscle strength are usually normal. Depression is common among these patients, and 50% of them develops dementia, like Alzheimer's. Constipation, urinary hesitancy, seborrhea, and orthostatic hypotension (low blood pressure when they stand up from a sitting or lying position) are common among these patients because of autonomic nervous system dysfunction.

Is there a way to prevent Parkinson's disease?

Since primary Parkinson's disease is idiopathic (cause unknown), there is no way to predict or prevent it as yet. Scientists are now searching for a biomarker, a biochemical abnormality these patients might have in common, so screening diagnostic test might be developed to detect Parkinson's even before symptoms develop. PET (positron emission tomography) brain scanning may eventually lead to advances in our understanding about this baffling disease. Secondary Parkinsonism to a great extent is preventable by avoiding those conditions and drugs mentioned earlier that cause it. One general health rule that applies and must be observed especially in this particular situation, is stop abusing our mind and body by living a healthy lifestyle.

Do hand tremors presage Parkinson's disease?

The usual hand and finger tremors we see among older persons and some even among those who are younger than 40 do not necessarily mean those individuals will develop Parkinson's disease later in life. These so-called "normal" tremors or shakes do not indicate the presence of a disease. However, if they are so severe as to affect the daily normal use of the hands, a neurological evaluation might be in order.

What is the treatment for Parkinson's disease?

Drug therapy to replace the mission neurotransmitter dopamine, to stimulate dopamine receptors, to inhibit the major enzymes that break down the remaining dopamine in the brain, and drugs to control the involuntary movements, rigidity, and tremors is the standard treatment. Rehabilitation and physical therapy are most helpful. Since the inactivity due to Parkinson and the constipating side effects of the medications, high-fiber diet and stool softeners are part of the standard regimen.

How about surgery?

Surgery was once very common in treating Parkinson patients, but when Levodopa was discovered, this drug became so effective surgery was confined to only few cases. Most patients respond to anti-Parkinson medications, but these drugs may lose their efficacy over time. Stereotactic ablation (surgical cutting) and cryothalamotomy (insertion of supercooled metal probe into the thalamus [relay station deep in the brain]) to destroy the part of the brain that produce tremors results in significant improvement. Some patients enjoying sustained improvement for up to 4 years following surgery. Pallidotomy, another procedure using the same principle as above, is creating renewed interest among neurosurgeons. High-frequency electrical stimulation of the globus pallidus appears to be promising, and so with deep brain stimulation. These procedures are under further scientific evaluation. Fetal dopamine neuron transplantation is another exciting option under study.

Passive Smoking: More Deadly

What is passive smoking?

Secondhand smoke is the fume that one involuntarily inhales after someone who smokes exhales it (called mainstream smoke), or the fume that goes directly to the atmosphere from the burning tobacco (cigarette, pipe or cigar), called sidestream smoke. When nonsmokers breathe in this smoke or fumes from other people's cigarettes, cigars, and pipes, this is involuntary inhalation, called passive smoking, a more deadly source of lung diseases and cancers. Tobacco smoke contains about 4,000 (yes, four thousand) chemicals, 200 of them known poisons.

What are these poisons in cigarette smokes?

Some of them are benzenes, formaldehyde, and carbon monoxide, which are released into the air by smokers. Not only is the smoker inhaling these poisons but so is everyone around them. Smoking around people is similar to spraying known poison gas into the atmosphere, victimizing and posing even greater health hazards to nonsmokers as well, as the smoker enjoys his habit.

Is it true that secondhand smoke is more toxic?

Yes, it has been scientifically proven that secondhand smokes are more dangerous to health than firsthand smoke. The smoker, who inhales the (mainstream) smoke, "filters" it so some degree before exhaling it, but the nonsmoker around him/her inhales the "pure" and more dangerous sidestream smoke. Besides the tar and nicotine in secondhand smoke, there are several cancer-causing substances in secondhand smoke and in much higher concentration than in mainstream smoke. So the person who smokes in public, around people, is giving himself/herself a lower dose of poisons and giving his victims (family members, friends, and strangers) around him/her a higher and a more deadly dose of poison.

Does passive smoking cause cancer?

Yes, most definitely. Smokers developing lung and other cancers from smoking tobacco is a scientifically proven fact. In the United States, cancer victims of smoking and family members of smokers who died from cigarette-related illness have sued cigarette manufacturing companies and have won millions in awards. While they vehemently denied before, cigarette companies today have admitted in public that tobacco causes cancers and other lung illnesses. The courts have likewise ruled in a similar fashion in favor of victims of passive smoking (as in the airline stewardess's case). In 1986, the surgeon general of the United States reported that involuntary (passive) smoking can cause lung cancer in healthy nonsmokers. In fact, the US Environmental Protection Agency (EPA) has now classified secondhand smoke as a known carcinogen (cancer-causing agent).

Does passive smoking hurt children and infants?

More so. Young children and infants are more vulnerable to tobacco smoke and fumes. Pregnant mothers who smoke, pass these dangerous substances to the fetus, causing higher incidents of smaller babies, some with diminished mental acuity, or even wit retardation, most with babies that are prone to frequent respiratory infections and asthmatic attacks. Studies have shown that in their first two years of life, babies whose parent(s) smoke(s) at home have higher incidence of lung diseases such as bronchitis and pneumonia than babies of nonsmokers. Smoke also aggravates asthma in children and may even precipitate attacks. Parents, especially pregnant mothers, and all of us for that matter, should not smoke, but if we have too, we should do it outside our home, and away from people.

How bad is the situation among young children?

Studies have shown that even among children without asthma, acute respiratory illnesses occur two times more often to young children whose parents smoke around them as compared to those with nonsmoking parents. Passive smoking by children (secondhand smoke exposure) is associated with 150,000 to 300,000 cases of bronchitis and pneumonia each year in infants and young children less than 18 months old. We should not be doing this to our children. Let us satisfy our smoking habit, if we must, without endangering the lives of our family members and other people.

How about secondhand smoke at the workplace?

The US Surgeon General's Report of 1996 established that the simple separation of smokers and nonsmokers within the same air space may reduce but *not* eliminate the risk of exposure to environmental tobacco smoke. In view of this, an increasing number of state and local laws now restrict smoking at the workplace. The idea behind this law is that the preferences and rights of both the nonsmokers and the smokers should be considered whenever possible. However, when these choices conflict, the health and the preferences of nonsmokers should prevail and come first. More and more private companies, on their own, are also adopting policies that restrict smoking and protect nonsmokers.

Providing a smoking area in the same building with one ventilation system is like designating a urinating area in a swimming pool.

Other disadvantages of smoking?

Besides the health hazards among smokers, and to those people around him who are forced to inhale secondhand smoke, tobacco smoking leads to environmental pollution. Burning tobacco causes bad odors, which cling to people's clothes, hair, skin, and even curtains, etc. In an air-conditioned room, the air-conditioning demands can jump as much as 600 percent in order to control the bad odor of tobacco, which also lingers on. The bad odor is due to the burned chemical that penetrate our skin and the fabric of our clothes. The habit, which used to be so glamorous and very "in" is now "out" and considered "dirty." It is also expensive and very offensive to nonsmokers. The prediction is that someday, smoking, in view of all these health hazards, will be tabooed and smokers will be outcasts.

Do smokers know the dangers of smoking?

Yes, most, if not all, smokers know the dangers of smoking; but not as many know and accept the hazards of passive smoking. A recent Gallup poll conducted by the American Lung Association revealed that majority of both the smokers and nonsmokers know how dangerous smoking is to the health of the smokers and the people around him/her. To be around people who smoke is to expose yourself to the dangers of secondhand smoke, the two most significant of which are cancer and emphysema.

What can be done about secondhand smoke?

Both the smokers and nonsmokers have their rights. Smokers have the right to smoke, even if smoking is bad for their health. People have the right to commit suicide. In the same token, nonsmokers have their rights also. They have the right to protect themselves and their children from unwanted cancer-causing smoke. Someone's enjoyment should not be allowed to hurt others. Unless everybody in the same household are smokers, every home should be smoke-free.

Steps that could be taken: (1) Let family, friends, and coworkers know that you mind if they smoke around you. (2) Put "No Smoking" signs in your home, car or office to make people aware. (3) Support legislation to restrict smoking in public places, like workplace or restaurant, movies, busses, and other public places. (4) Propose nonsmoking resolutions in your social/civic organization meetings. (5) Encourage management, unions, and companies where you work to establish policies to protect nonsmokers on the job, and help promote the concept of a smoke-free families in your community. After all, we have the right to protect ourselves from poisons and cancers.

Pelvic Inflammatory Disease

The much dreaded pelvic inflammatory disease (PID) is an infection and inflammation of the upper genital tract among women, usually involving the cavity of the uterus (endometritis), fallopian tube (salpingitis), cervix (cervicitis), ovaries (oophoritis), and the surrounding tissues in the pelvis.

What is the incidence of PID?

The true statistical incidence of PID is not known because the illness cannot be diagnosed for certain by relying on the clinical signs and symptoms, which could be manifestations of other diseases. Also, most of these women do not have symptoms.

How prevalent is PID?

Pelvic inflammatory disease is the most common gynecologic reason for hospital admission in the United States, accounting for 49 out of 10,000 recorded hospital discharges. In England and Wales, about one out of every 62 women (1.6%) between the ages 16-45 is diagnosed to have PID. But since most are asymptomatic, this statistic underestimates the true prevalence. In developing countries, a crude estimate can be gained from hospital admissions: 17%-40% in sub-Saharan Africa and 15%-37% in Southeast Asia, 3%-10% in India.

What are the risk factors?

The risk factors associated with PID mirror those for STDs (sexually transmitted infections in general: young women, poor socioeconomic status, lower educational attainment, behavioral problems, STD, new or multiple sexual partners, use of IUD (intrauterine device for birth control), and instrumentation of cervix and uterus (as in abortion).

What bacteria cause PID?

Neisseria gonnorhoeae is the most common cause of PID. This organism can also cause urethritis (infection of the urethra where urine comes out from), migratory polyarthritis, endocarditis (inflammation of the inside of the heart). The other one is *Chlamydia trachomatis*, which causes severe cervicitis.

What are the signs and symptoms?

If symptoms are present, they are usually lower abdominal pains, fever, vaginal discharge, and/or abnormal uterine bleeding. Symptoms commonly occur during or after menstrual periods. The cervix is inflamed, red, and easily bleeds. The discharge could be yellowish-green. In many cases, acute abdomen happens, which require abdominal exploration.

How does the infection start?

Following unprotected sexual intercourse with partners who are infected, the infection ascends from the cervix. The epithelial (tissue lining) damage caused by the bacteria (especially *Chlamydia trachomatis* and *Neisseria gonorrhoeae*), allow opportunistic organisms to enter the tissues and aggravate the infection. If untreated, the PID spreads within the abdominal cavity, forming abscesses (pockets of pus) and possible blood poisoning and shock and even death.

What is the prognosis of PID?

Pelvic inflammatory disease has a very high morbidity. About one out of five (20%) of affected women become infertile, 20% develop chronic pelvic pain; and among those who are lucky enough to successfully conceive, one out of ten (10%) develop ectopic pregnancy. Amazingly, clinical signs and symptoms of PID resolve and subside in many of these women, but the damage has already been done. Those few with milder infection may escape permanent damage.

How about recurrent PID?

Recurrent pelvic inflammatory disease is associated with 4 to 6 times increase in permanent, irreversible, damages to the fallopian tubes that leads to sterility. The diseased and scarred inner lining of the tubes adversely hinder the normal travel of ova (eggs) from the ovaries (where the ova are produced) all the way to the outer third of the tube where one egg is supposed to meet the one penetrating sperm, following copulation. This is why infertility is most common among PID patients.

What are the complications of PID?

Besides infertility, there could be tubo-ovarian abscess in 16% of these women, where the tubes and the ovary are infected and full of pus, causing acute severe abdominal pains necessitating hospitalization. Some develop what is called Fitz-Hugh-Curtis syndrome, presenting as right upper quadrant abdominal pains associated with acute salphingitis, due to perihepatitis (inflammation of the liver, which could also form abscesses).

What is the treatment for PID?

The primary objective of the treatment includes complete control and resolution of the infection and prevention of infertility and ectopic pregnancy. In view of this, prompt, aggressive, and vigorous antibiotic therapy is initiated immediately, soon after the cultures/sensitivity are obtained to determine the bacterial cause and what antibiotics would be effective. But as always, as in the case of most illnesses, prevention is the best strategy for a healthier life.

Peptic Ulcer Disease

What is peptic ulcer?

Peptic ulcer, as the second part of the name suggests, is a "wound, an open sore," an excoriated area in the mucosa (inner wall) that penetrates the muscle layer of the stomach or of the duodenum (the first part of the small intestine attached to the stomach). The symptom is typically burning, gnawing, or hunger pains in the epigastric (stomach pit) area, often relieved by food or antacids.

What causes peptic ulcer disease?

There was a time when stomach acid hypersecretion (due to stress, spicy food, alcohol, tobacco, etc.) was universally accepted in the medical community as the cause of peptic ulcer disease. Two brilliant physicians, Barry Marshall and Robin Warren, were ridiculed by their colleagues in the scientific world for postulating that peptic ulcer disease was caused by a bacterial infection (*Helicobacter pylori* organism). Dr. Marshall ingested the organism himself and produced acute peptic ulcer disease, proving to the medical community that his postulate was correct. Multicenter studies following his treatise proved that he was right. Marshall has radically revolutionized the understanding of the disease, its diagnosis, and most importantly, its treatment.

How did this change the treatment?

Before Marshall's discovery, gastrectomy (cutting part or whole of the stomach out) was very common as a treatment for peptic ulcer disease. Today, with appropriate triple antibiotic therapy, peptic ulcer disease is effectively managed, transforming a former surgical disease to a medical disease. Occasionally, however, surgery may still be needed for severe bleeding peptic ulcer disease; but this is not as common today, with proper antibiotic treatment.

Do aspirin and arthritis medications cause peptic ulcers?

Yes, aspirin and NSAIDs (nonsteroidal arthritis medications) are known to cause peptic ulcers and severe bleeding. The irritation is both local (on the mucosa of the stomach) and systemic (inhibiting prostaglandin production adversely affecting mucosal defenses and thinning the blood), leading to ulcerations and hemorrhage.

Is alcohol bad for those with peptic ulcer?

Yes, most definitely. The same thing is true with cigarette smoking, chocolate, tea, coffee, spicy foods, which are also irritants for the stomach. They increase hydrochloric acid production in the stomach, which bathes and damages the stomach mucosal lining, making it more susceptible to the *H. pylori* bacteria. Milk, which used to be prescribed decades ago as a part of peptic ulcer therapy, is now avoided since it also causes "rebound" acid production and retards ulcer healing.

Do children develop peptic ulcers?

Yes, but it is relatively uncommon among children compared to among adults. About 15% to 20% of abdominal pains in children are due to peptic ulcer. Most primary peptic ulcer disease in children are seen in the ages between 8 and 17. The pains usually wakes the child from sleep and are sometimes aggravated by eating. About 25% of these pediatric patients have bleeding ulcers. Peptic ulcer due to *H. pylori* infection is not very common in children. Any persistent abdominal pains in children warrants prompt medical consultation.

How is the diagnosis made?

After a good history-taking and physical examination, the physician can already make a strong presumptive diagnosis of peptic ulcer disease. Fiberoptic gastroscopy (a lighted magnifying flexible scope passed through the mouth down to the stomach used to view its inside) is today a part of the state-of-the-art investigative tool in the diagnosis of peptic ulcer disease or malignant tumor (cancer) of the stomach. Bacterial cultures may likewise be taken to check the presence of *Helicobacter pylori* organism. Through the scope, cytology (microscopic examination for cancer cells), cultures for bacteria, and tiny biopsies may be done to make a diagnosis.

What are the possible complications of peptic ulcer disease?

Hemorrhage is the most common complication, leading to vomiting of blood or blood in the stools, coloring them black; anemia; weakness; or even dizziness and syncope (passing-out spells). Perforation of the wall when the ulcer "eats" the entire thickness of the stomach wall, creating a hole, allowing stomach contents to spill into the abdominal cavity causing peritonitis (severe inflammation and infection). Inflammation from peptic ulcer involving the stomach outlet into the duodenum can cause spasm and scar that blocks this outlet, causing vomiting. Stomach cancer has been reported 3 to 6 times more common in peptic ulcer due to *H. pylori infection*. Gastric lymphomas have also been linked to this bacteria.

Are TUMS and Rolaids safe for ulcer pains?

TUMS, Rolaids, and other over-the-counter self-proclaimed "treatment" for peptic ulcers or hyperacidity are quite popular among lay people. These will not cure hyperacidity or peptic ulcers. If the symptoms persist, it is most prudent to seek medical consultation. Remember, peptic ulcers can have life-threatening complications if not properly treated, and cancer of the stomach must be ruled out as the cause of the symptoms.

What is the treatment?

For Peptic ulcer due to *H. pylori infection*, the combination of bismuth, metronidazole, and tetracycline cures about 80% of this infection, leading to ulcer healing. Proton pump inhibitors capsules, H2 blocker pills, and antacids are other adjunctive modalities of the comprehensive regimen many physicians use in conjunction with the triple antibiotic therapy above.

How about surgery?

Surgery used to be very common for peptic ulcer disease. With the discovery of *H. pylori* infection as the major cause of peptic ulcer disease, surgery has declined precipitously. Today, surgery is relegated to the complications, like uncontrollable bleeding, perforation, gastric outlet obstruction, suspected cancerous peptic ulcer, and symptoms refractory to medical treatment. With this new triple antibiotic therapy, even the complications of peptic ulcer disease have been reduced significantly.

Dangers of Potato Chips

The Environmental Law Foundation (ELF), based in California, has filed notices with the attorney general of the state against the following potato chip companies: Lay's potato chip maker PepsiCo Inc., Pringles maker Proctor & Gamble Co., Cape Cod potato chip parent Lance Inc., and Kettle Chips maker Kettle Foods Inc.

This civil action is intended to alert the public thru proper product labeling that potato chips contain high levels of acrylamide, a toxic and cancer-causing chemicals substance, according to the Office of Environmental Health Hazard Assessment. This chemical is formed when starchy foods are fried or baked at high temperatures. When meats are cooked at high temperatures, the cancer-causing heterocyclic amines are produced.

The ELF has listed the following offenders on "how their potato chip brands exceeded the required warning levels for acrylamide—Cape Cod Robust Russet: 910 times; Kettle Chips (lightly salted): 505 times; Kettle Chips (honey dijon): 495 times; Pringles Snack Stacks (pizza-flavored): 170 times; Lay's Baked: 150 times.

Those companies who distribute, market, or sell, their potato chips without such warnings are in violation of California law, California Proposition 65.

It is really safer and healthier to eat food in their raw state. While sushi, for instance, is not enjoyed by most people, properly prepared and uncontaminated raw fish and boiling water-blanched seaweed are a couple of the healthier foods there are. Of course, celery, carrots, cauliflower, cucumber, tomatoes, broccoli, *sinkamas*, salad greens, and other fruits and vegetables are best eaten raw.

In the meantime, while we are developing our taste for raw or minimally processed foods, we can shy away from the obvious "unhealthy ones" in the market, like red meat, potato chips, French fries, processed meats, and all soda drinks.

Prediabetes: A "Warning"

What is prediabetes?

Prediabetes is a condition where a person has a blood sugar level that is higher than normal and is at high risk of developing diabetes mellitus but has not reached the blood sugar level threshold that would change the condition into full-blown diabetes. Patients with prediabetes have impaired glucose tolerance and an increased risk of heart attack and stroke, just as diabetics. Within 10 years, prediabetics develop type 2 diabetes unless proper measures are taken to prevent it. Prediabetic stage is a "warning" and is the best time to diagnose the condition in order to ward off diabetes itself.

What other factors increase risk?

Besides being overweight or obese and not exercising daily, which are major culprits, the other factors that increase the chances of developing prediabetes/diabetes are (1) age—older than 45, although data today show that more younger people are getting the disease; (2) genes—those with a parent, sister, brother with diabetes; (3) family background—Afro American, Asian American, Pacific Islander, Hispanic American/Latino; (4) abnormal blood cholesterol levels—HDL (high-density Lipoprotein) is 35 or lower, and triglyceride is 250 or higher; (5) blood pressure 140/90 or higher; and (6) gestational diabetes—women who give birth to at least one baby weighing more than 9 pounds.

When should one have a blood sugar test?

Routine blood sugar level should be tested when one reaches age 35, unless the person has some symptoms suggesting possible diabetes (frequent thirst, frequent urination, excessive hunger) or has a strong family history of diabetes, in which case the blood sugar level should be tested earlier. One practical diagnostic test (even for prediabetes) is to have a 2-hour postprandial (two hours after a meal) blood sugar test. If the level is 140 or higher, the person has at least a prediabetes condition, which will lead to diabetes, if not managed promptly. Hemoglobin A1C is another test that could be of great help.

How much weight loss is needed?

This study has shown that a weight loss of 5% (about ten pounds for most of the prediabetics) amazingly reduced the risk of developing diabetes by 58%. There was even a greater risk reduction of 71% among those who were 60 years and older. The idea is, of course, to maintain a normal weight and do daily exercises. The formula, to be effective, calls for both regimens.

Don't these measures also help diabetics?

Most definitely, yes. Maintaining normal weight and a regimen of daily physical exercises have been shown in various research studies decades ago to help better control blood sugar level among diabetics and therefore reduce or prevent the severely disabling complications of diabetes. But it is only lately, with this massively convincing large study, together with the other similar clinical investigations, that scientists and clinicians have proven that the condition called prediabetes can actually be prevented from developing into frank diabetes by losing excess weight and doing daily exercises, two very practical and simple enough measures that can prevent a dreadful, debilitating, and expensive disease.

What are the major complications of diabetes?

Diabetes type 2 is today the leading cause of new blindness, kidney failure, peripheral nerve damages, and leg amputations. This does not include its aggravating impact on coronary heart disease and stroke. Indeed, it is a miserable and debilitating illness worth preventing with all our effort and care and determination. After all, diabetes, to a significant extent is preventable in many cases.

How can diabetes be prevented?

Preventing the onset of diabetes could be as easy as losing weight among those who are overweight plus doing daily physical exercises. The Diabetes Prevention Program in the United States has impressively shown that these two lifestyle changes alone can ward off diabetes in about 60% of people with prediabetes, among them the 10 million overweight Americans who are otherwise poised to develop the disease. With this new tool in our fight to prevent prediabetes from turning into horrible diabetes, it behooves all of us to use this new promising scientific knowledge to our advantage as early as now. After all, diabetes is a dreadful disease.

Pregnancy and Women's Health

James M. Brown III, MD, and Rachel Chua, MD, both fellows of the American College of Obstetrics and Gynecology based in Lake Charles, Louisiana, are our specialist consultants for today. They will discuss various topics on pregnancy and women's health, inspired by queries emailed to us by our readers.

Mother's Diet and the Fetus

In general, women who are overweight have an increased risk of health issues including blood clots, gestational diabetes, and hypertension, all of which can lead to complications in pregnancy and delivery. Also, women who come into pregnancy with poor glycemic (diabetic—blood sugar) control have a higher risk of neural tube defects as well as other birth defects, including cleft palate, cleft lip septal anomalies, hydrocephalus, and limb reduction and miscarriage. The reason obstetricians routinely check all women for gestational diabetes is because poor glycemic control typically leads to bigger babies and more complicated deliveries requiring C-sections. Shoulder dystocia, where the shoulder could not pass thru the birth canal, is one of the complications and is an emergency.

Also, if a baby is used to a certain amount of glucose coming across the umbilical cord, its pancreas will try to produce insulin to control the glucose. The baby will then store the sugar and gain weight. At delivery, when the cord is cut and the flow of glucose from the mother to the baby is interrupted, the baby pancreas may still continue to produce insulin and causing a precipitous drop in the blood sugar. This is dangerous to the brain of the newborn. When detected, intravenous glucose is provided immediately until the pancreas is able to regulate its insulin production.

Normal-weight women who regularly feast on junk food and sweets in the early pregnancy gain weight more easily and so with the fetus. It has been shown in rats that when a pregnant mother ate a diet that was high in sugar, fat, and salt, their offspring was more likely to have high triglycerides and cholesterol and be at a higher risk of heart disease. They also had higher glucose and insulin levels and were at a higher risk for type 2 diabetes.

It is essential for women to maintain a normal weight, especially when they are planning to get pregnant or are pregnant.

Foods to Avoid During Pregnancy

Pregnancy instinctively suppresses the immune system to a degree to prevent rejection of fetus as a "foreign body." As such, pregnant women are more prone to infection and should avoid foods that are not cooked, such as sushi, raw oysters, or even steaks that are grilled rare or medium. Well-cooked items are safer for pregnant women. Processed foods are also unhealthy for both the mother and the fetus. And so with high-cholesterol and extremely spicy foods. Fish is good for both, but because of mercury concern in fish and its effects on the fetus, the variety of fish that usually have high mercury content should be avoided also. As a rule, the larger the fish, the greater mercury it contains, because it eats up a lot of smaller fishes with mercury in them.

Reported information from the Natural Resource Defense Council obtained by the US Food and Drug Administration and the Environmental Protection Agency:

Particular fishes with highest mercury content are Marlin, orange roughy, swordfish, tilefish, king mackerel, big eye/ahi tuna. Those with high level are Chilean sea bass, bluefish, grouper, Spanish mackerel, yellowfin tuna, albacore tuna.

Those with lower mercury level are striped and black bass, carp, Alaskan cod, white Pacific croaker, halibut (Pacific and Atlantic), lobster, mahimahi, monkfish, freshwater perch, sablefish, sea trot, snapper, chunk light canned tuna. Suggestion is to eat no more than 6 oz serving per month of this.

The seafoods with lowest mercury level, which may be served two 6-oz servings per week, include: anchovies, butterfish, catfish, clam, crab, crawfish, croaker, flounder, haddock, herring, hake, north atlantic mackerel, chub, mullet, oysters, ocean perch, salmon (canned, fresh), sardines, scallops, american shad, shrimps, sole, tilapia, freshwater trout, whitefish, and whiting.

Warning: definitely dangerous for the fetus and the mother are cigarettes and alcohol, regardless of the amount. These chemicals can cause mental retardation, impaired growth, weakened immune system, and a host of respiratory and other illnesses.

All of us in general, and especially pregnant women, should minimize salt intake and avoid canned foods, like vegetables and processed meats, which contain high levels of salt as a preservative. Luncheon meats are to be avoided for the same reason. Besides their high salt content, processed foods are unhealthy in themselves as shown by scientific studies. It is also prudent for pregnant (even expectant) mothers to watch their weight and limit their intake of carbohydrate (bread, cakes, ice cream, sweets, etc.) and avoid junk foods like potato chips, French fries, and fast foods in general.

Medications to Avoid

The pills for the treatment of high blood pressure known as ACE inhibitors, when taken by pregnant women during the first trimester, carries a 7% teratogenic effects (causing congenital developmental malformation) in the fetus, almost 3 times more than the 2.6% risk in the general population. This teratogenic risk includes cardiovascular and brain malformations and other deformities in almost any organs. Beta blockers apparently increases risk of fetal growth restriction. Calcium channel blockers and Aldomet appear to be safe.

The first generation oral hypoglycemic agents for diabetes (sulfonylureas, such as tolbutamide and chlorpropamide) crossed the placenta and were felt to have possible teratogenic effects, hence avoided. The second generation glyburide crosses the placenta very minimally and is now being used more commonly during pregnancy to control gestational diabetes. The pill Metformin is being used more commonly, and some studies suggest that those women who take metformin throughout the pregnancy have lower risk of gestational diabetes. "I still use insulin for the majority of my diabetic pregnant patients . . . And where indicated, my diabetic and hypertensive patients are monitored with serial ultrasounds for growth and fetal well-being," says Dr. Brown.

Use of antiseizure meds still worries obstetricians worry because of the risks of cleft pallet and lip. "But we always strive to find the safe balance for these women for effective control of their disease," Dr. Brown stresses.

The proton pump inhibitors, like nexium and protonix, are considered safe for women with reflux.

Hormone Replacement Therapy

What's new in hormone replacement therapy (HRT) is more terms of mode of absorption rather than introduction of new hormones. Trend is definitely more toward transdermal absorption (thru skin) to bypass first pass effect through the liver. It appears to be better for patient compliance. The patches could be discreetly worn on the hip, abdomen, or extremities and conveniently changed once or twice a week.

The patches come in estrogen-only form or in combination estrogen/progestin form. There are a number of creams and gels (Estrogel, Elestrin, Estrasorb) that are applied to the arm or leg daily for estrogen-only replacement that also avoid first pass liver metabolism. Vaginal estrogens in pill, cream, or ring forms also provide the benefit of transdermal absorption of estrogen, but is not available yet in combination with progestins. Some of these are only approved for vaginal atrophy and have to be used several times a week such as Vagifem tablets, Premarin cream, and Estrace cream. Femring is approved for vasomotor symptoms as well. It is a small flexible ring that is inserted vaginally by the patient. It provides slow release of estrogen for 90 days.

The current new approach in hormone therapy limits the prescription only to those women who are symptomatic and the use of lower-dose therapy. Even the duration of therapy is now limited by clinical indication at follow-up instead of indefinitely.

"Since there are medications available today for treating osteopenia and osteoporosis, we also don't use estrogen anymore for these conditions, especially for women who do not have postmenopausal symptoms," according to Dr. Rachel Chua.

Tumors of the Uterus

Typically, uterine fibroids/myomas (tumors of the womb) are benign (not cancerous). In view of this, the rule "If they don't bother you, we won't bother them" is generally assumed, especially since they are such a common finding. Usual symptoms of symptomatic fibroids are bleeding and/or pain, and for these reasons, they are treated regardless of size and age of the patient. Type of treatment will depend on the woman's age, pregnancy plans, and surgical risk factors, including body habitus and medical history.

However, menopausal women with an enlarging fibroid need to be aggressively treated due to increased risk of malignant transformation from benign fibroma to leiomyosarcoma, a form of cancer.

If a patient is not done with childbearing, the uterine fibroids can be removed either hysteroscopically (for fibroid within the uterine cavity) or laparoscopically (for fibroids that are subserosal on the outer surface of the uterus).

If a patient is done with childbearing, hysterectomy is the choice, especially if there is pathology of the ovaries as well. As for giant fibroids, laparoscopic vaginal hysterectomy is still an option, with the advent of the Morcellator. Robotic hysterectomy is state of the art, which allows vaginal removal of an enlarged uterus and its cervix thru a laparoscope, saving the woman from a large abdominal incision.

This husband-and-wife team successfully performed robotic hysterectomy recently to remove a 16-week-size uterine fibroid (about the size of a large cantaloupe). Prior to the availability of robotic surgery, this would have required opening the abdomen.

Medical treatment for fibroids with Lupron is used only preoperatively to decrease blood loss. A treatment offered at some larger university settings is uterine artery embolization, blocking the artery with a clot, to cut off the blood supply to the fibroid to reduce its growth and size. This procedure is performed by an interventional radiologist.

The progressive advances in medicine and surgery, which are mind-boggling, are a welcome boon to people's health and well-being around the globe.

Processed Foods and Cancer

Did you know how many hotdogs are consumed each day in the United States alone? Roughly 633 hotdogs are eaten by Americans per second, or 37, 980 every minute, almost 2.3 million an hour.

A Lot of Dogs

According to Janet Riley, president of the National Hotdog and Sausage Council, USA, Americans eat twenty billion hotdogs a year. This does not include those sold at ball games, which is about 30 million during regular pro season.

Calories

Hotdogs, also known as franks, are popular because it is inexpensive, convenient to eat, and has lower calories than pizza or hamburger. A hamburger, depending on its size and condiments with it, could provide 350 calories or have as high as 800 to 1,000 calories. A slice of pizza has 272 calories, while hot dog has only 148.

Quality of Food

While calorie intake is vital to our health and being appropriately conscious about how much we eat positively impacts our well-being and our longevity, the quality of what we eat is also very important. As they say, we are what we eat.

Processed Foods: Unhealthy

Medical statistics on the relationship of nutrition/diet and health/ diseases and longevity show that a meal with processed foods (canned or frozen, especially meats, like hotdogs, bacon, ham, etc.) is most unhealthy. Eating processed foods has been linked to the development of cardiovascular and metabolic diseases, like hypertension, heart disease, stroke, diabetes, and various forms of cancers, most notably cancer of the pancreas and the gastrointestinal tract.

Foods manufactured are processed to preserve their texture, color, aroma, nutritive value, prevent bacterial growth, and to maximize their "shelf" life. This goes true with either canned or frozen food items. To achieve all these, various strategies are employed. The two common ones are the use of chemical preservatives and additives, and controlled heat sterilization.

What in the processing technique or in the chemical additives and preservatives used is hazardous to health has not been fully determined, but the statistics are too overwhelming to ignore. The association between the illnesses mentioned above, and the regular ingestion of processed foods is very significant.

There is no question that *fresh*, unadulterated, is best!

Killing Us Softly

In general red meats, eggs (the yellow yolk), and other high-cholesterol and high-fat food items harm our body. The adverse effects on our various organs happen so slowly, taking decades before illnesses and symptoms manifest themselves, that we do not feel sick or threatened immediately and thus continue consuming these great-tasting foods regularly. Metaphorically speaking, these foods are slow poisons which are killing us softly.

Healthier Option

The proven healthier alternative is a diet composed of fish, vegetables, fruits, nuts, grains, wheat, and other high-fiber foods. The high omega-3 contents in fish in general and the phytochemicals in vegetables, especially the green leafy ones, and the other antioxidant flavanoids in this regimen, are all beneficial in their boosting effects on our immune system and on their protective action for our cardiovascular and gastrointestinal health. Coupled with controlled carbohydrate and calorie intake, daily physical exercises, and stress management, this gastronomic option is healthier, a lifesaver, and one which maximizes people's potential longevity.

Prostatic Cancer

The American Cancer Society estimates that more than 232,000 men in the United States will be diagnosed with prostate cancer this year, and about 30,000, or roughly 13%, will die of it. This figure is in addition to the existing 2 million who have already been diagnosed to have it. Prostatic cancer is one of the most common cancers in man around the world, killing one almost every 19 minutes, and a new case is discovered every 2 and a half minutes. In the Philippines it is one of the top five cancers among men, and in 2005 alone, about 4,000 new prostatic cancer cases were found.

What is a prostate?

The prostate is a gland in men that is shaped like a walnut, roughly about an inch and a half in diameter, located underneath the urinary bladder and in the area behind the pubic bone and the base of the penis. The male hormone testosterone produced by the testes ("balls") along with sperm, stimulates the prostate to secrete part of the semen (whitish, thick, cloudy fluid) in which the spermatozoa (sperm) wiggles and travels.

Does cancer of the prostate cause symptoms?

Cancer of the prostate does not cause symptoms early because the malignant tumor usually develops in the outer portion of the prostate and therefore does not cause blockage of the urethra. Even without symptoms, this form of early stage of the cancer may be detected during a medical examination. This is the reason why a regular checkup, including a digital (finger) rectal prostate examination (once or twice a year), is very important among men who are 40 years and older, even those without symptoms, to catch prostate cancer before it spreads. Blood (serum) PSA level is also an important test for prostate cancer. When symptoms occur, the cancer may already be advanced.

What is a PSA Test?

PSA stands for prostate-specific antigen, which is done by radioimmunoassay methods and is the most sensitive marker for monitoring progression of prostate cancer and response to therapy. Its precise role in early detection is still being evaluated. PSA is elevated in 25% to 92% of those with cancer of the prostate and 30% to 50% of those with benign prostatic hyperplasia. Transrectal ultrasound (TRUS) could provide a preliminary diagnosis by means of soundwaves and confirmed by guided-needle biopsy of the prostate for a more definitive histologic tissue diagnosis. The other routine initial tests include urinalysis and blood tests, urine flow test, IVP (intravenous pyelogram) kidney X-rays, and cystoscopy ("telescopic" examination of the urethra and the bladder, done through the penis).

What about for cancer of the prostate?

Localized cancer of the prostate gland may be *cured* by radical retropubic prostatectomy (RRPP), with an incision done in the lower abdomen, about 4 inches above the front base of the penis. However, if there is extensive local spread, if the patient is too old or in poor health, or if there is already metastasis (distant spread of the cancer, usually to the bones), RRPP is not the preferred modality. In these cases, hormone control therapy, irradiation (X-ray IMRT treatment) or bilateral orchiectomy (removal of both testicles) may provide palliation (improvement but not a cure). Radiation for control of pains due to spread of the cancer to the bones may provide relief. Chemotherapy after failure of hormone treatment has been found to be ineffective.

What is the prognosis of these patients?

The ten-year cure rates among patients with localized (with no spread) cancer of the prostate treated by radical prostatecomy or radiation therapy is about 65%. In other words, ten years after the treatment, 65 out of a hundred are still alive and well. Those patients who are not candidates for the radical prostate surgery or for irradiation may respond for several years to adequate hormonal control and/or orchiectomy. The prognosis among those with metastases is obviously worse, but treatment may provide a long-term palliation.

Red Meat and Cancer

A diet high in processed meat (sausages, luncheon meats, etc.) may increase the risk of carnivores developing pancreatic cancer by almost 70%, reported a recent major study that was published in the *Journal of the National Cancer Institute* and released to the public in October 2005.

The report showed "an average of 41 cases of pancreatic cancer were diagnosed per 100,000 people each year among those who ate the most processed meat compared with 20 cases among those who ate the least."

This research, which included 180,000 individuals, also found that individuals who ate even nonprocessed red meats—including pork, beef, and any other red meats—had a 50% higher risk of having cancer of the pancreas. While this is 20% lower compared to those who ate processed meats, 50% increase in the risk is still too high for comfort, since pancreatic cancer is a very painful and fatal disease with no known cure.

Scientists think the culprit carcinogen (cancer-causing agent) may not be the saturated fat in red meats but the nitrate-based preservatives and the cooking method, like charcoal grilling and broiling. Apparently, the cooking method and the nitrate preservatives each play a great role as carcinogens.

While the saturated fat in fresh (no preservative) red meat appears not to be linked to pancreatic cancer in this study, other studies have shown that people who eat red meat regularly have a higher risk for developing cancer of the colon, breast and other cancers in general, compared to those who minimize eating red meat. Red meat also causes a quick rise in the cholesterol blood level, a condition that increases the risk for the development of heart attack and stroke.

In 2005 alone, 32,180 Americans and 60,000 Europeans were found to have pancreatic cancer, a disease that is often diagnosed late because they are not readily obvious clinically. Less than 5% of these patients live for more than five years after the cancer is first detected.

Other risk factors include smoking, family history of cancer of the pancreas, obesity, diabetes, age (older ones), gender (male), ethnicity (African), exposure to certain dyes, pesticides, and chemicals related to gasoline. *Helicobacter pylori* infection that causes the common ulcer of the stomach is also a predisposing factor. African Americans appear to have higher incidence of pancreatic cancer and poorer prognosis than whites.

Abdominal ultrasound, CT scan, and endoscopic ultrasound are some procedures, together with some blood and liver function tests, that aid in the diagnosis of pancreatic cancer.

The treatment of pancreatic cancer varies according to the stage of the malignancy. The management includes surgery, radiation, chemotherapy alone, and chemotherapy with a targeted treatment. The Whipple procedure is the most popular surgery for cancer of the head of the pancreas. Modern advances in surgery today have allowed resection of pancreatic cancers which were considered unresectable in the past. Completely resected pancreatic cancer provides the best opportunity for a longer term survival, albeit still not a cure.

The most common drug used is gemcitabine (Gemzar); but recently this drug, in combination with erlotimib (Tarceva), has proved useful in advanced cases. Chemotherapy may be used in combination with radiation, which uses high energy X-rays to shrink the tumor or slow its growth.

The other option is biological and targeted therapies, which "enhances the body natural immune system to stop tumor growth, changing cellular signals that permit tumor growth, making tumors more susceptible to an immune system attack and blocking the process that change normal cells into cancer, thereby stopping the abnormal growth behavior of a tumor."

Smoking is one of the most significant risk factors, besides eating red meat. For prevention, minimizing red meat ingestion, abstinence from cigarettes, maintaining a normal body weight, daily exercises, and eating a lot of vegetables, fruits, and whole grains have all been found to significantly lower the risk of the development of pancreatic cancer, not to mention heart disease, stroke, other forms of cancer, and even Alzheimer's.

In cardiovascular illnesses, like heart attack and stroke, in metabolic diseases, like type 2 diabetes and in most cancers, lifestyle and personal behavior are the greatest factors in the causation of these maladies; and these killers are therefore preventable.

As always, as far as our health is concerned, the ball is in our court. How we play it will determine the quality of our life and our future.

Red Wine and Health

Is wine really good for our health?

Yes, most particularly red wine. But this will, of course, depend on other considerations and factors. We do not recommend any alcoholic beverages to pregnant women; persons who are alcoholics or have history of addiction; those with liver, gastrointestinal, or other diseases where alcohol is contraindicated; those who are allergic to it; poorly controlled diabetics, etc. Persons with a health problem should first consult with their physicians before ingesting alcoholic beverages.

Why is red wine better?

Red wine has been singled out as cardioprotective (good for the heart) because its skin contains *phytochemicals*, such as *resveratrol*, that help protect the plant's self-defense system and *proanthocyanidins (OPC) and cathechins,* which are also powerful antioxidants. And these same substances have been found good for humans. Studies at the University of California, Davis, and Cornell University have confirmed the beneficial effect of these potent antioxidants that aid in preventing cancer and heart coronary heart disease. Also, the alcohol in it has some sedative and euphoric effects when wine is taken in moderation; and these are healthy for the psyche, especially in these stressful times.

Are all red wine the same?

No, not all red wines are alike or equal as far as the amount of *resveratrol* they contain. Research on seventy red wines from New York rated the Pinot Noirs (Pino Nwahs) to contain the highest amount of this *phytochemical*, with an average content of 13.6 micromoles per liter, about twice found in Cabernet Sauvignon (Cabernay Sow vin yong), Merlot (Merlo), and Cabernet Franc. The specific wines and vintages with very high level were the '97 Pinot Noir from Benton-Lane Winery in Oregon and the '98 Noble Muscadine from Dennis Vineyards in North Carolina. Large commercial wineries manipulate their wines more and reduce the *resveratrol* and other antioxidants as a result; small wineries utilizing the old European technique produce wines with higher *resveratrol.*

Why the difference in *resveratrol* contents?

After analyzing several hundreds of wines in his laboratory at Cornell, Professor Emeritus Le Creasy found that "wine produced in dry climates, like California central valley had lower *resveratrol* level than from the same variety of grapes grown in humid climates like New York."

How about white wine?

Resveratrol is found in grape skins and *OPC and C* in the grape seeds. In red wine, the skins and seeds are included in the fermentation for at least 2 to 3 weeks, while white wine is made from juice that is pressed from the grapes, where the skins and seeds are not included in the fermentation, This explains why only red wine has a significant level of *resveratrol, OPC, and C.*

Are the more expensive red wines better?

No, not necessarily. A Pinot Noir imported from France, which is much more expensive, is not a better "health drink" than a Pinot Noir from New York. An older vintage variety, which, again, is more pricey, might taste better in most cases, especially for connoisseurs, but not necessarily superior in its antioxidant value. Most wine-drinking families drink regular red table wine, but the choice is so personal and according to one's taste. Mine is Pinot Noir when available, Cabernet Sauvignon, second, and Merlot, third.

Is red wine also good against degenerative diseases?

Yes, according to Professor Susan Ebeler of the UC-Davis, "There's increasing evidence that red wine contains components which may impart important health-protective effects against a number of degenerative diseases."

At what age should one start drinking red wine?

In Italy and France, preteens are already allowed to imbibe "a little" wine with dinner. I am not advocating the same for us because our laws have set a legal drinking age, but I am not sure that this European practice is unhealthy at all. As a matter of fact, available medical evidence suggests that drinking a glass or two (not more than 3) red wine is a lot healthier than drinking a couple cans of beers or a shot or two of hard liquor. Medically speaking, allowing our children to smoke cigarettes, not exercise, or eat red meat, eggs, and other high cholesterol foods day in and day out is certainly and definitely more unhealthy and dangerous than allowing them to drink a little red wine with dinner in a disciplined manner.

How much is "not too much"?

The generally recommended "healthy medical dose" for adult is between one and two (at most 3) *wine glasses* of red wine with dinner. I qualified the type of the glasses because drinking more (improperly using larger or taller glasses) is not necessary to achieve the health benefit from red wine. Wine has to be enjoyed, not endured. So take it as a fun drink and not as a "prescription medicine."

How about beer and hard liquor?

Beer and hard liquor do not impart the same health benefit as red wine does. They are social drinks that people over the centuries have developed a taste for, basically imbibed at parties. If a person drinks alone regularly or has to drink to be sociable, then there is something wrong. While ingestion of alcohol at a gathering makes most people less inhibited, a little "euphoric," and friendlier (and thus appear to be more sociable), one should not feel he/she needs a drink to be sociable. Using alcohol as a crutch is not healthy.

What is the drug action of alcohol?

Ethanol (ethyl alcohol) is the potable form of alcohol found in alcoholic beverages, unlike methanol (methyl "wood" alcohol), which is an industrial solvent and a poison. Antiseptic rubbing alcohol is isopropyl alcohol, certainly not for drinking. The mode of action of ethanol is on the central nervous system. It is a sedative and a depressant, although a small amount (one to two drinks) might appear to act like a "stimulant." The effect varies in each individual. The same amount could make one "the life and soul of the party," make another sleepy, and bring out aggression and violence in others.

Does drinking improve sexual performance?

Ethanol may make one feel carefree, excited, and merrier; but it does not directly improve sexual prowess. In Macbeth, act 2, scene 3, Shakespeare wrote alcohol "provokes the desire but takes away the performance." After a glass or two of red wine and a romantic situation and an appropriate ambiance, Shakespeare might be wrong; but after 3 or more, he will most likely be right. Again, it depends on the personal tolerance of the persons involved.

What is the French Paradox?

While the Frenchmen eat a lot of "unhealthy" cholesterol-rich foods and many of them smoke, the incidence of heart attacks and the mortality rates from heart attacks among the French males, according to the popular 1970 studies, appeared much lower than those of Americans and Scandinavian men. The favorable results among the French were likewise found among Italians and the Swiss. The obvious difference in these five cultures and societies, said the researchers, was the habit of drinking red wine with the meals among the people of France, Italy, and Switzerland. Perhaps, we should add our country to this list.

Any rule of thumb for healthy drinking?

Without being fecitious, the best drink consists of at least 8 glasses of filtered water a day. But where alcohol is concerned, red wine (Pinot Noir, when possible) is my personal choice, a glass or two with dinner (certainly not more than 3), without chasing it with beer or hard liquor! Just like anything in life and in health, moderation is the key, especially to what I will call "therapeutic drinking."

In the meantime, here's—a votre sante!

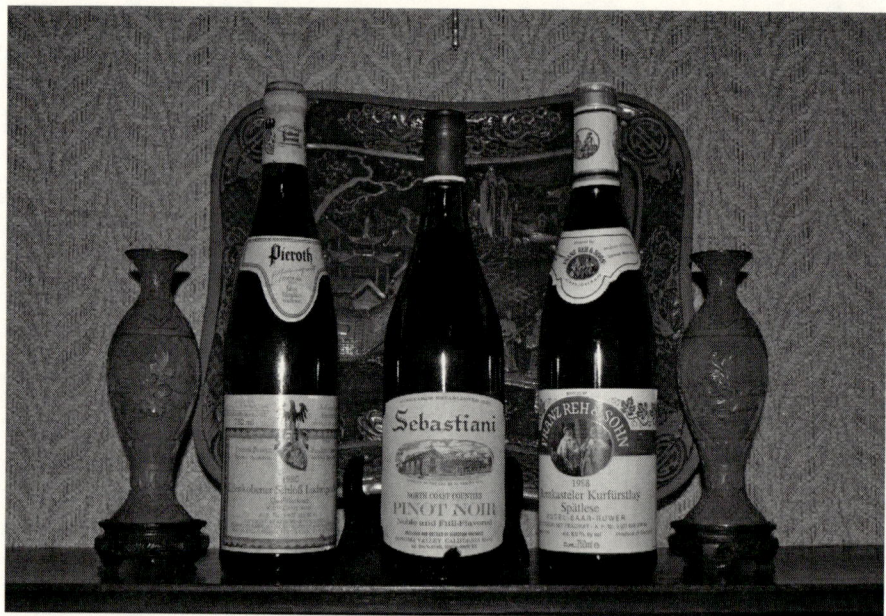

Red wine with dinner, exercise, dieting, and watching the waisline
are a prescription for health and longevity.

Refractive Surgery

What is refractive surgery?

Refractive or vision correction surgery is an operation on the eyes to correct error of refraction, like nearsightedness, farsightedness and astigmatism, to eliminate the use of prescription eyeglasses or contact lenses.

What are the various procedures available today?

The advent of Excimer laser in 1988 ushered in a new revolutionary era in vision correction. It provided added lifestyle choices made possible by the freedom from, or dependence on, prescription eyewears. That important technological advance resulted in major treatment modalities not possible before then. The three popular procedures for refractive surgery today are LASIK (laser assisted in-situ keratomileusis or laser vision correction), PRK (photorefractive keratectomy) and Intacs (corneal ring segments) implants.

What is Excimer laser?

Excimer laser is a computer-controlled ultraviolet beam of light that reshapes the cornea (outer window of the eye), resulting in the light focusing more directly on the retina at the back of the eye. Excimer laser gives out a cool or nonthermal (not hot) light beam, making it ideal for corneal surgery, eliminating the possibility of thermal burns to the surrounding tissues. Each laser pulse is so accurate it achieves disruption and removal of the molecular tissue bonds between the corneal cells up to 0.25 micons (or 0.00004 of an inch), which improves the vision. Usually, only about 50 microns of tissue (about half the thickness of human hair) are removed to achieve the correct amount of vision correction.

What does each procedure involve?

In LASIK, a thin layer of the corneal (outer covering) stroma is fashioned using a microkeratome (cutting) instrument, and this tissue is set back in place after the laser procedure is done. LASIK reshapes the corneal tissue *underneath* the surface of the cornea, while PRK uses laser to remove the epithelium, a thin protective "skin" *on top* that covers the cornea, before the actual corrective treatment is performed. For Intacs, two tiny incisions and tunnels are made on the outer edges of the cornea; and the Intacs (half-moon or C-shaped) ring segment is implanted in each tunnels, and a suture is placed.

What are Intacs?

Intacs are two mini half rings, made of biocompatible plastic that has been safely used for about five decades in cataract operations and in contact lenses. Intacs permanently corrects error of refraction when placed within the outer edges of the eyes as described above.

What are the benefits of these procedures?

The corrective surgery decreases or eliminates the dependence on glasses or contact lenses, increases safety while indulging in outdoor or sports activities, provides more convenience, improves vision 24 hours a day, and in some people, it may improve self-esteem, the look, or satisfy vanity.

Is general anesthesia used for this?

No, only topical anesthesia is used for these procedures. Eye drops to numb the eyes are instilled prior to the surgery. This is enough to prevent the patient from feeling any pain during the operation.

Does this correct aging vision?

Error of refraction in the elderly, usually starting from age 40, is called presbyopia. The 3 procedures mentioned above will not correct presbyopia. Those undergoing any of those vision correction surgery will still need reading glasses.

Are there potential risks and side effects?

Just like any surgery, these vision correction procedures have possible risks and side effects. Following the surgery around 5 to 25% of patients will have some haziness of vision that is aggravated at night. It peaks at 8 to 12 weeks after treatment and in almost all of the cases, this problem resolves with eyedrops and the natural healing process. Some patients may notice halos or glare when looking at bright lights or at night. A few of them may feel increased intraoccular pressure, and many will experience some discomfort that is relieved by home pain killers like acetaminophen (Tylenol). Infection is rare but possible. It is best to discuss all the details about the recommended procedure, advantages and disadvantages, timing and sequence of surgery, possible risks and complications with your ophthalmologist performing the procedure.

Can this procedure be done on a pregnant woman?

Because of the nature of the procedure, these laser-assisted procedures may *not* be done during pregnancy, until three months after delivery and breastfeeding. After the procedure, the patient should wait 6 months before becoming pregnant.

Who are candidates for this vision correction?

Those age 18 or older, with otherwise healthy eyes, with mild to moderate nearsightedness (-1.00 to-14.0 diopters), farsightedness (+1.50 to +4.00 diopters), and astigmatism are good candidates for LASIK or PRK. For Intacs, the best patients are those with nearsightedness (-1.00 to-3.00 diopters). These procedures will provide better vision without eyeglasses or contacts, but none of them will give perfect vision. A realistic expectation is very essential with this refractory surgery.

Restless Leg Syndrome

What is restless leg syndrome?

Restless leg syndrome (RLS) is condition where the individual develops a strong, irresistible urge to move their legs whenever they sit or lie down. This may be accompanied by uncomfortable sensations in their legs, which RLS patients described as painful, tingling, crawling, pulling, or creeping. This entity has been known for at least a few hundred years, but it was only in the 1940s when it was officially named.

When do the symptoms of RLS occur?

The symptoms are precipitated by prolonged sitting or inactivity, or while the individual is traveling, attending a long meeting, watching a movie, or at a concert, or even while trying to relax or trying to sleep. Typically, the symptoms begin or worsen in the early evening and at night. Stretching or walking may provide some relief as long as the activity continues.

Does RLS impair sleep?

Yes. As a matter of fact, sufferers usually seek medical attention because of inability to get enough sleep, not realizing RLS is causing the disruption in their sleep. Many have been treated as a sleep disorder. The right diagnosis could be missed by the physician if his/her index of suspicion for RLS is low, leading to severe frustration among patients and physicians alike.

Are men more affected by RLS?

No, restless leg syndrome affects more women than men and can start at any age. Studies show that more than 50% of those with RLS have a family member with RLS also.

What could mimic RLS?

Some conditions that could be confused with restless leg syndrome are calcium deficiency, varicose vein leg discomfort, leg pains among those taking anticholesterol drug Lipitor, blockage of arterial circulation in the leg from hardening of the artery and/or diabetes mellitus, and fibromyalgia. There are also other neurological and metabolic entities that could cause leg discomfort.

How is RLS diagnosed?

Basically, through medical interview and physical examination (to rule out other possible causes), by deduction and elimination process. Laboratory tests, such as blood tests, X-rays, etc., are not diagnostic, but may be useful in discarding other diseases on the "suspected" list of possibilities. This is why keen awareness and a high index of suspicion on the part of the attending healthcare provider are essential in making the accurate diagnosis. RLS could be a very elusive culprit.

Are referrals necessary?

In this day and age of medical sophistication and specialization, a testament to the obvious fact that no one individual can know everything, a RLS sufferer may be referred by the initial attending physician to other specialists. While this may not be a welcome inconvenience and added expenses for the patient, sending the patient to specialists is an honest act of concern and dedication on the part of a physician for the ultimate benefit of the patient. This holds especially true for RLS, a baffling condition that could really challenge the diagnostician.

What is "therapeutic diagnosis"?

When the preponderance of evidences point to a certain disease entity but the physician is still not 100% certain because of lack of a laboratory diagnostic aid and objective confirmation, the physician may try to treat the patient with a medication that best suits the clinical picture. This trial, if successful, not only improves or cures the patient, but also confirms the diagnosis the physician suspected. While this is not the usual scenario, sometimes the physician is left with no choice but to rely on his training, experience, and diagnosis skills in treating his patient, when laboratory tests are not helpful or are impotent.

Is there a drug available for RLS?

Yes. A "new" drug has been approved by the US-FDA in May 2005 for the treatment of restless leg syndrome in the United States. It's actually an old drug being used for the treatment of Parkinson's disease and now found effective for restless leg syndrome also. The medication is known by the brand names Adartel and Requip (chemical name: ropinirole).

A Killer in Our Kitchen

Quietly sitting in our kitchen is a good friend but a bad enemy, a killer, when "abused." We are not talking about fire or boiling water, or knives, or even bacteria. We are referring to an old friend from times immemorial: table salt (sodium chloride).

Most of us eat more salt than our body needs. Some of us ingest 3-4 times more than the recommended daily allowance in a day. In the United States, the RDA for sodium is between 1,100 and 3,300 mg for adults; but statistically speaking, the average salt intake in the USA is between 4,000 and 5,000 mg a day. The British are healthier in their RDA, which is called recommended nutritional intake (RNI), set at 1,600 mg. One teaspoon table salt is about 2,400 mg sodium.

Overdosing on Salt

Sodium deficiency is uncommon, so there is no reason to be afraid of not getting enough salt. Shaking the salt habit is healthier. Only those who do strenuous or prolonged physical exercises, like athletes and marathon runners, who sweat a lot, and people with severe diarrhea or other conditions that cause dehydration may need extra salt. Ordinarily, we do not, because the foods we eat already contain enough. As a matter of fact, usually too much. Salt overload is unhealthy and eventually takes its toll as years go by. Salt is indeed, without exaggeration, a silent killer lurking in our kitchen.

The foods that contain more than enough sodium include processed foods (cured meats, fish, and vegetables), canned goods, fish sauce, soy sauce, shrimp or anchovy paste, dried fish, soft drinks, salted dried plums, and salty recipes. Some individuals even combine some of these foods and condiments.

While salt is an essential part of our body, a vital ingredient fundamental for normal physiology, excess amount harms our cells, tissues, and organs. Medically speaking, 500 mg (about a fifth of a teaspoon total) a day should suffice for our daily nonstrenuous activities. The *iodized* version of sea salt or regular salt is the recommended version for our use.

Since salt adds taste to food, it is easy to be addicted; and the saltier the food we learn to eat as children, the more our taste buds crave for it as adults. Our threshold increases, and pretty soon, what is normal tasting for us actually tastes too salty for persons used to eating salt in moderation and more so to those on low-salt-diet.

The Diseases Excess Causes

Those with hypertension (high blood pressure) should use less than 1,500 mg of sodium a day or limit their intake to no more than 3/4 of a teaspoon a day. Eating more than 1,500 mg a day almost instantly raises the blood pressure a bit even among individuals with normal blood pressure and elevates the blood pressure much higher among hypertensives. Low-salt diet also makes high blood easier to manage and control.

What is not a common knowledge is that excess salt intake is linked to Alzheimer's, osteoporosis, obesity, kidney disease, diabetes, sleep apnea, and cancer. Among those who habitually use the salt shaker even before tasting the food, the incidence of hypertension, heart attack, and stroke are also much higher.

Why Salt Is Addictive

Eating more salt than what our body physiology needs alters our brain chemistry. When we ingest salt or salty foods, it triggers the release of a substance called dopamine, which is a neuro (nerve) transmitter associated with our brains "pleasure center," inducing addiction, much like what happens when one indulges in smoking or drinking alcohol, without control and moderation.

More Dangerous Than We Think

A Japanese study revealed that salted food intake is associated with a 15% increase in the risk for developing cancer, like stomach cancer and cancer of other organs. Excess salt also leads to faster calcium loss, which leads to osteoporosis and bone fractures. This bad habit also causes insulin resistance, leading to, and aggravating, diabetes. Some clinical research found that excess salt ingestion among people with high blood "are up to 600% more likely to develop stroke-related dementia." Salty foods also lead to injury to the inner lining cells of arteries causing arterial blockages and kidney disease.

The American Medical Association and countless medical practitioners deplore this excess, and "AMA estimated that a 50 percent reduction in sodium usage in processed and restaurant food could save 150,000 lives every year." Unless one is doing a lot of exercising and sweating, around 500 mg is enough and will ward off a variety of health complications associated with high blood pressure.

Beware of Salt Traps

Some of the common salt traps include: the most obvious is the saltshaker (which is safer in the condiment shelf, together with the soy sauce and fish sauce, than on the dining table), canned goods (vegetables, about 1,000 mg sodium per can), and processed foods (bacon, 200 mg sodium per slice; one hot dog, 600 mg sodium), which are better left in the grocery stores. Frozen foods may contain as much as a whopping 4,000-5,000 mg sodium (good for 8 to 10 days supply of sodium), all in one frozen meal! Fresh foods are definitely healthier when properly prepared. Diet or light foods mostly have high salt content to make these less-than-appetizing foods more palatable. Reading the food label for any sodium content will give one a clue. Any ingredient that has the word sodium in it is salt.

Herbs, Condiments to the Rescue

Watching our salt intake does not mean bland or joyless meals. One can be creative using healthier substitutes, like pepper, chives, basil, thyme, oregano, rosemary, curry, lemon, mustard, vinegar, etc., and end up with most tasty and satisfying meals, which are healthy as well. The natural salt in every food items provided us by Mother Earth's fields and gardens is enough a chemical preservative, together with some of those condiments, for our body to ward off diseases, including cancer, and achieve health and maximal longevity. Any excess salt we take only tends to undermine our well-being and shorten our life.

Reeducating Our Taste Buds

We have about 10,000 taste buds (gustatory calyculi), located on top of the tongue, under the tongue, inside our cheeks, roof of the mouth, and even in our lips. Those in the lips are the most sensitive to salt.

Since the taste buds are made up of an average of about 100 receptor cells each, which are replaced by new ones every ten days or so, we can reeducate them by consistently eating less and lesser salt until we hit our goal of eating no more than half a teaspoon a day total (including the salt already in the foods we eat).

The simple strategy of *not* using the salt shaker is a good start. Adding pepper, or other nonsalty condiments as substitutes, would be a great second step. And the third, and most important, ingredients in this recipe to a healthier self are determination and will power. For the privilege of having good health, this "sacrifice" is definitely worth it.

There are no official RDA for infants and children. Since exposure to the bad habit of eating excess salt can start early in life, it is prudent for parents to set a good example for their children and guide them accordingly toward a healthier lifestyle.

Salt is good. Salt is life. But in excess, salt is a killer, no matter how subtle it may be. To play it safe, let's keep salt on our side, as a friend.

Sexual Sterilization

What is tubal ligation, and what is vasectomy?

These are two surgical procedures for permanent birth control. Tubal ligation is sterilization for women, where the fallopian tubes are ligated (tied by sutures) to prevent the ova (eggs) from being transported to the uterus. Vasectomy is sterilization in men, where the vas deferens (two tiny tubes, one connected to each testicle where semen is formed) are cut to prevent the semen from being ejaculated.

Are these procedures permanent?

While very rare and practically unheard of, there are case reports in the medical literature of spontaneous recanalization (where the cut channels, either vas deferens or fallopian tubes, rejoined together on their own to reestablish the channels), making pregnancy possible once again. However, for all intents and purposes, once vasectomy or tubal ligation is done, these should be considered permanent sterilization.

How common and how safe are these procedures?

In the United States, where family planning is seriously practiced, one partner is sterilized in about 1/3 of all married couples. So in 33% of all married couples, either the husband had a vasectomy or the wife had a tubal ligation or a hysterectomy (removal of the uterus). These surgical procedures, like any operations, are not devoid of possible complications; but they are very safe. Vasectomy could be done in about 20 minutes in a surgeon's office, under local anesthesia, and the patient walks out a few minutes thereafter. Tubal ligation is a more extensive surgery requiring general anesthesia and where the gynecologist has to open the abdomen, or (more recently) doing the ligation through laparoscopy (a lighted and seeing "telescope" is used through small incisions in the abdomen, the procedure seen and monitored live on a video screen). This simpler procedure does not require overnight hospitalization, hence it is very popular.

Can vasectomy and tubal ligation be "reversed"?

Yes, reanastomosis (hooking the cut ends together) of the vas deferens of the fallopian tubes can be done, even after several years following the original procedures. Since the vas deferens are smaller in caliber, the reconstructive operation is more tedious and difficult compared to reanastomosing the fallopian tubes, which are larger structures. Pregnancy rate after reconstruction of the fallopian tubes is about 50-80% and the vas deferens about 45 to 60%.

Is a man sterile immediately after a vasectomy?

No, about 15 to 20 ejaculations are usually needed after vasectomy before sterility is achieved. Semen analysis follows the procedure, and the man is not considered sterile until he subsequently produces two sperm-free ejaculates.

Does vasectomy make a man impotent or less potent?

No, vasectomy does not cause impotence or a decrease in libido or sexual desire. Most medical literature reports the opposite. Following the procedure, men appear to have more sexual drive and potency. Part of this could be due to the sense of security and freedom vasectomy confers on them and their partners. Tubal ligation does not reduce libido either, and it also gives the women similar sense of security and peace of mind.

Does vasectomy protect the man from venereal disease?

No, vasectomy does not protect anyone from catching sexually transmitted diseases. This is a myth that must be dispelled once and for all. Without prudence and without proper protection, any man, with or without a vasectomy, is equally susceptible to venereal diseases.

Who should be sterilized for contraception, the male or the female?

After a careful consideration of all ramifications—religious, medical, psychological, social—following a consultation with the physicians, the husband and wife should make the joint decision as to who should undergo the sterilization procedure. Vasectomy is a lot simpler procedure and equally effective. However, if the gynecologist found an intra-abdominal condition in the woman which needs to be explored, tubal ligation might be the choice, while the abdomen is open during surgery. Tubal ligation is also done following a Cesarean section when the delivery is the last one desired by the couple. Since there are other factors and issues involved, it is best for the couple to discuss this matter in detail with their physicians beforehand.

What is the advantage of a hysterectomy over tubal ligation?

Elective hysterectomy (removal of the uterus) is an acceptable means of sterilization when other chronic conditions of the uterus exist, like severe dysmenorrhea, cervical dysplasia, or menorrhagia. Although a more extensive surgery than tubal ligation, hysterectomy has long-term advantages: it is 100% effective as contraception, the absence of menstrual disorders, and the prevention (or preclusion) of possible development of leiomyomas (benign uterine tumors) or uterine cancers. Again, the expert advice of the gynecologist is most essential in this matter.

What are the other contraceptive methods?

The contraceptive regimens (in their order of popularity) are oral steroid pills, condoms, spermicides, withdrawal, diaphragm, periodic abstinence, and intrauterine devices (IUDs). A new modality, polysiloxone capsules containing levonorgestrel that are implanted under the skin, was first introduced in 1991. Pregnancy rates are less than 1% per year for oral contraceptives, IUDs, and subdermal implants and about 5% per year for the five sex intercourse related methods listed above. It should also be noted here that sometimes condoms could have holes in them, damaged by rough handling or poor storage conditions. In these cases, the condom will not be as effective in preventing pregnancy or sexually transmitted diseases.

What causes failure in contraception?

There are many factors affecting failure rates in the nonsurgical contraceptive methods, like the level of education, degree of motivation, age, strength of character, etc. These are inversely related to the failure rates. In general, the partners who are more mature, more educated, with greater strength of character and higher degree of motivation have lower failure rates. Sex drive, especially in the young, where the hormones are at their peak level, is such a powerful force that contraception has always remained a dilemma and a challenge to the family planners. Nature is not easy to tame.

Sexually Transmitted Epidemic

How many STDs are there?

There are more than 28 sexually transmitted diseases. The more common ones include herpes, hepatitis B, gonorrhea, chlamydia, human papillomavirus (HPV), syphilis, and HIV-AIDS. STDs result from the transfer of microorganisms (infectious "bugs") from one person to another during sex. Some of these STDs may also be transmitted by blood transfusion, thru infected syringe and needles, or even by birth (mother-to-fetus in the womb).

How prevalent are STDs?

In the United States alone, about 15 million Americans are infected with at least one of these sexually transmitted diseases each year. Two-thirds of the victims are persons under age 25, including the 4 million teenagers who get the infection each year.

Can a one-night stand lead to STDs?

Yes, most definitely. A single encounter or a one-night stand can lead to infection with any of the sexually transmitted diseases, if one of the partners has the infection and an intact condom or protection was not used. Thirty-three percent (one in 3) sexually active young people will be infected by this dreaded STD by age 24. Those infected with STDs do not develop any degree of immunity to subsequent STD infections.

Does promiscuity increase the risk of STDs?

Most definitely, yes. The more sex partners one has, the more exposure he/she has in getting HIV or other sexually transmitted diseases. The partners are not guaranteed to be free of infection. Some may not even be sure or intentionally hiding the truth. If one had sex with a person with HIV, the chances of getting AIDS is very high. And today, there is still no cure for AIDS. It is, indeed, a death sentence.

Do persons with an STD have symptoms?

Most victims of an STD have no initial symptoms or signs. The symptoms usually appear when the infection becomes worse. HIV may not even be detected for years, then AIDS explodes like a bomb.

Which STD is most common?

Chlamydia is the most common STD in America, where more than 4 million persons are infected annually. This bacterial infection usually does not have symptoms, but may cause burning urination and discharge of pus from the vagina or penis. If not treated among women, it may cause PID (pelvic inflammatory disease) leading to infertility and ectopic (tubal) pregnancy. Chlamydia can also cause infertility among men and frequently coexist with gonorrhea, requiring two different treatments.

What is hepatitis B?

Worldwide, chronic hepatitis B is one of the leading causes of death, killing more than one million people annually. The disease is spread by contact with an infected patient's semen, blood, or other body fluids. A pregnant woman with hepatitis B can transmit this to her fetus. Some victims may not symptoms at all. Vaccine to prevent hep B is available. For those infected, antiviral medications are used; but when the damage to the liver has set in, liver transplant may be needed.

What is "the clap"?

This is the street name of gonorrhea, the bacterial infection that infects around 800,000 people in the USA annually. Infected men may have thick whitish pus discharge from the penis, and women may have yellowish or bloody discharge from the vagina, and both may have burning during urination. In women, this could cause PID and sterility. The infected pregnant mother can transmit the infection to her baby as it comes out of the birth canal, allowing the bacteria to target the baby's eyes, causing blindness.

Is genital herpes common?

About half a million cases of genital herpes in the United States alone are diagnosed each year. This viral infection comes from direct sexual contact with an open wound or even by skin or oral contact with the herpetic sore on the genitals. The initial sign might be itching, burning, tingling in the genital area, followed by painful blisters, lasting for 2 weeks to a month. When the sore heals from treatment, the virus hides in the nerve cells of the body, and the ailment recurs 1 to 6 time a year. Herpes is incurable and increases the patient's risk of HIV infection. As a joke goes, "unlike love, herpes is forever."

Is there a cure for HPV?

None. Human papillomavirus, which causes genital warts, is incurable and may recur even if the warts are removed. More than one million new cases are found each year in the US. The warts are white, pink, or gray cauliflower-like lesions in or around the vagina, on the cervix (mouth of the womb), on the penis, or around the anus. In some cases, this viral infection increases the risk for certain cancers.

How prevalent is HIV/AIDS?

Worldwide, about 1% (one out of a hundred) persons has human immunodeficiency virus (HIV) infection; and although asymptomatic (no symptoms) for years, the HIV-infected person is a prime candidate to develop AIDS (acquired immune deficiency disease). The virus targets and destroys the person's immune system; and when this happens, even relatively minor infections worsen rapidly, go out of control, and kill the patient. The months before death is a stage of severely miserable and agonizing existence for the victim. AIDS is the leading cause of demise among persons ages 24 to 44. In Africa, HIV/AIDS are rampant, sex partners infecting each other and mothers transmitting the HIV to fetus in the womb, in epidemic proportion. The virus is transmitted thru semen, breast milk, vaginal fluids, blood, and any body fluids that has blood. With this deadly infection around today, indiscretion and carelessness could translate a few moments of pleasure to a lifetime of "eternal" hell.

112,000 Bacteria on Our Skin

No, that is not a typo. Scientists in the new Human Microbiome Project at the National Institute of Health have sequenced genes from 20 skin sites of volunteers and "found that bacteria hailed from 10 different phyla, 205 genera, and 112,000 individual bacteria," using a sophisticated molecular technique of microbial DNA analysis. So you and I have this much germs crawling on our skin.

The variety discovered was much greater than previously known, with the forearm showing 44 species of bacteria on average, amazingly greater than those in the belly button and the armpits. The skin behind the ears had the least diverse, with 19 species on average.

Three areas of the skin were studied: dry, moist, and oily. The dry areas included the inside surface of the midforearm, the palm, and the buttock. The oily skin is between the eyebrows, beside the nose, inside the ear, the upper chest, and back. The moist sites were inside the nose, the armpit, the inner elbow, between the middle and ring fingers, the side of the groin, the top fold of the buttocks, behind the knee, the bottom of the foot, and the navel (belly button).

The study also revealed that "dry and moist skin had a broader range of microbes than did oily skin."

"Our work has laid an essential foundation for researchers aiming to treat or prevent skin diseases . . . We hope this will speed efforts to understand factors involved in eczema, psoriasis, acne, and other disorders affecting the skin," stated research leader Dr Julia Segre of the National Human Genome Research Institute in the US, as reported in the journal *Science*.

The four genera of bacteria that appear to be permanent resident of the skin are staphylococcus, streptococcus, propionibacteria, and sorynebacteria, accounting for more than 50% of the microbial population on our skin. The others appear to be more transient or vary from time to time.

Some scientists believe that these bacteria on our skin and those in our digestive tracts or elsewhere in our body, have evolved with us, and that "microbes are not accidental, but have been living in animals for a billion years." Some of these are good bacteria that help in our body physiology, providing protective layer on our skin or in our digestive function.

Unless indicated and prescribed by physicians, antibiotics (oral or topical) are harmful to the good bacteria in our body. This is why many patients on long-term antibiotic treatment for infections develop diarrhea, and abuse of antibiotics also leads to bacterial drug resistance to therapy.

The popularly used hand sanitizers and alcohol dry the hands and skin. Washing with plain water, or with soap and water (not strong detergents), are still safer and more economical. The use of skin moisturizing lotion after each cleansing is highly recommended to maintain the protective integrity of our skin.

While we do not want the bad bacteria on our skin or in our gut, "oversanitizing" our skin, our body, is more dangerous than the bugs themselves. Practicing good habits and discipline, like not touching our face because our fingers are loaded with germs and washing our hands before and after each meal, after holding public doorknobs, escalator banisters, etc., are prudent ways to cut down bacterial or viral skin, respiratory, and gastrointestinal infections.

The old-fashioned hand-washing (especially including our forearms), even up to 8 times a day following various activities, and showering daily are still healthy habits that simply maintain good hygiene and the proper balance of the bacterial flora on our skin and in our body.

Skin Care: A must for everyone

Wrinkles, also known as rhytides, are folds or creases in the skin, resulting from loss of elasticity and skin turgor associated with aging and with years of daily exposure to the ultraviolet rays of the sun. But a major factor is the lack of proper skin care, which should include the frequent use of skin moisturizers. This healthy daily practice should not be a monopoly of women. Men also have skin that needs good care every day, part of which is the use of moisturizers two to three times a day like women do. After a shower, a significant amount of the natural oil in the skin is washed away. This is where the use of facial and body moisturizers becomes most beneficial to the skin of the individual.

What is skin photodamage?

Skin photodamage is a spectrum of changes in the skin caused by chronic exposure to the ultraviolet rays of the sun. They include hyperpigmentation, telangiectasia, wrinkles, and tactile roughness. The prevalence of skin disorders that are linked to ultraviolet light exposure goes up with age, and the changes develop over several decades. Asian women, who prefer not to expose themselves to the sun, have younger-looking skin, compared to their American counterpart who sunbathe and "worship" the sun. Prolonged exposure to the sun and even the indirect sun reflection (from the sand, water, or from any surface) are harmful to the skin.

Does smoking cause wrinkles?

Yes, cigarette smoking is an important factor that contributes to the development of wrinkles, especially on the face. Smoking hastens facial wrinkle formation even among the young and also speeds up the aging process. The other extrinsic factor is exposure to ultraviolet rays of the sun. The intrinsic factors are hormonal status, aging, and intercurrent diseases.

What do these factors do?

The etiologic factors listed above contribute to the thinning of the epidermis (outer layer of the skin), fragility of the skin, loss of elasticity, and formation of creases and lines, wrinkles. Facial wrinkles in men and women are more common among smokers compared to nonsmokers. Among postmenopausal women, the fall in the estrogen level contributes to the development of, and increase in, wrinkles.

How about CO2 laser?

Carbon dioxide laser has been found to be of little benefit in removing or lessening facial wrinkles in 6 months compared to chemical peel, which is a bit superior, according to one small randomized clinical trial. Erythema (excessive redness) is noted to be equal in both regimen. It has also been found that there is no difference in perioral (around the mouth) wrinkles between CO2 laser treatment and dermabrasion. There was more erythema with CO2 laser.

Are cartilage preparations beneficial?

There is no convincing evidence that oral preparation of cartilage polysaccharide was truly effective in reducing wrinkles, although some manufacturers claim that their product is. One study shows the topical (cream) form was beneficial in reducing fine wrinkles at 120 days. The final word on the antiwrinkle properties of cartilage polysaccharide has not been said yet.

Is Tretinoin effective for wrinkles?

Under the supervision of a physician, the use of topical tretinoin for 6 months has been found to be efficacious in significantly reducing fine wrinkles, but not coarse wrinkles. Usual short-term complications include burning, itching, and erythema. Skin feeling occurs in all users, and this peaks at 12-16 weeks. The idea is to replace the old skin with the "new" skin. Isotretinoin, on the other hand, has been found in two randomized trials to be effective in improving both course and fine wrinkles in 36 weeks among those with mild to moderate photodamage. The downside is the severe facial irritation that happens as a complication in about 5-10% of individuals on isotretinoin.

How safe are these medications?

Tretinoin and isotretinoin and other drugs have been used by dermatologists and plastic surgeons extensively; and under their supervision these medications have apparently been safe. We strongly recommend that these and other "antiwrinkle" medications be used only under a physician's supervision.

Are facial moisturizers beneficial?

While facial moisturizers do not remove wrinkles, they can delay wrinkle formation by keeping our skin healthier and a bit more resistant to damages caused by dry and neglected skin. Even the skin turgor appears to be firmer among those who use facial moisturizers. A well-"hydrated" skin makes for a more youthful-looking face. Besides living a healthy lifestyle, which includes, among others, a low-fat, low-carbohydrate, high-fiber diet of fish, vegetables, nuts, and grains, and daily exercise, hygiene and skin care every day are a must for everyone. Medically speaking, the daily use of facial moisturizer and body lotion is not cosmetic vanity but a physiologic necessity.

Do We Need Sleep?

Is sleep important?

Yes, sleep is essential to health and survival. No animal can remain healthy and live without sleep. Sleep is also important in keeping ourselves looking good, hence the phrase "beauty sleep." The rest and benefit our body gets from sleep depends on many factors, including our emotional state. Sleep provides our body our much-needed physical and mental rest. This is the time when we revitalize our system, recharge, and reenergize our "power pack" in preparation for the following day's activities. Rest maximizes the regenerative and repair processes for our cells in the body. Adequate sleep keeps the wrinkles at bay. People who lack sleep grow older and look older prematurely. The value of sleep should never be ignored.

What are the kinds of sleep?

There are two types of sleep. One is nonrapid-eye movement (NREM, which is 75% to 80% of total sleep time) which normally initiates sleep and ranges in depth from 1 to 4 (4, being the deepest level) with commensurate difficulties in arousal. The other is the rapid-eye movement (REM, which makes up the 20% to 25%).

What is the difference between the two?

In NREM, the EEG (electroencephalogram: brain waves) are slow. The muscle tone, respiratory rate, heart rate, blood pressure are lowered. In REM, other the respiratory rate and depth are increased, but the muscle tone is even less than in NREM. The blood pressure varies and could be elevated, especially at dawn, near the waking stage. In normal sleep, the REM follow NREM in each of 5 to 6 cycles.

How much sleep does one need?

Infants need about 20 hours of sleep a day. They wake up only to feed every 3-4 hours and go right back to sleep, because their basal metabolism is faster. They churn energy at a higher speed for growth and development. As we grow older, the need for sleep becomes less. Somebody 60 years or older might wake up after 4 hours of sleep and level 4 sleep disappears. However, we recommend at least 8 hours of sleep for any adult. And if practical, a siesta or a catnap in the early afternoon is beneficial. One feels energized even after a very short nap.

Why do some people have insomnia?

Insomnia or difficulty in sleeping may be primary (long-standing with no obvious physical or emotional cause) or secondary (due to aches and pains from any source, depression, anxiety, withdrawal from cigarette, alcohol, or drug, etc.).

Should insomnia be treated?

Any condition that affects our health, sense of well-being, and comfort should be treated. There are now sleeping aids that are safe and can be taken regularly, provided it is done under medical supervision. And insomnia, after properly diagnosed and the etiology determined by the physician, could be a simple matter of sociopyschological adjustment or using hypnotics (sleeping pills) or mild tranquilizers that will spell the difference between feeling great or feeling tired and lousy every day. The key here is medical consultation and evaluation to rule out any hidden serious illness causing the insomnia.

What is sleepwalking?

Somnambolism, or sleepwalking or sitting, or other complex behavior during sleep, is most common among late childhood and adolescence. The eyes are open but without evidence of recognition. The person may mumble repeatedly and walk almost normally, except that they may hit chairs, tables, and other obstacles without realizing it. There is no accompanying dream, and their EEG (electroencephalogram) shows a state of wakefulness than sleep. When they wake up, they do not remember the episode.

What is hypersomnia?

This is a condition where a person regularly sleeps about 25% or more than usual, to the extent that it interferes with his/her socioeconomic functions. This could be caused by excessive use of sleeping pills or by a tumor in the brain affecting the hypothalamus or brain stem. When this abnormal increase in absolute sleep persists, it must be investigated.

How is this different from narcolepsy?

Narcolepsy is a rare syndrome of recurrent attacks of sleep, sudden loss of muscle tone, sleep paralysis, with initial REM sleep pattern, instead of the normal NREM. Sleeps occurs anytime, suddenly, uncontrollably, to a person, wherever he/she is, whether talking to another or attending a conference, etc. The attacks may happen from a few to many times a day, from a few minutes' to hours' duration.

What is sleep paralysis?

Sleep paralysis is an occasional occurrence (just when falling asleep or right after waking up), the person wants to move and for a moment could not move at all. This is temporary and can be due to a feeling of terror and happens in normal children and adults. No treatment is needed for these episodes, except eliminating the cause of the "terror" in the few cases where this is the cause.

Why do people snore?

Snoring is caused by the vibration of the uvula (small appendage that hangs down at the back end of the roof of the mouth, the upper palate), the softer part of the roof (soft palate), the back part (base) of the tongue, and the vocal cords. Snoring happens when the soft palate and the structures in the area adjacent to it (which normally are taut and firm) become limp and sagging, especially as we grow older. The structures could be so sagging as to block the upper airway, causing, not only snoring, but sleep apnea. Allergies, causing nasal congestion and leading to mouthing breathing, can also cause temporary snoring. Sleeping prone or on the side, with the head of the bed raised, could help reduce snoring. Taking sleep medications, tranquilizers, alcoholic beverages can also aggravate snoring (and apnea) among those who snore. We recommend snorers not take any of these.

Are all sedatives and hypnotics safe?

No, not all sedatives and sleeping pills are safe. Some are too potent, some are too crude and ill-refined, and some have worse side effects than others. If too strong for you, the sleeping pills can hurt you seriously. Many of them can cause addiction also. It is not safe to buy over-the-counter medications without physician advice and supervision. Your medical caretaker can recommend to you the sedative or hypnotic best suited for you and your condition.

Are We Getting Enough Sleep?

"Most American adults sleep poorly," according to a study of the National Sleep Foundation on 1,506 adults which was reported in Washington by the Associated Press. The findings are obviously applicable to most of us in general.

Lack of sleep translates to lesser mental acuity and concentration, poorer health, greater driving hazards, reduced productivity, and diminished sex drive.

Sleep experts recommend a minimum of 7 to 9 hours of sleep in 24 hours. The survey showed that adults sleep an average of 6.9 hours a night. The few minutes to 3 hours of sleep deprivation is enough to cause problems.

Seventy-five percent of adults reported they frequently have difficulty in sleeping, like problem in initiating sleep, waking up often during the night and/or snoring, waking up too early, and feeling unrefreshed and tired. Many also stated that they ignored the problem, and some do not even think they actually have any sleep deficit. Only about 50% of those surveyed stated they were able to sleep well most of the time. Twenty five percent thought their sleep problem had adverse effects on their daily routines.

Richard Gelula, the chief executive officer of the Sleep Foundation, said there's a link between sleep and quality of life. "People who sleep well, in general, are happier and healthier," said Gelula. "But when sleep is poor or inadequate, people feel tired or fatigued, their social and intimate relationship suffers, work productivity is negatively affected, and they make our roads more dangerous by driving while sleepy and not fully alert."

Obviously, the quality of sleep, besides the number of hours, is very important. Chris Drake, senior scientist at the Henry Ford Sleep Center in Detroit and cochair of the 2005 poll task force, stated that some of the nation's sleep habits can be attributed to an "always-on-the-go society."

The commercial world of today stretches business to 24 hours a day, with 24-hour pharmacy, restaurants, casinos, supermarkets, etc., so people tend to stay up late, watch late night shows on television, surfing the web on the Internet, etc. All these reduce people's time to sleep. And some people even need more than 9 hours of sleep to feel refreshed and rested.

This study also showed (1) sixty percent of adults stated they have driven a vehicle while drowsy from lack of sleep the past year, and 4 in 10 reported they have had an accident or near accident because of tiredness or falling asleep at the wheel. (2) Seventy five percent claims their partner has a sleep problem, snoring as the most common complaint. (3) Four out of ten of those surveyed reported lack of sleep adversely affected their sexual relationship, having lost interest in sex, having poorer performance, or having sex less often. (4) Seventy percent claimed that their physician never asked them about their sleep.

The recommendations of the National Sleep Foundation and experts in the field are abstinence from any stimulant, coffee, and alcohol before bedtime and to seek medical help if they think they are having sleep problems and/or snoring, or not getting enough rest at night.

Lack of sleep reduces the normal recharging time of our body battery, our energy source, causing a negative chain of reactions in our physiology and body chemistry. This leads to physical and mental stresses to our system. All these alter the normal homeostasis (internal balance) within us, weakening our immune system and increasing our risk of developing metabolic diseases, hypertension (high blood pressure), stroke and heart attack, among others, or aggravating existing illnesses.

Adequate sleep and rest are essential to health.

Snoring and Sleep Apnea

What is sleep apnea?

Usually associated with snoring, sleep apnea means the cessation of breathing during sleep. This breath-holding initially lasts for 10 seconds and progresses to 20 to 30 seconds, and each episode is immediately followed by gasping for air. This cycle could repeat itself several times (20 to 100 times per hour) the whole night long. The snorer is totally oblivious of all this, and only the roommate is aware of this bothersome snoring and scary sleep apnea.

How prevalent is sleep apnea?

The incidence is about 2% among middle-aged women and 4% among men of that age group, which is similar to the incidence of diabetes and asthma. Sleep apnea is a primary risk factor for hypertension (high blood pressure).

What are the types of sleep apnea?

There are two types: central sleep apnea (CSA) and obstructive sleep apnea (OSA). CSA is much less common, less than 10% of cases comprises this group, and is due to the brain's failure to send a signal for the person to breathe. This can happen among individuals with cardiac or neurological diseases. In OSA, part of the back of the throat collapses and blocks the airway during sleep, preventing airflow to the lungs. This causes decreased oxygenation and a low blood oxygen level, which alerts the brain to transmit a "wake up and breathe" message to the sleeping person.

What effects does sleep apnea have?

The person wakes up with a dry mouth and throat, perhaps with a headache, and a lousy feeling akin to a hungover. There may also be fatigue and sleepiness throughout the day, together with some memory deficiency, poor attention and concentration, and bad mood—all signs of lack of sleep, due to sleep apnea. The psychological stress of all this impacts negatively on the individual. The recurrent transient hypoxemia (low blood oxygen level) and daily impairment of sleep are added risk factors for the development of hypertension and coronary heart disease.

Does singing lessen snoring?

Singing helps tone the flabby muscles of our upper airways, the soft palate, in particular. Singing exercises for 20 minutes a day appear do the trick for some. Belting out a few songs, even off-key, every day in the family room or in the shower might annoy your housemate; but it will at least please her in bed every night when you snore less.

Are "snore stoppers" effective?

"Snore aids" advertised in the various media, such as nostril clips, nasal or throat sprays, magnetic wristbands, do not work to stop snoring, much less cure sleep disorders. Only those fraudulent vendors who make bundles of money by duping the ignorant public could sleep well, minus their conscience. One contraption, the jaw sling, which prevents the jaw from dropping while the person is asleep, shows promise for some snorers, but uncomfortable to wear.

What is the nonspecific therapy?

Weight loss for those who are overweight can minimize the episodes of sleep apnea. Avoidance of sleeping pills, sedatives, and alcohol, all of which increase the frequency and duration of sleep apnea, is most essential. Lying flat on the back induces sleep apnea for a lot of people. This could be avoided by placing a pillow at the back and lying on the side.

What are the various treatment regimens?

The three modalities are: (1) physical or mechanical, (2) surgery, and (3) non-specific therapy. The specific prescription depends on the medical examination and laboratory findings. The physical or mechanical treatment works only when used as the patient sleeps and apnea returns when the regimen is not utilized. There are two forms: continuous positive airway pressure (CPAP) and dental/oral appliances. CPAP, the most commonly prescribed, uses a snugly fitted face mask where continuous positive pressure air is blown into the nose, forcing the airway to stay open for proper breathing. Dental/oral appliance, which is fitted by an orthodontist, uses a device that moves the lower jaw forward to cause an under bite, which opens the airway.

What is the surgical treatment?

Surgery removes tissues, like nasal polyps, adenoids, tonsils, and any oropharyngeal deformities that causes obstruction to airflow. One of them is called uvulopalatopharyngoplasty, which excises tissues at the back of the throat. The success rate is low, between 30 and 60%; and it is hard to know which patients will benefit from it, side effects and eventual outcome. The others are tracheostomy (creating a hole in the windpipe for those with severe obstruction, which is not too common), surgical reconstruction for those with deformities, and surgery to treat obesity, which contributes to sleep apnea.

What medical conditions contribute to sleep disorders?

There are many impairment of sleep due to a variety of medical ailments, like emphysema, congestive obesity, heart failure, diabetes, stroke, and others conditions associated with pains like cancer, arthritis, acid reflux in the esophagus (food pipe). Anxiety disorders and depression are also associated with sleep disturbances. Consultation with a sleep specialist is critical for proper diagnosis and management of these disorders.

Sleep Less and Get Fat

A new study conducted at the Eastern Virginia Medical School in Norfolk showed that people who sleep less tend to weigh heavier than those who sleep more.

The clinical investigation, which included 1000 subjects, reported that "total sleep time decreased as the body mass index (a measure of weight based on height) increased." Whether this means heavier individuals tend to sleep less, and vice versa or having enough sleep makes it easier for people to control and maintain their normal weight was not clear.

The authors of this study warn that "this does not establish a cause-and-effect relationship between restricted sleep and obesity (but) future investigations demonstrating success in weight loss via extensions of sleep would help greatly to establish such a relationship."

"We've put so much emphasis on diet and exercise that we've failed to recognize the value of good sleep," said Fred Turek, a physician at Northwestern University in Chicago, who wrote a related editorial in a recent issue of the *Archives of Internal Medicine*, where the study was published.

Some earlier researches have shown sleep deprivation to cause a decline in an appetite-suppressing protein hormone called leptin and increase in another hormone (ghrelin) that causes a craving for food . . . in addition, neuropeptides in the brain governing sleep and obesity appear to overlap.

In another study involving more than 8,000 adults, researchers found that those who sleep only six hours a day had 23 % risk of getting obese; five hours, 50%; and for those who sleep less than 4 hours a day, 73%, compared to those who sleep 8-9 hours a day.

"It is now critical to determine the importance of lack of sufficient sleep during the early formative years in putting our youth on a trajectory toward obesity . . . a trajectory that could be altered if sleep loss is indeed playing a role in this epidemic," Turek's editorial said.

The alarming rise in obesity, especially among children, a subject we have written about in this column the past several years, is now an epidemic in many developed countries, especially in the United States, where "supersizing" of hamburgers, French fries, high-calorie, high-sugar beverages, and other high-carbo food items have dominated the fast-food chains. As "admirers and followers" of trends in food and fashion, etc., in the United States, Asians are now facing the same overweight and obesity dilemma.

What is alarming is not the negative aesthetic effect of obesity or of being overweight, but their multitude of dangerous implications on the health and longevity on the victims. Insufficient sleep has been shown in other previous studies to lead to a "cascade of metabolic, cardiovascular, and general medical disorders"; but the lay public has somehow not made the connection yet. Hopefully, this recent study will help convince people that enough sleep (minimum of 8 hours a day, which does not have adverse effects or possible complications anyway) is essential, not only in weight control but in maintaining our health and well-being and in warding off illnesses in general.

However, I would like to remind ourselves that adequate sleep is only one-fifth of the total equation for a healthier, happier, more productive, and longer life. The other four are (1) a healthy diet: high-fiber, high-grain, low-fat, low-cholesterol, low-carbohydrate, low-salt; (2) daily exercises; (3) stress management and relaxation; and (4) abstinence from tobacco and strict moderation in alcohol intake.

Slimming Tea: A Hoax

What are slimming teas?

Slimming teas was a term designed by unscrupulous manufacturers who claim that drinking them would lead to loss of weight. These teas are marketed as a diet aid for weight control, and some even vendors even say they are good for the skin.

How did this all start?

This same unsupported claims have been around for centuries, where herbal teas were described to have properties that cause loss of weight thru their effect on the metabolism, appetite, and by directly dissolving fats. Chinese, Mongolian, and Italians have long believed herbal teas were effective for weight control. African herbal teas are advertised similarly, with the added claim that they reduce water retention and "cleanse the system of toxins." Like some Chinese teas, these African teas have senna leaves in them, which have some purging effects.

Are these teas effective as a diet aid?

The claims that herbal teas or teas in general cause loss of weight and therefore effective as diet aids are false. There are no scientific basis to show that these teas contain any ingredient that would curve or suppress the appetite or cause so much increase in metabolism to lead to weight loss. If one drinks teas only as a way to lose weight, the only thing the person will lose is money, not weight.

However, if one drinks tea often daily, without sugar or cream in it, and drinks it as an alternative (as a substitute, *not* in addition) to high-calorie snack, or if one drinks tea for breakfast and lunch instead of eating those meals (which some people do to control weight), obviously this will lead to less calorie intake and therefore cause weight loss. This same good effect could also be achieved by eating apples or other fruits for breakfast and raw vegetables for lunch and have a moderate dinner. This is the healthier way to diet. To this, of course, one has to do daily regimented exercise routine.

Does drinking tea alone control weight?

Most definitely not. If you are overweight and continue to eat the same amount of calories, drinking teas, herbal or not, even a gallon a day, will not lead to weight loss. In order to control weight properly and safely, the calories must be reduced and physical exercise increased.

Does cutting down on carbs lead to weight loss?

Yes, cutting down on carbohydrates, like soft drinks, rice, bread, cakes, ice cream, can lead to weight loss, because these are sugars that have high glycemic index and easily add pounds to the body. Totally eliminating rice 3 meals a day, for instance, will dramatically cause weight reduction, provided the rest of the (total) foods ingested daily do not exceed 1,000 calories. Tough? Yes, but this is the safer and lesser expensive way to control weight compared to spending your hard-earned money for appetite suppressant drugs or the so-called miracle diet pills or potions that are actually very dangerous.

Is purging a good way to lose weight?

No, this is a dangerous way to lose weight. When one takes a laxative or any substance that has a purging effect, excessive water and electrolytes are lost through diarrhea, which is harmful to the kidneys and other vital organs. Kidney and liver failure and heart rhythm disturbances could ensue. Deaths have been reported in this type of abuse.

Why does a person gain weight to begin with?

This basic understanding is important, if one is to be able to control or maintain body weight safely. It is a matter of calorie intake and output. If one eats more calories than he/she expends with physical activities each day, the excess calories will add pounds to the body mass. If we fill up a balloon with sugar and keep adding to it, the balloon will keep on swelling and become heavier and heavier. But if we create a hole in the balloon that will allow sugar to leak out as fast as we pour more sugar into it, the balance in the "input and output" will keep the balloon from becoming larger or heavier. In essence, if we exercise off the calories we take in, we can maintain our desired weight. If we are too heavy, then we must exercise more and eat less until we find that ideal balance of intake and output of energy.

So, are teas bad for us?

No, not at all. As a matter of fact, teas, especially green teas, are good antioxidant for our body. As we have reported in this column before, teas contain a lot of flavanoids, like garcetin, kaemptenol, myricetin. Studies have shown that regular intake of these compounds by drinking tea (especially the green variety) reduces the rate of acute heart attack by 40% and also significantly lowers risk of a fatal heart attack. Unlike teas, coffee, cola drinks, and other caffeine-rich beverages have adverse, albeit subtle, effects on health. But for weight control, teas are not miracle drugs and will be effective only (as we stated above) if taken in lieu of food.

Smoking and Cancer

Smoking causes lung cancer besides other malignancies and cardiovascular diseases that maim, kill, and hurt our society. In the United States alone, more than 500,000 people die each year from smoking related illnesses. These are preventable deaths! Smokers are about 10 times more prone to die premature deaths than non-smokers. This unnecessary loss of lives is at an immense direct cost for non-smokers as well in terms of increased in health insurance premiums and taxes, not to mention personal and family tragedies in all shapes and forms.

As we have alluded to in a previous column, secondhand smoke is even more dangerous. Innocent bystanders are forced to inhale cigarette smoke at their workplaces or in public places, thus increasing their health risk. The Environmental Protection Agency engineers have shown that even the best available ventilation and air-moving equipment were unable to reduce carcinogenic (cancer-causing) air contamination to a safe level for a non-smoker sharing work space with a habitual smoker. Physical isolation of the tobacco addict is most essential as shown by these scientific studies.

Tobacco use leads to four times as many excess deaths annually compared to all other drugs and alcohol abuse combined, ten times more than all automobile fatalities per year, twelve times more than deaths from AIDS, and much more than all the American military casualties (in all wars) in this century put together. That's how dangerous and damaging tobacco is to the human body and to society as a whole.

At the beginning of the past century, lung cancer was almost an insignificant health problem for the world. It became a minor problem in the 1930s (death rate of 5 per 10,000). Today, it has become the main killer among men and women. Since women started "really" smoking in the 1950s, "because it was glamorized in ads by actresses and models as a sophisticated and fashionable habit," lung cancer in females has increased at least sixfold, an alarming rate, with death rate comparable to that in males. Women also have added risks: osteoporosis, thrombophlebitis (vein inflammation and blood clot formation), arthritis, infertility, cervical cancer, and menstrual irregularities. Pregnant smokers face miscarriages, stillbirths, low-birth weight, and SIDS (sudden infant death syndrome) babies. Almost 30,000 female lives are snuffed out every year as a result of smoking. Of the 4 billion cigarette-related deaths in the world each year, about half a billion are women. It is now the top killer among women. Today, one woman dies from cigarette-related illness every three minutes! Indeed, "you've come a long way Baby!" (as a cigarette ad once proudly proclaimed).

But what is puzzling and bothersome to me is the great dichotomy with which our society (and most especially the government!) deals with the cigarette-health risk issue. On one hand, they are most vocal and vigilant against the so called illegal drugs and other substances that pose a moderate public health dilemma, promulgating most aggressive laws and heavy criminal sanctions against their production, distribution, or use. On the other hand, society and the government have long subsidized with tax monies the production and distribution of tobacco, which is by far the country's most serious and deadly substance. Yes, our government and society are peddling drugs, not the moderately dangerous ones but the most deadly one. The one that makes lives miserable. The one that kills the bread winner or the mother in the family, victimizing the children and their future. The one that separates loved ones. The one that destroys hopes and dreams.

But the tide appears to be changing, at least in the United States. The courts in Northern America have eventually scratched the surface in bringing about some justice, albeit delayed, in the tobacco death arena. Dying or dead smokers have successfully won handsome awards from some giant tobacco companies, who, finally, after more than seven decades, have officially admitted that tobacco is an addictive drug, carcinogenic, and can kill in more ways than one and that they had known this fact for decades but had lied about it. The color of money obviously lures even the color blind among our unscrupulous politicians.

Having said that, I strongly feel that people who wish to smoke (or to jump off a cliff or off a tall building to hurt or kill themselves) have the right to do it. That is their constitutional right, and while I am against tobacco as an individual and as a physician, I shall defend the right of the cigarette afficionados to smoke where it is allowed, since there is no law against smoking per se. The only exception to that right, or any other right under our constitution, is when its exercise adversely affects or conflicts with, or curtails, the rights of others. The smoker has the right to smoke and enjoy it, but he does not have the right to force or expose his loved ones, his friends, or strangers, to the more dangerous and more carcinogenic fumes coming from his cigarettes. This is where the lines have to be drawn, morally, socially and legally.

It is beyond my comprehension why we, the people, tolerate our government supporting these merchants of a deadly poison called tobacco, one substance that continues to maim and kill our family and fellowmen in epidemic proportion. Could the overriding reason be the millions and millions of dollars the tobacco lobbyists are pouring into the campaign chests of compromising politicians, making the latter afraid to snuff out the tobacco industry, and we, the people, on the other hand, simply don't care?

The situation is terrible and frustrating, and we must be fuming mad!

Smoking Damages
DNA Instantly

For cigarette smokers and those who may be tempted to start, here's a bit of truly disturbing new information from the American Chemical Society.

New research revealed that tobacco smoke causes genetic damage within minutes of inhalation of cigarette smoke, not years. The adverse effects are almost instantaneous as the smoke gets into the lungs. This new finding corrects the old notion that smoking took years to initiate damages to the body.

According to the study in *Chemical Research in Toxicology,* there are toxic chemicals in tobacco that cause damage in DNA linked to cancer development among smokers. Lung cancer due to smoking kills more than 3,000 lives every single day around the world. There are almost 20 other cancers caused by tobacco use.

Mental Effects on Children

Secondhand smoke (involuntary or passive smoking) has been found to cause physical and mental aberrations among children. These helpless victims of parents or family members who smoke can suffer recurrent respiratory tract infections and psychological disturbances as they regularly inhale secondhand smoke in their environment.

Children exposed to the toxic substances from secondhand smoke are more prone to develop hyperactivity, bad behavior (conduct disorder), and other mental health disorders, as reported by Mark Hamer, PhD, from the University College of London, published December 6, 2010, in the *Archive of Pediatric Adolescent Medicine.*

Scary Data on Smoking Risks

Here are some chilling data on the devastating and deadly effects of smoking:

- There are 4,000 chemicals (600 of them poisons, 69 cancer-causing) in every stick of cigarette, toxic chemicals like those found in paint stripper, toilet cleaner, rocket fuel, lighter fuel, chemicals in moth balls, the poison used in the gas chamber, and other toxins.
- Smoking causes almost 1/3 of all cancer deaths in the world.
- Smokeless tobacco-50 times worse than regular cigarettes.
- Passive smoking—responsible for about 6,000 lung cancers among nonsmokers and 35,000 deaths from secondhand smoke-related diseases per year.
- More than half a million are killed each year in the USA alone by smoking-related illnesses,10 times more than car accidents, 12 times more than AIDS.
- And a lot more than all the military casualties in all wars in this century put together
- One person in the USA dies of a heart attack every minute (mostly smokers).
- One dies of other smoking-related illness every 3 minutes!
- Smoking has orphaned billions of children around the globe, greater than all the wars combined has caused.
- Smokers die 13-14 years earlier than nonsmokers.
- Risk of dying from lung cancer among smokers compared to nonsmokers: 22 times greater in men and 12 times greater among women.
- Since 1950, lung cancer deaths among women have increased 600%.
- Smokers have three times risk of dying from heart attack.

- Tobacco use is the leading cause of preventable deaths.

California study (1988-1998): A light, a ray of hope, *if* we follow this example.

- Death rates dropped by 12% for cancers of the lung, pancreas, bladder, and oropharynx, when smoking dropped from 22.8% to 18.4%. (In 2000, it was down to 17.1%.)
- Consumption dropped from 127 packs per day to 69 packs, a 45% decline. National average dropped by 25%.

The wonders of quitting are truly remarkable, and they provide smokers who want to kick the habit great hopes for their future, as illustrated hereunder:

Twenty minutes after quitting:

- Blood pressure drops to normal.
- Pulse rate drops to normal.
- Heart rate drops to normal.
- Circulation has already improved.
- Body temperature of hands and feet increase to normal.

In 24 to 48 hours:

- Chances of heart attack begin to decrease.
- Nerve endings in nose and mouth begin to regrow.
- Ability to smell and taste are enhanced.
- Mucus begins to clear from the lungs.

One year after quitting:

- Excess risk of coronary heart disease is half that of a smoker's.

Five years after:

- Lung cancer death rate decreases by half.

After ten years:

- Lung cancer death rate is now equivalent to that of a nonsmoker.
- Precancerous cells are replaced by healthy cells.
- Risk of other cancers (mouth, throat, bladder, etc.) decreases.

At fifteen years:

- Those who kicked the habit are now at *no* more at risk of heart disease than if you had never smoked!

All medical evidences available today make one thing absolutely clear: Tobacco is a poison. It maims and kills. Smoking is slow suicide that could end in a miserable death for the smoker and devastation for his/her family. Isn't it time to quit taking this poison?

Statin plus Fish Oil

Cardiovascular diseases are the number one killer in most developed countries in the world today. In the United States, one person dies of heart disease every 34 seconds; in the Philippines, one every 9 minutes. Each 24 hours, more than 2,500 Americans die from heart disease, and every 20 seconds one person in the United States suffers a heart attack. The nations with the highest deaths from heart disease are Bulgaria, Czechoslovakia, Hungary, Poland, Romania, and the former Soviet Union. The ones with the lowest are Canada, Japan, France, Spain, Switzerland. And these statistics do not even include stroke and those who succumbed to the complications of these illnesses.

The main culprit pathology is none other than fatty accumulation on the inside walls of the arteries to the heart, brain, kidneys, aorta, and legs. Except the aorta, which is connected to the heart as an outflow pipe whose diameter is about an inch, and the leg arteries which are about 1/3 to 1/4 the size of the aorta, the diameter of the arteries that supply the heart and the brain is only about 2 to 3 millimeters, like spaghetti.

Whenever we eat animal fats (from red meats, eggs, dairy foods), our blood thickens; and as the thick blood runs through the arteries, its coats the inner walls of these arteries, much like "brushing thick paint" on the walls of these arteries 24/7, all the year round, for decades, all the years of our life. The coats of blood on the wall gets thicker and thicker and harden like cement, reducing the caliber of these tiny noodle-size arteries or even blocking them completely, cutting the blood oxygen and nutrition supply to the heart muscles. This eventually leads to a heart attack.

A study, called JELIS, was done on 12,000 subjects, 6,000 of them on cholesterol-lowering drug called statin alone and the other 6,000 taking statin plus omega-3 in the form of EPA (eicosapentanoic acid) fish oil (1,000 mg capsule twice a day containing 1,800 mg of EPA). While those on statin only showed significant lowering in stroke and heart attack events, those on the combination therapy fared even better, with an additional 16% reduction, a statistically significant added benefit. Reducing the LDL with statin and increasing the HDL with omega-3 is indeed an excellent strategy. (JELIS stands for Japan EPA Lipid Intervention Study at Kobe University, published in the *American Heart Journal* in 2003 and revisited in 2006.)

As far as cholesterol level is concerned, clinical research has found that for every 1 mg decrease in LDL (low-density lipoprotein, the bad cholesterol), there is a corresponding 0.7% lowering in cardiovascular risk; and for every 1 mg increase in HDL (high-density lipoprotein, the good cholesterol), there is resultant reduction in CV risk by 2%. There is no question that cholesterol plays a major role in the development of arteriosclerosis (hardening of the arteries) and consequent cardiovascular diseases, like hypertension (high blood pressure), stroke, and heart attack.

In today's clinical setting, the combination of statin and omega-3 is a very popular option taken by physicians, not only for their patients but for themselves and their family. Many cardiologists prescribe vitamin D3, and a mild blood thinner, like aspirin, on top of statins and omega-3, as an overall preventive measure against cardiovascular diseases. Of course, this regimen, in order to be effective, must include low-fat, low-cholesterol diet (of fish, vegetables, soya, grains, nuts, fruits), daily exercise, abstinence from tobacco, and disciplined moderation in alcohol intake. Any single item in this treatment "recipe," if used alone, disregarding all of the other essential "ingredients" enumerated above, is doomed to fail. While our knowledge and abilities as physicians are not perfect and still limited, the advances in medical science and technology over the past half a century have confirmed the benefit from this multifaceted prophylactic approach in dealing with the multifactorial malady, called cardiovascular diseases, the treacherous killer of the modern man.

The Stem Cell Controversy

What is the controversy about?

Scientists, working on mouse models have discovered that stem cell therapy could possibly help cure many common diseases that afflict man today. Some of these include stroke, spinal cord injury, heart diseases, Parkinson's, Alzheimer's, osteoarthritis, retinal degeneration and blindness, rheumatoid arthritis, liver and kidney diseases, burns, type 1 diabetes, and muscular dystrophies. While the goal of the stem cell research is unquestionably laudable and its potential benefit to mankind tremendous, the controversy centers on its ethical, moral, religious, legal, and social ramifications. Basically, the grave concerns are where the stems cells will be harvested from (adult, fetus, or embryo) and the possible misuse and abuse of this new technology. And I could not agree more. This evolving science merits a deep soul-searching introspection and a serious, intense, and thoughtful deliberation to arrive at a morally, ethically, and medically sound stem cell treatment protocol that will also ensure the protection of the unborn, besides healing the sick, and at the same time preserve the dignity of humankind it seeks to serve.

What are stem cells?

The building block, the foundation cell, for every cell, tissue, and organ in the body is the stem cell. Stem cells are undifferentiated, with no "specific assigned task as yet." This has been likened to a blank computer microchip that could be "programmed to perform any number of special tasks." Subjected to proper conditions, stem cells will develop into specialized tissues and organs (heart, liver, kidneys, etc.). Also, stem cells are "self-sustaining and can replicate themselves for long periods of time."

What is its practical benefit to man?

With its unique characteristics, stem cells can provide the cells to replace damaged or diseased tissues with new living cells that will regenerate into healthy, young, normally functioning tissues, in the treatment of condition like Alzheimer's, Parkinson's, etc., as listed above, where specific parts of the organs have been damaged and rendered "nonfunctioning" leading to the development of the disease.

Organ donation is available today, but the organ supply is very limited; and the procedure is expensive, arduous, and usually complicated by rejections of the transplanted organ(s). This is where stem cell therapy has a great advantage in, according to researchers.

Where are stem cells harvested from?

We all came from a single cell, medically termed zygote, which is the product of fertilization. The zygote divides into two cells, and each of those two divides into another two cells, and so on. After about five days of conception, about 150 of those cells form a hollow ball called blastocyst, which measures smaller than a grain of sand and contains two types of cells: trophoblast and inner cell mass. The inner cell mass is made up of embryonic stem cells, which can form all cell types, differentiating into specific tissues and organs later in the development of the fetus. Stem cells could also be found in adult body, like bone marrow stem cells from the bone marrow. Identification of adult stem cell in all vital organs has not been completed as yet. Researchers are now finding ways to induce stem cells already present in the body to grow and produce the right cell types to replace damaged ones. Some specific sources also found to have stem cells are the umbilical cord, amniotic fluid, and baby teeth.

Is adult stem cells therapy now in use?

Yes, adult stem cell replacement (like bone marrow transplantation with a matched donor), has been a well-proven effective treatment and cure for some blood cancers (leukemia, lymphoma) and other blood disorders. It has also been shown that cells from the bone marrow can give rise to similar specialized cells found in many other tissues like blood, kidney, pancreas, liver, muscles, and brain. Someday, we will be able to isolate our own bone marrow cells, pretreat them, and reintroduce them back into our system to renew or repair cells in various diseased organs in our body. More amazing than that is the prospect for stem cells to "grow" new organs, like heart, liver, kidney, etc., and solve the current problem of shortfall of organ donors and save millions and millions of lives around the world today.

But society as a whole, as early as this stage of this scientific evolution, has the moral responsibility and obligation to safeguard this new technology and protect itself and the helpless, from potential criminal exploitation of stem cell therapy for financial gains or other heinous or depraved motives.

Stomach Cancer

What is the usual type of stomach cancer?

The most common variety is adenocarcinoma, usually found in the body of the stomach and in the area between the esophagus (food pipe) and the stomach. The word *adeno* stands for "glandular" cell type as seen by the pathologist on microscopic examination.

How prevalent is stomach cancer?

This varies among countries and by sex. Per 100,000 Japanese population, for example, it is about 80 men and 30 women, white American men, 11, white American women, 7, British men, 18 and British women, 10. There has been an impressive decline in incidence in North America, New Zealand and Australia since 1930 but the reduction has been slower in Europe. The incidence also seems higher among those with Type A blood. In the USA, cancer of the stomach is relatively more common among Japanese American and Hispanic groups. The death rate in the USA for gastric cancer is between 14,000 and 15,000 a year. Sixty to 70 cases of these are men.

Is this cancer related to stomach ulcers?

Lifelong stomach ulcer caused by infection with *Helicobacter pylori* appears to be strongly associated with cancer of the stomach and so with poor intake of antioxidant vitamins A, C, and E (and folic acid and calcium also) and vegetables and fruits. The chronic inflammation in *H. pylori* infection may also be a contributing factor in the formation of gastric cancer among these patients.

What are the other etiologic factors?

Smoking is strongly related to cancer of the proximal portion of the stomach. This is one unhealthy habit people should stay away from because cigarettes are deadly, killing hundreds of thousands slowly and "softly." This type of gastric malignancy is also associated with obesity, gastroesophageal reflux, high-fat intake, and seen more among the more affluent people. Those in the lower socioeconomic bracket has been seen to be more prone to distal stomach cancer.

How about eating smoked or salted fish?

Eating dried salted fish and smoked foods (or the nitrates in them) have been suspected to increase the risk of stomach cancer. There seems to be a higher incidence in Asia, particularly in Japan. Currently, however, we find no absolute proof in the medical literature that confirms this; but I would still advise caution here. As far as a good daily dietary regimen is concerned, there is nothing better and safer than fresh fish, vegetables, fruits, high-fiber foods, and abstaining from red meat and eggs, which are high in cholesterol and fats and low in fiber. Red meat has been implicated as a causative factor in colon cancer and other cancers.

What are the symptoms to watch for?

They vary from person to person. Most do not even have obvious symptoms before they are discovered. The symptoms could be a sense of indigestion, upper stomach discomfort, gassy bloating feeling, loss of appetite or pain on eating, loss of weight, tarry (blood in) stools, anemia, weakness and fatigue, depending on the stage of the cancer. But any of these symptoms may also be caused by other illnesses, which may not be as serious and are curable. This is the reason why a regular medical checkup and seeing the doctor early are important practices to prevent serious illnesses. If in doubt, consult your physician.

How serious is gastric cancer?

Without surgery, invasive cancer of the stomach is fatal. From the day it is diagnosed, the mean survival rate is less than 6 months. That's how fast this type of malignancy kills.

How early could this cancer be detected?

Because many do not have obvious symptoms, gastric cancer may have spread before it is diagnosed. In the USA, greater than 50% of patients recently diagnosed already have metastasis (spread) to regional lymph glands or to other vital organs.

What is the survival rate?

In the United States, the 5-year survival rate (the number of patients alive after 5 years) is 90% (nine out of ten) among those where the tumor is confined to the mucosa (stomach lining only) and 20% (one in five) among those with large tumor and lymph node spread.

Is it true the survival rate is higher in Japan?

The 5-year survival rate in Japan for gastric cancer is about 50% for those with advanced stage of the disease, compared to 20% in the USA as stated above. The reason is unclear. It is postulated that the stomach cancer of those who were born and lived in Japan might be a "different" kind of pathology and that there are other unexplained factors as well. But what is interesting is that the type of stomach cancer among Japanese who were born and have been in the United States for a while behaves like the gastric cancer among white Americans. Obviously environmental factors do play a role.

What is upper GI endoscopy?

This is an examination of the food pipe and stomach, using a flexible fiber-optic lighted and magnified scope (about the caliber of the little finger), that is passed through the mouth, down the throat, the esophagus, and to the stomach, to view any pathology and do a biopsy, if needed. Endoscopic ultrasound is another recent diagnostic tool and is very helpful in assessing the condition of the esophagus and stomach, and also for any lymph node or regional spread of the cancer.

What is the treatment?

When stomach cancer is diagnosed, complete surgical excision is the best option, if maximal survival rate is to be achieved. But this is not always feasible, depending on the stage and anatomy of the disease. Subtotal gastrectomy (removing part of the stomach involved in the cancer) has been found to have the same survival rate benefit compared to removing the entire stomach. No difference in the 5-year survival rate or postoperative mortality.

How about chemotherapy?

Current clinical evidence has shown that adjuvant chemotherapy (surgery plus chemotherapy) versus surgery alone significantly increase survival rate. In other words, it is not any better than surgery alone. It also found that those who had adjuvant chemotherapy had much more postoperative complications. There are various current chemotherapeutic agents that have not been fully evaluated thus far. But ongoing researches continue. Hopefully, someday soon, the "perfect" regimen will come along. Better yet, a vaccine to prevent gastric cancer. In the meantime, let us stay away from unhealthy habits and prevent diseases from coming our way, especially deadly cancers.

New Stool Blood Test for Cancer

Is it normal to have blood in your stools?

Blood in the stools is never normal. If the stool has blood in it, it is either from a bleeding from a ripped mucosa (lining) of the rectum (from passing very hard stools when constipated), or from a bleeding polyp, a more serious condition, or even cancer. Traces of occult blood (not obvious to the naked eye) may be from taking iron pills or red meat or raw fruits and vegetables, vitamin C, or aspirin (which causes blood thinning and some microbleeding in the guts in some people). Women who are menstruating when the stool sample is taken may have either frank red blood or traces of blood in the stools.

Why be concerned about it?

As we have alluded to above, blood in the stools could be a sign of a serious illness in the gut. Bright red blood (and/or occult blood) could be from constipation as mentioned, from hemorrhoids, anal fissures, or from a colon condition (from chronic inflammatory disease to colorectal cancer). Black tarry stools (blood undergoing digestion and transit from higher gut down to the rectum) could mean bleeding in the stomach (like from inflammation, ulcer, or cancer). There are other possible causes of blood in the stools. Since cancer is a serious illness, and since this is common, it is important to make sure it is not present.

What test could be done to find out?

The diagnostic procedure is called fecal occult blood test (FOBT), a noninvasive way of detecting the presence of occult (hidden or not obvious to the naked eye) blood in the feces. There are two popular tests: Guaiac smear test, available from hospital outpatient laboratory or the doctor's office and interpreted by a medical practitioner; and the InSure test. This is done as a screening test and should be done even if there are no symptoms as a prophylaxis measure.

Who should be tested?

For people age 50 and older, the American Cancer Society recommends the FOBT be performed every year. The test is done earlier than 50 (also once a year) if the person has any symptoms or any of the following: a family history of colorectal cancer or polyps or hereditary colorectal cancer syndrome, or a personal history of colorectal or adenomatous polyps or chronic inflammatory bowel disease. The test does not carry any risk.

How accurate is the FOBT?

Fecal occult blood test is very accurate when it comes to detecting occult blood in the stools, although there could be false positive results (where the test shows positive result but there is no active bleeding present). According to an Australian study, the relative sensitivity for detecting cancer was 39% for the Hemoccult test and 85% for the InSure test. For cancers and advanced adenomas combined, the sensitivity was 50% for the Hemoccult test and 77% for InSure. Both tests had a false-positive rate of about 4%.

What's this newest test for occult blood?

The "new" fecal test for occult blood is called InSure (manufactured by Enterix), an immunochemical technology that is superior to the standard guaiac (Hemoccult) test for screening tool for colorectal cancer, according to Sheillah C. Gentile, MD, Diplomate of the American Board of Family Medicine, of Munster, Indiana. InSure was released in 2003 and wildly used today. It is much more sensitive and more specific in diagnosing colorectal malignancy. Also, with InSure, the stool sample is taken by swirling a brush (that comes with the kit) around water in the toilet bowl after defecation, unlike Hemoccult which requires collection of stools on a sheet of tissue provided, from which the specimen is taken, which people consider "gross" and messier. With InSure, only 2 stool samples are needed, versus the Hemoccult, which requires

3 samples. But more importantly, with InSure, one does not need dietary and medication restrictions as with the guaiac Hemmoccult. It is certainly the new preferred and more convenient and more specific test for occult blood.

Why is colorectal cancer a silent killer?

Cancer of the colon and rectum is the second leading cause of death in the United States, many times undiscovered till too late. It kills more every year than prostate cancer and breast cancer combined. People's neglect in monitoring their own health accounts for this unfortunate statistics. Actually, early detection could make this deadly disease preventable in many instances. In 90% it is actually preventable and curable after its early diagnosis. Statistics show that only about 40% of those who need to be screened for colorectal cancer actually see their physician for such screening.

How much role does prevention play?

In colorectal cancer, just like in many forms of cancers, prevention plays a vital role. A healthy lifestyle, including daily exercises, abstinence from cigarettes, moderation in alcohol intake, eating a high-fiber (a lot of vegetables, fruits and nuts and grains, and minimal red meat) diet, helps greatly to minimize the occurrence of colorectal cancer. Fecal occult blood test annually and colonoscopy every five years for screening for those 50 and over are highly recommended to assure early detection and higher cure rate of this malignancy, if found. A simple and inexpensive test for occult blood in the stools could make the difference between life and death. In majority of cases, colorectal cancer and death from this malignancy are preventable.

Stroke or CVA

What is stroke?

Stroke, medically termed cerebrovascular accident (CVA), is a medical condition where a portion of the brain is deprived of oxygen and the patient develops partial or full paralysis of one side of the body and/or blindness in one eye and/or slurred speech or even becomes confused, comatose, or even dies, depending on the severity of the stroke.

What causes oxygen deprivation to the brain?

The brain could be deprived of oxygen when the artery supplying blood to a particular area of the brain is blocked by a clot (embolus) that has traveled from the heart or from the neck (carotid) artery or blocked by hardening of the artery in the neck or in the brain, or when an artery in the brain ruptures and causes bleeding in the brain. Any condition that cuts the blood (oxygen) supply to the brain would cause a stroke.

What is temporary stroke?

Temporary stroke, medically called transient ischemic attacks (TIA), is a situation where a small clot travels to the brain and blocks the blood supply to a portion of the brain; and somehow the small clot dissolves, allowing the circulation to the brain to resume. Spasm of an artery supplying the brain, that later relaxes, could also cause this temporary TIA.

Could blindness result from a stroke?

Yes, blindness could be a part of a stroke, or it could also be a part of TIA. This type of blindness is what is medically termed "amaurosis fugax." The blindness happens to the same side where the blood clot is. If the blockage is in the right side of the neck (carotid) artery, the blindness occurs in the right eye.

How about the muscle paralysis?

The paralysis, or muscle weakness, happens to the opposite of the blocked (carotid) artery. If the right carotid artery is the one blocked, the paralysis affects the opposite side (the left) of the face, arm, body, and leg.

What happens after a stroke?

Depending on the severity and extent of arterial blockage, the patient could have symptoms ranging from mild slurring of speech to total inability to talk (aphasia), with or without paralysis, which could also range from mild (paresis) to severe paralysis (absence of muscle strength). The more severe case could lead to coma or even death. Those who survive are candidates for various levels of physical therapy, speech therapy, or rehabilitation or even vocational therapy, depending on the degree and nature of the stroke.

Does high blood pressure lead to a stroke?

Not all people with high blood pressure develop a stroke. Those with uncontrolled or untreated high blood pressure have a high probability of developing a stroke. They are more prone to have a stroke, especially from a ruptured artery because of the tremendous high pressure inside the artery.

How does one prevent a stroke?

Anybody older than 30 years old must have a complete medical checkup by his/her physician. Patients with stroke or heart attack are getting younger and younger. The physician can analyze the risk factors affecting his patient and prescribe a good preventive regimen or start managing whatever illness is found. The earlier the diagnosis of a condition is made, the better the chances of treating it successfully and avoiding a more complicated course.

What are the other preventive measures?

Living a good and healthy lifestyle is the key. This includes a healthy diet of fish, vegetables, fruits, fiber cereals, multivitamins; staying away from eggs and red meats, like pork and beef; regular physical exercises, even simple brisk walking 4 times a week or more; no smoking; knowing how to relax and enjoy life; having a regular medical checkup about once a year.

Is ballroom dancing a good form of exercise?

For cardiovascular fitness, ballroom dancing is one of the best forms of exercise. This activity eases the mind, gives pleasure to the soul, and exercises all the muscles of the body. The dancer does not even consider this to be "work" or "exercise," hence he/she enjoys it better than any other aerobic exercises. Time flies by and before you know it, you have lost a lot of calories and have exercised your body and heart to the maximum . . . in a pleasurable way.

What are the diagnostic tests?

There are various tests available for the early detection of conditions that could lead to a stroke. The simplest is a good medical checkup by your physician, who will listen for a special abnormal sound (bruit) in your neck (carotid) arteries. The presence of a bruit (swishing sound) indicates severe obstruction in the artery. If this is found, a Doppler ultrasound of the carotid artery is ordered to find out if a blockage is present and how severe. If this shows definite blockage that is very severe (70% or higher), surgery could be done to remove the blockage. If the Doppler test is not clear, a CAROTID ARTERIOGRAM (a dye test) is done for a more definitive diagnosis. This dye test will tell for sure if the blockage is severe, how severe it is, and whether surgery is needed.

How safe is the surgery for carotid artery blockage?

Surgery for the blocked carotid artery is very safe. The risk is less than 1%. Since blockage of the carotid (neck) arteries is one of the commonest causes of stroke, this procedure (carotid endarterectomy) is a common routine procedure, especially in the United States and Europe. The surgery itself takes about an hour or so, and the patient usually goes home either the following day or two days after surgery.

How do I find out if I have a blockage in my carotid artery?

The initial step is to see your physician, who will examine you. If there is a bruit (swishing sound) in your carotid artery in the neck, he will refer you to a cardiovascular specialist, who will perform the necessary tests to find out for sure if you indeed have a blockage in your carotid artery or not. If you yourself hear a "swishing" sound in your neck, consult a physician right away.

Drug Improves
Stroke Outcomes

A tablet of a common household remedy, aspirin, is now a routinely prescribed initial immediate treatment for an impending acute myocardial infarction (popularly known as heart attack) among most patients. The blood-thinning ability of aspirin prevents a severely blocked coronary artery of the heart from closing completely and totally cutting off the blood supply to the cardiac muscles. This simple therapy bides time for a more definitive management in an emergency room or acute coronary care unit setting.

Medical science, in its wisdom and experience, pursues new, more effective, and safer drugs; but it also looks back and zooms in old drugs for potential good side effects or previously undiscovered actions, then "recycles" them. Such was the story of the new indication for, and use of, aspirin for acute heart attack. Some new drugs or new actions of older drugs were discovered serendipitously.

And now comes the good news that another common drug, an antibiotic that has been on the market since 1967, when given 6 to 12 hours after an acute ischemic stroke (caused by cut-off in blood supply to the brain from arterial blockage) resulted in significant improvement in the clinical outcomes.

The drugs is minocycline, a semisynthetic, second-generation derivative of the antibiotic tetracycline that has already been found to have significant protective effect on the brain in animal models of Parkinson's disease, Huntington's disease, multiple sclerosis, and amyotrophic lateral sclerosis.

The new study, conducted by Yair Lampl, MD, and his associates, at Edith Wolfson Medical Center and Tel Aviv University, Israel, reported the encouraging preliminary findings, which were published in the October 2, 2007, issue of *Neurology*. "The improvement was already apparent within a week of the stroke," Dr. Lampl stated. The investigation involved a small number of subjects, 152 patients randomized, 74 received minocycline, and 77 placebo.

The American Academy of Neurology considers this "very exciting because many people who have had a stroke cannot be treated if they don't get to the hospital within 3 hours after symptoms start, which is the time frame for currently available treatments."

The neuron-protective effect is said not to be from minocylines' antibiotic property but from its "anti-inflammatory action, causing a noted reduction in microglial activation, matrix metaloproteinasee reduction, nitric oxide production, or inhibition of apoptotic cell death," reported the study.

Dr. Philip Gorelick, MD, from the University of Illinois College of Medicine, told Medscape that "the study by Lampl and colleagues provides an exciting possibility for neuron-protection" and that "minocycline [is] a multipotential neuron-protectant in acute ischemic stroke."

As a general principle of management of any acute medical/surgical emergency, the physician would like to be able to institute an immediate regimen that would minimize the initial damaging effects of the injury, giving the patients a window of opportunity to receive definitive treatment and, their body, the maximal ability to fight the acute medical condition.

While these preliminary findings are most encouraging, a much larger double-blind, randomized clinical study will be needed to confirm this new promising discovered effects of this antiobiotic, its safety in stroke patients, and learn the optimal does of minocycline needed and the time window for its use, etc.

This very stringent requirement of science and regulatory agencies like the US Food and Drug Administration is a glaring example of how proprietary drugs are evaluated and tested before their release to the public, not only for efficacy, but for patient safety, as compared to a lot of the advertised pills, potions, juices, lotions, herbals, with ludicrous claims of miraculous cure for multiple diseases, using anecdotal success stories and (obviously paid) testimonials, mostly with no scientific basis.

Sudden Infant Death

What is Sudden Infant Death Syndrome?

Sudden infant death syndrome (SIDS) is an unexplained and sudden death of an infant under one year of age. It is a major cause of death in infants in this age group, mostly occurring between one month to four months old. Otherwise known as "crib death," SIDS strikes nearly 5,000 babies in the United States each year. The incidence has gone down significantly.

What causes SIDS?

Nobody knows the etiology (cause) of sudden infant death syndrome. It is called a syndrome because medical science still has not found what causes it, or why it occurs, in spite of more than 30 years of scientific research.

Does smoking increase the risk of SIDS?

Yes, the risk of SIDS among infants, who is in the same house as a smoker and therefore exposed to secondhand smoke, is much higher. No one should smoke around the baby. Babies and young children, who are around smokers, have more colds and other diseases. Even their chances of developing cancer when they grow up could be significantly increased.

Does this happen to healthy babies?

In majority of cases, the infants were healthy, and death happened suddenly and quite unpredictably, usually during sleep.

Is overfeeding the baby a factor?

While overfeeding was not found to be factor in SIDS, it is always best not to over feed the baby. The pediatrician's feeding recommendation should be followed and strictly adhered to. If there is any question or doubt, do not delay asking the pediatrician about it.

How does SIDS kill the infant?

Nobody knows for sure, but it appears that the baby is suddenly unable to breathe or stops breathing, resulting in respiratory arrest and ultimately cardiac arrest. The causative mechanism for this event is not clear either. One can suspect that the upper airway somehow suddenly becomes blocked. Why? Science does not know.

Anything new on SIDS?

Yes, over the past several years, research has learned a very important lesson that can help reduce the risk of having SIDS: *keep the babies on their back when they sleep.* Keeping the infants on their back when they sleep has tremendously reduced the incidence of crib deaths. The old teaching was that the babies should sleep on their tummy. That advice was abandoned because of the observation that the prevalence of SIDS was very low among those babies who slept on their back and higher among those who slept on their stomach.

Does sleeping on their back lead to choking?

No, this is not true. There is no evidence that sleeping on their back increases the chances of choking among these babies. As a matter of fact, as we have stated above, the risk of SIDS is a lot lower among babies who sleep on their back. Millions and millions of babies around the world now sleep on their back and doctors have not found an increase in spiting up, vomiting, or choking.

Can all babies sleep on their back?

No, there are babies who have health conditions that require them to sleep on their tummy. They include, among others, birth defects, babies who spit often after feeding, breathing difficulty, heart or lung problems. The individual situation is best discussed with the pediatrician. Aside from these, all other infants can, and should, sleep on their back.

Can the baby sleep on their side?

Yes, one alternative position is to let the infant sleep on the right side. Make sure the baby's right arm is forward to prevent the infant from rolling over to the stomach. The side position affords *less* protection from SIDS than sleeping on the back. The on-back position is the best. Again, consult your pediatrician on this matter for advice.

Can the baby sleep right away after feeding?

All infants do. That is why after feeding, the baby should be held with head up (almost sitting position on the lap of the mother) and burping is induced. It is very important for the baby to burp (to let the air out of the stomach) to prevent discomfort of a bloated stomach and perhaps colic. After burping, the baby may sleep. Make sure the crib is flat and that the head part is *not* lower than the foot part, to prevent eructation or milk from the stomach flowing out to the mouth.

Can blankets pose a hazard to the baby?

Yes, if it is "free-floating" and not wrapped securely around the infant's body, the blanket or any other material, especially plastic bag or sheets or toys, can pose a danger to the baby when any of them cover the face or put in the mouth, causing choking and asphyxiation. The crib must be clean and free of any of these potentially dangerous objects.

Is "tummy time" allowed?

When the baby is awake, he/she can be placed on the stomach, but make sure someone alert and responsible is watching the baby at all time. Some "tummy time" while the baby is awake is deemed healthy for the infant.

Any strategy to reduce SIDS?

Things pediatricians and SIDS experts advise parents and babysitters to do to help reduce the risk of SIDS include: (1) Early and regular prenatal medical check-up reduces the risk of SIDS. (2) The mother should not smoke or drink alcohol during or after pregnancy;.(3) *The baby, from day one, must always sleep on its back,* and not *on its tummy.* (4) The baby must sleep on a firm (but not hard) mattress or surface. (5) Don't use fluffy blankets or comforters under the baby. (6) Don't let the baby sleep on water bed, pillows, sheepskin, or other soft materials that can smother the child. (7) Do not put any stuffed toys or any toys in the crib, which could suffocate the infant. (8) The temperature in the room should be warm but not too warm (between 68 and 72 degrees Fahrenheit. (9) Babies of mothers who smoked during pregnancy have higher risk of SIDS, and babies and children must never be exposed to secondhand tobacco smoke. (10) Breast-feeding the baby will help boost the child's immune system and keep the baby healthy.

Should mothers fear SIDS?

Practically all babies are born healthy, and they stay that way. While the awareness of sudden infant death syndrome is important, to prevent it from occurring by lowering the risk, mothers should not allow the fear of SIDS spoil their joy and pleasure with the new baby. SIDS are now not as common as before, following the strategy outlined above.

Adolescent Suicide

How prevalent is adolescent suicide?

Statistics gathered between 1952 and 1992 in the United States show adolescent suicide among those 15-19 years of age has tripled (386% increase the past 40 years). Adolescent suicide is the third leading cause of death in the 15-24 age group, accounting for 13.7% (4,849) of all deaths, accident and homicide being the first top two causes. Among those ages 10-14, it has increased five times during the same period. Male to female ratio is 6:1, though females attempt suicide more frequently. Estimates of attempted versus completed (successful) suicide range from 50:1 to 200:1.

What is the most common method used?

Drug overdose is the most common method used, particularly among females. The most common one used in completed or successful suicide among adolescents is by firearms. In twelve years (1980 to 1992), the use of firearms accounted for 81% of the increase in overall suicide rates for those ages 15-19 and 64.9% among those 25 and younger. Most of the females who succeeded in killing themselves used firearms. Fifty percent of households in the USA own a gun.

What are the risk factors suicide?

Mental problem is a risk factor, especially major depression, psychosis, etc. Other factors include substance abuse, family history of suicide, sexual abuse, delinquency, gay and lesbian youth, runaways, juveniles in detention centers, halfway houses, prisons, group homes. Those high achievers who may have rigid perfectionist personalities and impulsive behavior are also at an increased risk.

What are the stressor events?

Stressors or precipitants that contribute to suicide are loss of a loved one through divorce, death, or breakup of a relationship; interpersonal or family conflicts. School problems, financial dilemma, and family violence are stressors that aggravate the situation because they lessen the much-needed support responses to an adolescent crisis.

Is pregnancy a risk factor?

Previously thought of as a possible risk factor in suicide among adolescents, pregnancy has been ruled out as a risk factor. In fact, fewer than expected happened during or following teen pregnancy. On the other hand, divorced teen girls, facing the harsh reality of financial and other unanticipated dilemma, are at an increased risk of self-destruction.

Can media coverage of suicide trigger one?

Yes, television, newspaper or radio coverage of suicide (or exposure to a recent suicide or suicide attempt in the community) can serve as a trigger for vulnerable adolescents to act on suicidal thoughts and plans. This is what is termed as "cluster suicides."

Is depression associated with suicide?

Clinical evidences show that depression is very strongly associated with suicide. The symptoms and signs include depressive mood; reduced interest or pleasure; isolation from family and friends; weight loss when not dieting, or weight gain; insomnia or hypersomnia (sleeping a lot); fatigue; diminished ability to think or concentrate; indecisiveness; irritability; unusually argumentative and temperamental behavior; hyperactivity; delinquency; school failure; repeated accidents or injuries; sexual acting out, etc.

Do these adolescents talk about it?

No, they do not volunteer information on their suicidal thoughts or intention, but these adolescents feel relieved when a confidant or a medical professional brings up the subject. When this comes up, it is best to ask questions in a nonjudgemental, nonthreatening, and direct manner, like, "Have you thought of suicide?" "Are you thinking about suicide now?" "Do you have a plan for doing it?" If answer is affirmative, "What is your plan for committing suicide?" A positive response indicates the need for more professional questioning and assessment of risk factors, and the plan of counseling or therapy is based on the degree of risk.

Does suicide run the family?

While genetic predisposition to suicide has a role in its etiology, the environmental factors (home, school, workplace, etc.), or so-called stressors and precipitants, appear to weigh a lot heavier in the equation, even in multiple suicide cases in the same family. Siblings from the same parents but exposed to different environment, stressors, and precipitants react and behave differently to various dilemmas in life.

What can friends and family members do?

Family members and friends who notice signs of depression and/or suspect suicidal tendency should show understanding and compassion without anger or condescension to the individual in distress. They should reassure the person that his/her current emotional condition is temporary and treatable. They should suggest professional help, but this should be done without intimidation or coercion. A "no-suicide" contract, where the adolescent pledges not to attempt self-destruction, is often helpful but cannot be totally and solely relied upon.

Should suicide info be kept confidential?

Most usually, the adolescent will swear to secrecy a friend or a family member, or a professional, about their suicidal tendency or thoughts. The temptation to accede to this request should be avoided, because suicidal intent is not something that should, or can, be kept confidential, if suicide is to be prevented. As a matter of fact, the family members should be advised as soon as the information is known in order for them to remove all medications, firearms, etc., from the home and make these inaccessible to the adolescent. This knowledge will also make the family members more understanding and supportive of the adolescent in crisis, who is hurting badly and really crying for help inside.

What is the best plan for treatment?

If suicidal tendency is suspected, a family member or a friend who is close to the adolescent may suggest professional help. Nowadays, a visit to the psychologist or psychiatrist is commonplace. One does not have to be "crazy" to see psychiatrist. Many politicians, head of states, businessmen, actors, and actresses routinely seek counseling for prophylaxis, to prevent, minimize, or learn how to handle stressors in life. The counselor will have interview sessions with the adolescent, the family members, and friends, most often separately, and make an assessment of the case and tailor the specific management regimen for the individual. Today, more than ever before, medical science has the mind-boggling sophistication to perform "wonderful miracles."

Hazards of Sunlight

What in sunlight is beneficial and harmful to us?

The sun and its light are not only beautiful but vital to our life and survival on this planet. Without the sun, life forms on earth will cease to exist as we know it today. About 75% of our body's supply of vitamin D is generated by our skin's exposure to sunlight (UV-B rays in particular). Abnormally low blood level of vitamin D increases the risk of colon and breast cancers and may also speed up. the growth of an existing or early melanoma. Of course, vitamin D can be taken by mouth. The harmful effects of sunlight come from its ultraviolet (UV) radiation, which could be dangerous to our health in more ways than one, depending on the amount of exposure and dose that a person gets.

What are the sun-related diseases of the eye?

Cataracts (cloudiness of the lens), which, in severe forms, could cause blindness, especially exposure to UV-B radiation; macular degeneration, the major cause of impaired vision in the USA for people older than 55; photokeratitis, a reversible sunburn of the cornea, also from excessive exposure to UV-B; pterygium, growth of pinkish tissues on the white of the eye, which may spread on the clear cornea and block vision. This results when one has prolonged sun exposure on the beach or snow without eye protection and can be very painful for 1-2 days, with temporary blindness.

How about adverse affects on the skin?

Excessive exposure to UV rays predisposes to skin cancer, which includes the face and the eyelids, besides skin in other parts of the body. There are three major types of cancers of the skin: basal cell carcinoma, the most common one; squamous cell carcinoma, second most common; and malignant melanoma, the most deadly, but fortunately, the rarest. Malignant melanoma spreads easily and often deadly if not caught early.

How prevalent are skin cancers?

This is an epidemic and is a global phenomenon. In 1978, in the United States alone, there were 480,000 cases of nonmelanoma skin cancers, rising to over one million in 1994, with a growth rate of 7% per year. In Canada, from 1970 to 1986, melanoma frequency rose 6% per year for men and 4.6% per year for women. Australia has the highest incidence of melanoma in the world. It is said that by age 75, two out of three Australians will have been treated for some type of skin cancer. In the United States, the estimated 30,000 cancer deaths each year could be prevented if Americans, who love sunbathing, do not overexpose themselves to the sun.

Do sunscreen skin lotions cause skin cancer?

It has not been proven beyond doubt that sunscreen skin lotions cause skin cancers. However, the increase in incidence of melanoma in Queensland, Australia, where use of sunscreen has long been aggressively promoted, even by medical firms, has been pointed out by researchers as "the first clue." It is also noted that the frequency of melanoma was the greatest in countries where chemical sunscreen have been vigorously marketed. Cedric and Frank Garland of the University of California cautioned that although sunscreens do protect against sunburn, there is no scientific evidence that they protect against basal cell carcinoma or melanoma in humans. The Garland brothers firmly believe that the use of chemical sunscreen is the primary cause of the epidemic of skin cancers. People who use sunscreen lotion tend to stay longer in the sun, with a false sense of security. Dr. Gordon Ainsleigh of California stated that the use of sunscreen causes more cancer deaths than it prevents.

Are babies and children also affected?

Sun and UV radiation exposure and the use of sunscreen have the same effects on babies and children. It looks funny when we see parents put sunshades (sunglasses) on their babies and children, but there is nothing funny about this practice. Babies and children are not immune to the risk of ocular injury from UV rays. The use of UV protective sunshades and brimmed hat or cap is recommended by pediatricians, not only to minimize glare and squinting, but to protect the eyes from UV radiation. Sunshades for children must be made of plastic and not glass for added impact protection. There are available baby and children sunscreen skin lotions, but check with your pediatrician before using them.

Are UV rays in tanning salons safe?

No, the radiation from the UV lamps in tanning salons are extremely harmful. The tan one gets from artificial tanning does not even have the protective effect of sun-induced tan, and like exposure to the sun, this could cause skin diseases mentioned above.

How do we protect ourselves from UV radiation?

Since UV radiation comes not only from the sun but is reflected from the ground, snow, sand, water, and other reflective surfaces, the use of wide-brimmed hat or cap will reduce the UV radiation to the eyes by 50%. Wraparound UV absorbing eyewear provides the greatest protection, because it also limits radiation from the peripheral rays. Polarized sunglasses or transition lenses reduce glare but do not, by themselves, provide protection from UV radiation.

Sunglasses and/or prescription lenses that absorb 99-100% of the full UV spectrum to 400 nm are the best for babies, children, and adults. Labels on sunglasses should be closely scrutinized to make sure that they say the lenses absorb 99-100% of both the UV-B and UV-A. If they do not have labels, do not buy them. Consumers must be cautious when the label claims the lenses "block harmful UV" but does not specify how much.

For skin cancer protection, do not rely on sunscreen skin lotion. The best is not to sunbathe for more than 20 minutes or so, and if you do, apply "physical" sunscreen lotion. Wear protective clothing and wide-brimmed hat when you go outside during sunny days. Avoid sun exposure between 10:00 a.m. and 3:00 p.m. if possible. Also, it has been shown that taking vitamin C, D, and E and selenium protects against the damages of UV rays by lessening the adverse effects of the UV rays on the immune system.

If one must absolutely be out in the sun, he/she must wear a "physical" sunscreen with an SPF of 15 or higher, which contains titanium dioxide, zinc oxide, or talc. "Physical" sunscreen works by reflecting the UV radiation rather than absorbing the sunscreen into the skin. Doubling the amount of the lotion or reapplying it later in the day does not confer added protection.

Lastly, if you develop any skin spots or notice any mole in your body to be growing larger or darker, or feel any lumps in your body, consult your physician without delay. If treated early and caught in time, most skin cancers are curable.

Is Sweet Potato Better Than Rice?

Sweet potatoes, which originated in Central America 5000 years ago, are one of the oldest vegetables known to man. After his first voyage to the New World, Christopher Columbus took sweet potatoes with him and introduced it to Europe in 1492. The Spanish brought sweet potatoes to the Philippines, Africa, and other Asian countries in the 16th century. Four centuries later, it reached the United States.

Potato is a root vegetable and comes in various colors: white, red, yellow, golden orange, and purple. The orange colored ones are called yams, popular as a regular item (like white potato and beets) during Thanksgiving in the United States, served with turkey, ham, roast beef, etc.

Asians have been so accustomed to eating rice as their staple that they simply consider or presume it to be better than sweet potato. However, scientifically speaking, sweet potato is superior to rice in many ways, nutritionally speaking. And cheaper also, cup per cup, about half the price of rice.

Scientific nutritional analysis, using one cup of baked sweet potato and one cup of boiled rice (with nothing added in either case) shows very interesting and enlightening data, summed up here (minus the boring detailed figures).

For one thing, rice has no vitamins A, B6, C, D, K, and riboflavin, which sweet potato does. It also has 5 times more fiber and 7 times more folate, compared to rice.

Sweet potato has about 20 times more calcium than rice and contains 30% more omega-3 and omega-6. It also has about 50 times more potassium and has more water content and about 11 more calories per cup.

A sweet potato has more vitamin A than a cup of carrots, more fiber than a bowl of oatmeal, and more potassium than a banana.

Sweet potatoes also contains various amino acids like, alanine, arginine, aspartate, glutamate, isoleucine, leucine, methionine, phenylalanine, tryptophan, tyrosine, and valine.

Anthocyanins

In some foods, like sweet potato, it has anthocyanin, which is a potent antioxidant, scavenger of the harmful free radicals in our system. Other items include blueberries, raspberries, red grapes, eggplants, beets, and also yellow, red, brown, and black rice—but not white rice.

Anthocyanins are the color pigments that give foods their deep rich red, blue, purple, as in some fruits and vegetables, or golden orange color as in sweet potato. Regular consumption of food items with anthocyanins provides some protection against hardening of the arteries, arthritis, and other chronic metabolic and degenerative illnesses, and even against cancer. Sweet potato for one also has anti-inflammatory properties.

Tetanus: Lockjaw

What is Tetanus?

Tetanus is a serious life-threatening condition that affects the brain and the entire nervous system caused by a toxin of a common bacterium, *Clostridium tetani*. The spores of this bacterium are practically not found in virgin soil but frequently present in cultivated soil. It is also found in the human colon, house dust, animal feces, warehouses, contaminated heroin, and even in operating rooms. Indeed, they may be found anywhere. Once the spores penetrate the wounded skin, they germinate and produce a toxin (tetanospasmin) that invades the bloodstream causing the illness.

Why is it called lockjaw?

Tetanospasmin, next to botulism toxin, is one of the most potent microbial poisons. Once the spores are in the bloodstream, they move inward toward the spinal cord at a speed of about 0.416 inch an hour, or about ten inches a day. After a week to 3 weeks, they start to cause short-circuiting of the nerve signals and block the ability of the muscles to relax. As a result, sustained muscle contractions develop, including lockjaw. The spasms of the facial muscles spread to the neck (causing nuchal rigidity, meaning stiffness of the neck), the hands, arms, and legs and also to the back, leading to severe (often fatal) breathing distress. Somehow, the spasms are initiated and aggravated by noise or touch.

How deadly is tetanus?

The mortality rate of tetanus is about 40% after it has spread, even in state-of-the-art medical centers. Each year, about one million infants die of tetanus because of poor hygiene. After the US immunization laws were legislated in the 1970s, the reported cases of tetanus dramatically dropped to about 50 cases annually (75% of these are adults who have never had immunization).

How does tetanus spores enter our body?

The tetanus spores enter our system thru animal bites, burns, ulcers, infected umbilical cords, contaminated surgical wounds, needle injection sites, and thru the commonly blamed "rusty nail." Wounds resulting from any dirty item which has been in contact with soil or animal dung are suspect. The incubation period (time span from exposure to appearance of symptoms) averages two weeks, although in some cases lasting to several months.

What are the signs and symptoms?

The initial presentation may include headache and depression, malaise and fever, followed by swallowing discomfort and difficulty opening the jaws. Then the neck becomes stiff, and the cheek muscles go into spasm, giving the face a sardonic grin (risus sardonicus). Irritability soon develops and the spasms involve the entire body, leading to painful involuntary contraction of all muscles. There will be restlessness, anorexia, and uncontrolled drooling of saliva. In a few cases, tetanus develops even without a previous history of a cut or a wound.

Can one get tetanus from a minor skin prick?

If the person is not immunized, yes, even from pricking a finger on a rose thorn or a tiny needle stick. A study from Great Britain reported that about 33% of tetanus cases in that country resulted from a very trivial injury the patients had not even noticed or remembered. This is why immunization is very important in preventing this fatal disease.

How fatal is the toxin?

The tetanus toxin is deadly poisonous (second only to botulism toxin). One-tenth of a milligram of tetanospasmin is the fatal dose for an adult. Once this toxin reaches the nervous system, it can no longer be neutralized by antibodies produced by immunization or even by antitoxin. Prognosis in these cases is almost always fatal. Again, prevention is the key.

Is this bacterium an anaerobe?

Yes, *Clostridium tetani* is an anaerobe, meaning it is killed off by oxygen and grows only in oxygen-free environment. This is the reason wounds are washed thoroughly with water (H2O) and hydrogen peroxide (H2O2) used by many to aerate the wounds, dilute the contamination, and kill the spores. This is also why deep penetrating wounds, where oxygen is least or absent, have a higher risk of developing tetanus among unimmunized individuals.

What vaccine is available to prevent tetanus?

DTaP immunization (used to be known as DPT) incorporates vaccines for the prevention of diphtheria (severe throat infection), pertussis (whooping cough), and tetanus. This is given when the infant is 2 months old, 4 months, and six months, a set of 3 shots. A fourth injection is given when the child is 12-18 months old, a fifth shot at age 4 to 6, and a booster tetanus-diphtheria (Td) at age 11 to 12 years old. Among adults, vaccination with Td is recommended every ten years. Adults who never had any immunization for tetanus will require a series of 3 injections of Td vaccine.

Can there be allergy to the vaccine?

Yes, it is possible for a person to be allergic to DTap or any other vaccines, or to any drug, for that matter. Your physician will guide you accordingly after a good history-taking and a thorough physical examination. The valuable benefits from immunization of any type is certainly worth the little risk getting it might entail. In general, available vaccines today are very safe.

How is the tetanus patient managed?

The main objective of the treatment is to tide the patient over the stage of the ailment preventing any deadly complications from occurring. The problems include asphyxia (suffocation) during spasm, exhaustion from generalized involuntary body spasms, pneumonia resulting from stomach contents backing up and into the lungs, and demise as a consequence of disorders of the control of vital brain functions like blood pressure, heart rhythm, and breathing. Penicillin and antitoxin are given plus a lot of supportive care.

Does the patient have to be on a ventilator?

Not all, but some cases may require a tracheostomy (a finger-size metal tube inserted thru the neck to the breathing pipe to allow patients to breathe better) and this tube is connected to a respirator, which will take over the breathing for the patient until he is able to breathe well on his/her own. The milder cases may respond to simple sedation and a quiet room to prevent spasms and not need a tracheostomy and/or a respirator.

Is it not too late to be immunized?

Unless one already has been infected with a full-blown tetanus, it is never too late to have prophylactic (preventive) immunization. The procedure is simple and most effective, and it behooves everyone to acquire this protection from a horrible and deadly disease, a fatal illness that is preventable. For a more specific and personal advice tailored to your individual situation and need, consult your physician. Your appropriate and prompt attention may save your life.

Tips on Drinking

Social drinking is the invention of modern society. And as long as it is done with grace and discipline and in moderation, the etiquette is totally acceptable. However, as far as calories go, alcoholic beverages contain one of the highest, per ounce. This is one reason why the choice of cocktails is important for those watching their calorie intake or weight.

The National Institute of Health reports that "the pounds put on during the holidays account for half of all the weight gained annually . . . and the unsuspected culprit is alcohol." While the observation is totally significant and relevant in the United States, it is today also apropos in other cultures around the globe, albeit, in general, less in Asia.

The Five Most Fattening Cocktails

1. Eggnog: 257 calories and 14 grams of fat, without alcohol, and more than 300 calories when you add distilled spirits.

2. Martinis: Many Martinis have 2-5 ounces of liquor and sugary syrups and can have 800 calories per drink. The "dry" martini, though, which is basically pure gin (or vodka) and a drop or two of vermouth plus a couple of olives may be around 200 calories. Without the olives and vermouth, it could drop down to 100 calories.

3. Hot Toddies: Hot toddy plus 2 ounces of liquor is about 200 calories. Adding creamy liquors, like Kahlua or Baileys, schnapps, or amaretto, it adds about 100 calories more, making it a total of 300 calories.

4. Margaritas: Whopping 400 calories per drink.

5. Mixers: An ounce and half (45 cc) of 80-proof spirits is roughly 65 calories, and together with 6 ounces of mixers (cola and other soda, plus syrups), the calories zoom at least a couple of hundreds.

Five Lower-Calorie Drinks

1. Champagne: The traditional drink for toasts is about 100 calories per drink, which is not too excessive for the waistline.

2. Wine Spritzer: With 3 ounces of club soda, the 3 ounces of wine to make the spritzer total about 60 calories and zero fat.

3. Wine: A glass of wine is about 100 calories. Great choice, especially the red variety.

4. Beer: Regular has about 150 calories and light beer, about 100 calories per can/bottle.

5. Gin or Vodka and Soda, or as a Dry Martini: One and a half ounces of 80 proof, with soda mixer or straight (without any mixer), have less than 100 calories and zero fat.

Choosing red wine is smart move, as it is good for cardiovascular health. Red wine has been singled out because the skin of the grapes where they come from contains *phytochemicals*, such as *resveratrol*, that help protect the plant's self-defense system, and *proanthocyanidins (OPC) and cathechins,* which are also powerful antioxidants. Studies at the University of California, Davis, and Cornell University have confirmed the beneficial effect of these potent antioxidants that aid in preventing cancer and heart coronary heart disease. Also, the alcohol in it has some sedative and euphoric effects when wine is taken in moderation; and these are healthy for the psyche, especially in these stressful times.

While drinking alcoholic beverages weakens our resistance (or makes us more susceptible) to other "temptations," like eating more and succumbing to additional high-calorie desserts (pecan pie, crème brulle, or chocolate mousse, etc.), the technique of drinking two glasses of cold water after each cocktail drink, used by experienced drinkers, not only ward off dehydration (caused by alcohol) but also helps in calorie and weight control.

Above all these tips, let us remember this vital one to avoid being a statistic: don't drink and drive!

Vegetables versus Lymphoma

Since man roamed the earth, vegetables have been hailed as a great health food. And even before modern science came out with the medical data proving their value, parents—especially mothers—around the world, from different cultures and traditions, had already been encouraging their children to eat vegetables.

In this new era of health consciousness, vegetables have once again been thrust to the center stage, under the spotlight, not only as a great food item, but one that has remarkable medical powers that bolster the immune system and prevent diseases, including cancers.

Recently, a Mayo Clinic study showed that eating lots of vegetables lowers the risk of non-Hodgkin lymphoma (NHL). This clinical investigation revealed the following eight findings, presented here verbatim:

- Those who ate a higher number of vegetable servings per week had a 42 percent lower risk of NHL than those who ate the lowest number.
- Those who ate the most servings of green leafy vegetables and cruciferous vegetables had a 40 percent lower risk compared to the lowest intakes.
- Those who had the highest intake of the carotenoids lutein and zeaxanthin had a 46 percent lower risk of NHL.
- Those who had the highest intake of zinc had a 42 percent lower risk.

The researchers postulated that vegetables contain antioxidants that help the body repair the damages in the DNA caused by oxidative stress, which is one of the risk factors for non-Hodgkin lymphoma. And eating vegetables at least 3 times a day, if combined with a healthy lifestyle that includes daily physical exercises, confers even a greater degree of immuno-protection. The antioxidants in vegetables also help neutralize the free radicals produced during exercise.

The following are some of the nutrients in vegetables that help lower the risk of developing non-Hodgkin lymphoma and cancers, in general: Lycopene, lutein, folic acid, zeaxanthin, gluoinolates (which are converted into isothiocyanates). Apparently, the protective substances induce a phase 2 detoxification pathways which minimize and help repair the damages in our DNA caused by our unhealthy and self-destructive lifestyle.

Besides preventing cancers, some vegetables appear to show some promise in treating some forms of tumors in experimental mice.

Di-indolylmethane (DIM) is a natural compound found in vegetables (like broccoli, cabbage, turnips, and mustard greens), which has not only been associated with cancer prevention, but more amazingly, with the potential ability to treat cancer. Obviously more extensive laboratory studies and, later, clinical application in humans are needed to validate this research observation.

While eating a lot of vegetables every day could protect us from diseases, including cancer, eating red meat and processed foods reduces the benefits conferred by the vegetables we eat. Besides being loaded with saturated fats and cholesterol, red meat and processed foods have also been implicated in the increased risk of developing heart disease, stroke, and cancer.

Man has always been searching for the formula for optimal health and longevity. The market is full of nonprescription herbal or "food supplement" pills, potions, and lotions, each claiming to be effective against a host of medical conditions as preventive or as a "cure." Not only are these items not approved by government sentinel agencies like the US-FDA and the BFAD, but they are cost prohibitive, ineffective, and potentially dangerous.

The manufacturing companies concerned hide behind the legal technicality by marketing their products, *not* as drugs, but as herbals or "food supplements" to escape the stringent requirements, although their infomercials state that their "health" products "are effective for" a variety of medical illnesses. If they have pharmacologic (chemical) effects, then they should be considered as drugs and be subject to the rigorous testing and clinical studies required for drugs, prior to their approval and acceptance as safe and effective for public consumption.

It is rather most unfortunate that the government appears to be simply powerless in dealing with the perpetrator companies and dealers and their unsubstantiated claims and deceptive practices, who are bilking the unsuspecting and ignorant victims of their hard-earned money.

Disease-inducing personal bad habits and unhealthy lifestyle include smoking; high-cholesterol, high fat, high-carbohydrate diet; inactivity (lack of physical exercise); alcohol abuse; and poor stress management. These factors, which are really within our control, are responsible for about 75% of all diseases afflicting man. Indeed, only 25% of these illnesses we have today are beyond our control. Most of our health problems are self-inflicted and self-induced and therefore preventable to a large extent.

Medical literature is full of data on clinical outcomes that justify this caveat: eating vegetables prevents diseases, while regular consumption of red meat and processed foods is associated with increased risk of debilitating and deadly illnesses, including cancer.

Vertigo: Dizziness

What is Vertigo?

Vertigo is the medical term for dizziness. It is a disturbance where a person experiences a feeling of movement in space (subjective vertigo), or a sensation that the objects are (the ones) moving around him/her (objective vertigo). Vertigo is usually accompanied by loss of equilibrium or balance. Vertigo can be debilitating and disruptive of normal daily activities, including sitting up or walking.

What are the causes of vertigo?

True vertigo—as distinguished from lightheadedness, faintness or other forms of dizziness—is caused by disturbance in the apparatus that maintains our body equilibrium (balance): the semicircular canal in our ear, the vestibular nerve, our brain stem, and our eyes. Overdose in medications, ear infection, anemia from gastrointestinal tract bleeding, and brain tumor are conditions that can cause vertigo. We normally feel a little out of balance when we close our eyes while standing still or walking.

What conditions or factors affect this apparatus?

Motion sickness, hysteria, otitis media (ear infection), obstructed ear canal, eye problems, Meniere's syndrome, intake of sedative or alcohol, multiple sclerosis and other nerve diseases, brain tumor, anemia, leukemia, and slow heart rate are some of the factors or conditions that cause vertigo.

Why do some of us feel lightheaded when we suddenly get up from a sitting position?

This common condition is called postural hypotension or orthostatic hypotension. Hypotension means low blood pressure. Postural means positional, and orthostatic means standing straight. The reason for feeling faint in the sudden change of position from sitting to standing is the blood is pulled down away from the brain by gravity, when one suddenly stands up. Going up on a fast elevator has the same hemodynamic effect.

What is Meniere's syndrome?

This disease is characterized by sudden episodes of dizziness, tinnitus (ringing in the ear), progressive deafness, accompanied by persistent nausea and vomiting. The vertigo persists for days or weeks, usually caused by vestibular neuronitis (inflammation of the vestibular nerve, the eighth nerve).

Why does a slow heart rate cause dizziness?

Bradycardia (heart rate below 60) may not be tolerated by some people (normal heart rate being 60 to 100 pulse beats per minutes), causing them to feel dizzy or faint or even passing out. The mechanism here is the slow heart rate means the heart is pumping or beating only 59 or less, and not enough blood goes up to the brain, resulting in fainting spells. Althletes or people who are physically conditioned, however, have a slower heart rate, some below 60, and tolerate this very well. As a matter of fact, this condition is healthier, because the heart does not have to work as hard as when it has to pump more than 60 beats a minute.

Can anxiety cause vertigo?

Yes, anxiety or anxiety neurosis or depression can cause a feeling of experiencing vertigo. This condition can cause almost any symptoms. However, in anxiety neurosis (psychoneurosis) it is more of giddiness or fear of losing one's balance while walking, rather than actual or true vertigo itself.

How about motion sickness, seasickness, or airsickness?

These are a variety of vertiginous conditions that are common among those with very sensitive or "weak" labyrinthine (equilibrium) apparatus. Some people are born this way. Others can tolerate (and even enjoy, without vertigo) fast carnival rides, like the high-speed roller-coasters, twirling, turning, and even upside down, because they have inherently strong labyrinthine apparatus. Astronauts, pilots, circus jugglers, high-rise construction workers, fast dancers, etc., are other examples.

Is prolonged motion sickness serious?

Yes, prolonged or excessive motion sickness, which is accompanied by vomiting may lead to dehydration, fall in the blood pressure (shock), loss of body mass, and even depression. History recorded such ordeals experienced by people, especially slaves, with poor vestibular apparatus, who were transported by ships from one country to another on journeys that took several months.

How can one prevent seasickness or airsickness?

Persons who are susceptible should choose to sit (on airplanes) over the wing section, and on a ship, in the midsection. Lying down or on a reclined position, with the head braced on a pillow, is best. Avoid reading and avoid alcohol intake. A very light diet helps. And so with avoiding looking at the waves while traveling by water. A well-ventilated cabin and going out on deck for fresh air help. To minimize or prevent motion sickness, your physician can prescribe "antivertigo" or "anti-motion-sickness" pills or patch.

For persistent vertigo (of more than a few days), it is prudent and best to consult your physician to rule out the possibility of an existing health condition, which could range from simple to serious. The earlier the diagnosis is made, the sooner the treatment can be initiated and the better the chances are for a successful cure or prevention of complications or a more serious stage of the disease.

Violence on Television

The cultures of corruption and of violence in society are close cousins, if not twins. They are intertwined. Where there is corruption, there is violence and vice versa. Violence is a symptom of a corrupt mind, and corruption is violence against fellow human beings and society.

Are we more violent as a society today? Do video games subliminally brainwash our young children's mind as they take pleasure in actively participating in virtual massive killings as an accepted form of entertainment? Do these violent games make these kids take violence and killings more lightly? Should parents and our legislators do something about this situation?

Studies have shown that watching educational and socially interactive children's shows on television have positive impacts on these children, not only in learning arithmetic or science but in social behavior, humanity, compassion, honesty, and responsibility.

On the other end of the spectrum, young boys and girls alike who watch violence on television have increased risk of aggression, including spousal abuse and criminal offenses as adults. Violence on any media adversely affects children's lives by eroding into their inborn and natural aversion to violence, making aggression, violence, and—in many cases—crime as acceptable social behaviors for them when dealing with their family and the public.

Adults are not immune to these negative effects. Most of us have heard the "*F*" word mentioned so many times in one sentence in shows and simply laugh at it.

Children learn from what they see and what they hear at home or in their world outside. They grow up with all those experiences, and they become the summation of what they learn. Whichever predominates rule their future.

We as parents have the grave responsibility of protecting our children from any form of harm, including negative influences, and of guiding them to become good, law-abiding, honest, productive, and compassionate citizens, making them a credit to society and to the human race as a whole.

Drinking and Blood Pressure

Mix binge drinking and high blood pressure, and you get a cocktail of medical conditions that shortens longevity. Indeed, binge drinking among those with hypertension increases the risk of death, compared to those persons with normal blood pressure. A lot of alcohol and high blood pressure are a lethal mix.

Binge drinking, which is a major public health issue, is defined as consuming a large amount of alcoholic drink in one single session. While it is a serious health problem, many drinkers are ignorant of the risks. Alcohol poisoning from binge drinking is not rare.

Published in *STROKE: Journal of the American Heart Association*, the South Korean study involving 6,100 subjects over twenty years found that "compared to people with normal blood pressure who did not drink, the risk of cardiovascular death in men, with high blood pressure was 3 times higher in general; 4 times higher if they consumed at least 6 drinks in one binge session; 12 times higher if they consumed at least 12 drinks in one binge session."

The American Heart Association defines moderate drinking as "a maximum of two drinks per day for men and one drink per day for women . . . a drink is defined as a 12-ounce beer, one 4-ounce glass of wine, 1.5 ounces of 80-proof spirits, or one ounce of 100-proof spirits."

When Gambling Hurts

Gambling as an entertainment has been with us even before civilization started. Cavemen had their own version of gambling. Today, we have casinos mushrooming around the world. Gamblers can bet online at the comfort of their home, using credit cards.

Gambling at home (mahjong, poker, blackjack, bingo, etc.) for charity or not, or gambling in casinos for fun, with discipline and limitations in terms of amount and time, can be refreshing, especially with friends. But uncontrolled frequent gambling, even at home with friends, especially with high stakes (no longer penny-ante friendly wager), is addictive gambling no less.

When one is helplessly hooked on gambling, a so-called "hidden illness," which the sufferer may not even realize, or has self-denial about it, or actually covering it up because of shame, then the fun has long stopped and the stage of addiction has set in. Many obsessive gamblers are also alcoholics, where weakness in the character appears to play a role, according to psychotherapists.

The strong uncontrollable urge to gamble dominates the victim, up to the point of giving up food, sleep, personal grooming, his job, his social life, and neglecting his family, in favor of gambling. Since habitual gambling is a losing game and a game of losers, soon the victim parts with all his money, his property, his self-respect, his friends, even his family. As the stress escalates, he resorts to more gambling in his desire to chase (win back) his loses. So he goes deeper and deeper in financial and emotional bankruptcy. Not a few of them ended up killing themselves, like a couple of physicians I have heard of.

Some of the signs and symptoms include changes of personality, attention, and responsibility; losing time from work or school; borrowing money or pawning or selling personal possessions; lying about amount and time wasted on gambling; gambling to escape problems; and having a sense of fear, depression, frustration, anger, hopelessness, and suicidal tendencies.

Addictive gambling is a disease; and like other illnesses, it could benefit from early attention, diagnosis, and prompt treatment. There are centers and support groups, which can help. Taking this wise and prudent step toward healing is one gamble the victim can bet on with his/her life—and usually win big!

Water "Ionizer"—A Scam?

As far as health is concerned, majority, if not all, of us, want the best health minus the sacrifices needed to achieve it effectively and safely. We want to be healthy without exercising, dieting, or abstaining from smoking and without disciplined alcohol intake. We want to have good blood pressure and good cholesterol level without skimping on our salt and fat intake and quitting cigarettes. We want to lose weight without cutting down on our calorie intake and exercising daily.

For expediency, any pill or juice or gadget that comes along with the claim that it is good for our health becomes a "must-buy" crutch, believing it will confer upon us good health and longevity without lifting a finger, moving a muscle, or getting off the couch and putting down the remote control and the potato chips.

Unfortunately, the manufacturers of these "health" lotions, potions, pills, juices, and gadgets are mostly interested in making their bank accounts healthy and least interested in the health of its consumer-victims. Otherwise, they won't continue to prey on the unsuspecting public and sell their useless products, which may even have severe long-term side effects. And organ failure and cancer are some of those possibilities!

It is one thing to pay for very expensive pills or juices or machines and finding out years from now that it was not effective. It is another to discover years down the line that its use has caused a debilitating or deadly disease.

Now comes the water ionizer, the "ionized" alkaline water it produces, the "special drinking water." Not only are these marketed waters and the ionizing machines expensive, but they are, according to scientists, "medically baseless and worthless." Most of the good effects these manufacturers claim for their products are available in healthy food items, like fish, fruits, bran, wheat, nuts, vegetables, and water purified by the most advanced multiple-stage reverse-osmosis filtration system. It might come as a surprise to many but boiled water, minus its sediments, is safer than some of this expensive drinking water. Using the commercially available home water filtration pitcher or the below-the-sink filtration system, and then boiling the water will even double the protection. This will certainly not cost $1500—$2500 like the ionizers.

When it comes to health, there is no better guide than our modern science, where extensive and rigidly controlled laboratory testing and double-blind, randomized, human clinical trials are the standard before any medication or device gets official approval and goes out to the market.

Anecdotal reports (usually solicited) or testimonials (usually from paid endorsers) are not scientific proofs. These are misinformation used to market the product with some semblance of "truth." Candidly, these are nothing but lies. If not approved by the US-FDA, RP-BFAD or any other similar national health agencies, any product is suspect. So, public, beware!

As far as the water ionizer is concerned, here is "the bottom line" as objectively explained in a detailed scientific paper, which aims to educate and protect the public:

> Here, in a nutshell, are few basic facts that anyone with a solid background in chemistry or physiology would concur with: (1) "Ionized water" is nothing more than sales fiction; the term is meaningless to chemists; (2) Most water that is fit for drinking is too unconductive to undergo significant electrolysis; (3) Pure water can never be alkaline or acidic, nor can it be made so by electrolysis; (4) Ground waters containing metal ions such as calcium and magnesium can be rendered slightly alkaline by electrolysis, but after it hits the highly acidic gastric fluid in the stomach, its alkalinity is gone; (5) The

idea that one must consume alkaline water to neutralize the effects of acidic foods is ridiculous; we get rid of excess acid by exhaling carbon dioxide; (6) The claims about health benefits of drinking alkaline water were not supported by credible scientific evidence; (7) There is nothing wrong with drinking slightly acidic waters such as rainwater. Body pH is a meaningless concept in this context because different parts of the body (and even individual cells) can have widely different pH value; (8) If you really want to de-acidify your stomach (at possible cost of interfering with protein digestion), why spend hundreds of dollars for an electrolysis device when you can take calcium-magnesium pills, Alka-Seltzers or Milk of Magnesia?; (9) Electrolysis devices or ionizers are generally worthless for treating water for health enhancement, removal of common impurities, disinfection and scale control.

To protect our health . . . and pocketbook, we must use our wisdom and due diligence.

Water Is Life!

Water crisis is threatening the world, and no country is immune to it. Many countries are already experiencing water shortage. As a matter of fact, the United Nation appears to be a notch more concerned about the progressive scarcity of clean water than about global warming. And rightfully so, because water is life, and no water means no life on earth. It is conceivable that water, rather than oil, will be the cause of future wars around the world.

Energy conservation is an essential environmental policy. While water has no calorie, it is, practically speaking, a form of "energy." Water conservation is taken very seriously in the well-developed countries like the United States and in European countries, where restaurants no longer serve water automatically but on request and where hotels encourage water-saving measures besides electrical power conservation, with a sign requesting unused towels be left on the shelves, etc. In desert cities like Las Vegas and those in other parts of the world, water conservation consciousness and practice are part of children's education and the daily life of the people. It only makes sense. Why waste water, or anything valuable for that matter, at all?

To avert a catastrophe

There are "three main plans to institute, which include water conservation, water justice and water democracy," according to Maude Barlow, cofounder of the Blue Planet Project and a vocal advocate of clean water for all, "in order for our planet to avert a catastrophe regarding this crisis that, according to the United Nations, should be our top priority."

In her book titled *The Global Water Crisis and the Coming Battle for Right to Water*, Barlow points out that "access to clean water is a human right," and exhorted the global community "to see beyond the borders to the moral courage necessary to conserve and share this precious resource, as well as working on a treaty like the one we hope to see regarding the climate crisis that sets goals for conservation, sharing of resources, providing technology necessary to developing countries that helps them with conserving through agriculture, infrastructure, and basic education."

Rainwater could be harvested from rooftops, from land surface, or from rock catchments and collected in pots, jars, barrels, etc., or in a more sophisticated reservoir like underground check dams, for future use.

An archaic technology could save the world

Water harvesting was practiced in the 9th or 10th century in the rural areas of South and Southeast Asia, and for almost 2000 years in Thailand. According to UNEP, 1982, "about 40 000 well storage tanks, in a variety of different forms, were constructed between 1970 and 1974 using a technology which stores rainwater and storm water runoff in ponds of various sizes. A thin layer of red clay is generally laid on the bottom of the ponds to minimize seepage losses. Trees, planted at the edges of the ponds, help to minimize evaporative losses from the ponds."

This centuries-old technology used by ancient civilization still offers our modern world of today a simple and practical way for almost every household or town to minimize the adverse effects of the predicted water crisis. Needless to say, water conservation (the wise and judicious use of water) is an essential part of the solution.

The popular systems have three major components: the catchment area, the collection device, and the conveyance system. An inexpensive filtration device is a fabric sack, used to remove particles before water enters the storage reservoir. A small chlorine dosage pump may also be used to sterilize the water. While rainwater linked illnesses have been reported to be few and insignificant, a treatment and filtration system may be added to ensure the water is safe for drinking. Boiling rainwater and throwing away mineral sediments is certainly a practical alternative, as a resort.

Crisis or not, rainwater harvesting and conservation today is a prudent and easy way to collect water for general use, help in protecting our environment, and, at the same time, save on our water bills too. Water is essential to life. Why waste it?

With the looming water crisis, it behooves governments and private sectors of all countries around the globe to formulate national policies to address the issue before an actual crisis dries up our wells and annihilate all living forms on earth. An intelligent, well-structured, preemptive, and prompt strategy today might spell the difference between survival and extinction of all life on this planet tomorrow.

Warning on Weight-Loss Products

If you are taking, or planning to take, any products (pills, potion or lotion, food supplements, or herbals) to help you lose weight, here is a wake-up call for you.

For at least the past three decades, we have been warning our readers about the dangers of weight control aids, especially those sold on the streets, in health food or herbal shops or organic food stores, marketed as "effective and safe."

In spite of the reported adverse side effects on various organs of the body, which have resulted in some deaths, these weight loss products continue to flood the market and people (ignorant and misinformed by the ads and infomercials) are duped into buying and using them. The fact that many of them are expensive may be a secondary consideration for some, but the real serious effects of these products are risks not worth taking. Besides, there is a healthier, safer, and more economical strategy available.

And now, once again, and even in a more forceful assault on the manufacturers of weight loss products, the US Federal Drug Administration (FDA) "has inspected some companies associated with the sale of these illegal products and is currently seeking product recalls," and "additional enforcement steps, such as warning letters, initiating seizures, injunctions, or criminal charges, are also possible," according to the agency report.

The FDA has expanded its warning list of weight-loss products from 28 to 69 in January 2009, from the original advisory issued by the agency December 22, 2008.

These weight loss products, according to the FDA, can cause important cardiovascular side effects from these components: sibutramine, phenytoin, phenolphthalein, and abumetanide. Some ingredients of some weight-loss products may even be carcinogenic (cancer-causing agents).

The FDA press release also noted that "One product, known as Phyto Shape, even contained rimonabant, the cannabinoid-receptor blocker that has been linked to neurological and psychiatric side effects . . . in 2007, an FDA advisory committee unanimously said no to rimonabant, and Sanofi-Aventis, the maker of rimonabant, eventually halted all clinical research with the weight-loss drug."

It is unfortunate that the public appears to be at the mercy of the well-designed but less than truthful commercials on these weight-loss products, especially the so-called food supplements and herbals, with their baseless claims about their efficacy and safety and obviously intentional omission of listing their adverse side effects, short term and long term. The ignorant and unsuspecting public swallows the advertisement hype and ends up spending hard-earned money for products that could cause health problems. Misinformed people also think that these products replace the need for dieting and exercising.

The safest (and lesser expensive) way to lose weight and maintain good health is to do daily exercises (aerobic exercises, dancing, tai-bo, normal-pace or brisk walking, swimming, etc.), and by cutting down calorie intake, to maintain the desired weight (monitoring the weight once a week, using it as a guide to dieting). Drinking a tall glass of water before eating also helps in reducing food intake. Avoiding carbohydrate foods (rice, bread, potatoes, cakes, candies, ice cream, and other pastries and sweets) will greatly help in weight control. Those who have given up most of these foods maintained their desired weight sooner and more permanently.

It is common to hear some people say they have not been eating a lot and still gained weight. Medical data show that all (100%) of the starved prisoners in any war in the history of the world lost massive weight, regardless of gender, physical built, family history, genetics, etc.

All lost weight, because of calorie restriction and hard labor (which is a form of physical exercise).

There is really no need for weight-loss pills, teas, and juices for safe and effective weight control for 99% of people who are overweight. Calorie control and daily exercises will do the trick. The 1% exception who have morbid obesity, not responding to calorie control and exercises, are possible candidates for gastric bypass surgery or Lap Band procedure.

To be more effective and lasting, normal weight maintenance must start from childhood. The old tale that fat babies and children are healthier is not true. Childhood obesity leads to early onset of serious diseases. And children as early as in their teens should have their blood cholesterol level checked, even once, to have a baseline data. Because of exposure to the junk food culture of red meats, eggs, fries, and milkshakes and other unhealthy items in fast-food chains, young children in various countries around the world have been found to prematurely have high cholesterol level. High cholesterol level among these young people is also associated with high risk of developing heart attack and stroke early, even before age 45. Pediatric experts have now lowered the normal value of blood cholesterol to be at 170, down 30 points from the former standard of 200.

One area where most of us parents have miserably failed in is in teaching our children to eat fish, vegetables, whole grains, nuts, and fruits daily, instead of a lot of carbs, red meat and eggs. This is the reason why today we have an epidemic (actually a pandemic) of obesity and hypercholesterolemia among children in well-developed countries and a severe increase in the global incidence of diabetes mellitus type 2, heart attack, stroke, and even cancer.

Advances in Women's Health

Our consultant for this topic, Anthony N. Gentile, MD, PhD, FACOG, of the Rosalind Franklin University of Chicago Medical School, is certified by the American Board of Obstetrics and Gynecology and of the American Board of Quality Assurance. He is in private practice in Northwest Indiana and Illinois. In today's forum, he discusses some interesting, and may be life-saving, advances in women's health.

Endometrial Ablation

Imagine a quick, minor, no-incision surgical procedure for women, performed in the office, which permanently stops heavy periods! That's what endometrial (inside lining of the walls of the womb) ablation means, "shaving off" the inside lining that is causing the abnormal and excess menstrual bleeding.

Most women will normally lose about 1/4 of a cup of blood with each period. About 20% of women will experience abnormal heavy periods during their reproductive years. This most often affects women in their 40s nearing menopause and often causes large losses of blood leading to anemia. There are many reasons for heavy periods, but the most common cause is hormonal imbalance. This imbalance is often related to obesity and anovulation (inability to produce eggs). Other serious causes may include cancer of the endometrium, endometrial polyps, bleeding disorders, and various medical disorders.

If the cause of the heavy periods is not correctable with medications and is not related to cancer or uterine tumors, etc., then endometrial ablation may be considered as a treatment. After the complete evaluation—which may include blood tests, pelvic ultrasound, and an endometrial biopsy—is done and pregnancy has been ruled out, endometrial ablation can be performed. The uterus and the ovaries are not removed. In about 20% of women, this procedure does not control the heavy bleeding, and further treatment or surgery may be required.

Oral sex and oral cancer

Women aren't the only ones vulnerable to human papillomavirus (HPV). This virus is now one of the leading causes of oral cancers in men! The news in the fall of 2010 about the health of 1988 Academy Award winning actor Michael Douglas has put the spotlight on throat cancer.

HPV, by all accounts, is the most common sexually transmitted germ in the world. Around 120 strains of HPV have been isolated from humans, about 40 of which are in the genital tract and are highly associated with cervical and vaginal cancers and warts. Strains #16 and #18 have been linked to oral cancer. Dr. No-Hee Park published a study showing that the mouth, cervix, and vagina all have the same type of cellular structure that are the target of HPV-16 and HPV-18.

Dr. Maura Gillison and colleagues from the Johns Hopkins Oncology Center studied 253 patients diagnosed with head and neck cancers. In 25% of these patients, the tumor tissue was HPV positive, and 90% of these positive HPV tissues had HPV-16 present. Their work and other recent studies have shown that men and women who reported having six or more oral-sex partners during their lifetime had a nearly nine-fold increased risk of developing cancer of the tonsils or at the base of the tongue. From 300 study participants, those infected with HPV were 32 times more likely to develop oral cancer compared to those with no virus. The other well-known major risk factors for oral cancers: smoking (3 times greater) and drinking (2.5 times greater) are in fact lower than the risk from HPV. There is a false perception that only women are at risk from HPV. Unlike cervical and vaginal cancer, this type of oral cancer is more prevalent in men!

Gardasil is a very effective new vaccine to prevent HPV types 6, 11, 16, and 18 infections. The vaccine is currently available to women between the ages of 9 and 26. Gardasil has not been tested against oral

HPV, but in principle, the vaccine may have an impact on oral cancers attributable to HPV. This is still awaiting study.

Mini Sling for Urine Leak

Urine incontinence or involuntary leakage of urine in adults affects nearly 25 million people in the United States, women being affected twice more often than men.

Won't it be nice to have a surgical procedure that takes only 7 minutes to perform, with less than 2 tablespoons of blood loss, and has an immediate cure rate of 92.3%?

Well, yes, luckily for women today, we have such a procedure. It's called the Mini Sling, using a mini mesh, instead of the technique that uses the old huge mesh for the repair. Dr. Gentile has done about three hundred of this procedure, and the success rate today has been rated as about 80%, but more widespread use of the procedure is needed for the final confirmation of the long-term effectiveness of this new technique.

The Mini Sling procedure requires a single vaginal incision with minimal dissection, has low rates of voiding difficulties, and has a very low complication rates.

Lifesaver Breast "Halo"

Imagine a screening test for breast cancer that can screen for the disease years before the cancer is palpable or detectable in a mammogram!

Breast cancer is one of the most common causes of cancer related death in women. More than 70% of breast cancers are first detected by the patient and often as a palpable lump. By the time a cancerous lump is palpable or visible in a mammogram, it has been growing in the breast for more than 5 years. More than 90% of breast cancers originate in the breast ductal tissues.

On October 6, 2005, the US FDA approved a new Papanicolaou (Pap) test system (Halo Breast Pap, made by NeoMatrix, LLC). This system is designed to collect nipple aspirate fluid (NAF) (somewhat like a breast milk pump) for PAP/cytological evaluation. The collected fluid can be used in the determination of normal, premalignant, and malignant cells.

Abnormal cells in NAF can be seen up to seven years prior to the presence of cancer on mammogram or self-examination. This system is not designed to be a diagnostic test, but rather, an aid in breast cancer screening.

Halo uses disposable breast cups to applying heat over a five-minute cycle while simultaneously generating mild compression on both breasts. Near the end of the cycle, gentle suction is used to retrieve ductal fluid. This is the first automated, noninvasive NAF collection device specifically designed for use in a medical office.

Laparoscopic Hysterectomy

Included in the advances in surgery is laparoscopic hysterectomy (removal of the uterus), that can now be performed through three small abdominal punctures and then have the patient return home to rest comfortably within 24 hours of the surgery and back to her normal activities in less than a week!

Hysterectomy is one of the most common major surgical procedures performed in the United States with over 600,000 performed annually. Most of these surgeries are performed by making a wide incision (cut) into the abdomen and then manually removing the uterus with clamps, sutures, scalpel and scissors. This technique has changed little over the past 50 years till now.

Laparoscopy is done by inserting a lighted telescope-like instrument (laparoscope) into the abdomen to view the abdominal and pelvic organs. The scope has built-in fiber-optic video camera, which allows magnified visualization of the inside of the abdomen and shown on a TV monitor for everybody in the operating room to view. New powered laparoscopic morcellators can cut up large tumors or other tissues into small pieces and pass them out of the abdomen through the small punctures. Laparoscopic coagulating instruments can seal large blood vessels and cut through them without injuring the healthy surrounding tissues. This also allows the surgeon to suture and tie knots while viewing the monitor.

Studies have shown that when LSH is performed by experienced laparoscopic surgeons, there is less blood loss, shorter operative times, comparable complication rates, and less scarring when compared to traditional abdominal hysterectomy.

Prenatal Genetic Test

Today's advances in medical science have brought pregnant women screening test that uses a single ultrasound of the fetal neck and two samples of maternal blood—performed at the correct intervals in pregnancy—that can predict the risk of a fetus having Down syndrome or Edward Syndrome (Tirsomy 18) with anear 95% accuracy. Other birth defects could also be detected early on.

In the United States, for every 100 newborn infants, 2 to 3 are born with major birth defects such as significant mental or physical problems. Birth defects can be caused by inherited genetic/chromosome errors or caused by exposure to harmful agents such as chemical, drugs, or radiation. For 70% of babies born with birth defects, the cause is unknown. The majority of birth defects occur during the first 12 weeks of life. Some birth defects may be detected early in pregnancy with special tests. Many birth defects are only detected at birth and others only much later in a child's development.

Every mother should be offered prenatal genetic screening, most especially those at higher risk. While most babies born with a birth defect have normal parents, sometimes there are risk factors that predispose the fetus to developing birth defects. For example: if the mother is 35 years old or older when the baby is due or if there is family history or a previous child with birth defects, then the risk of a birth defect in a future pregnancy is much higher.

Zinc toxicity from denture creams

On February 15, 2011, WebMD reported "an increasing number of mysterious nerve damage which turned out to be caused by overuse of popular denture products."

According to this revelation, "the culprit: zinc in Fixodent, from Procter & Gamble . . . and in Poligrip from GlaxoSmithKline," which became zinc-free May 2011. These two denture fixing creams are very popular among denture-wearers.

Zinc is an essential mineral in human physiology but in excess, it is toxic. The body balances zinc and copper level, and when one is low, the other one goes up. Too much zinc, for example, will lower the copper level, and vice versa. Zinc overdose leads to low copper level, which, in turn, "causes bone marrow suppression and degeneration of the spinal cord, usually resulting in crippling nerve damage, called the human swayback disease," says the report.

Other symptoms can include inability to sense pain, muscles weakness, excessive sweating, constipation, bladder dysfunction, twitching, hypersensitivity, and even paralysis.

Since one patient has died in Georgia and some patients became wheelchair-bound, determined to be caused by the denture cream, there have been a number of lawsuits filed against the two companies.

The great mystery behind patients developing spastic gait, weakness and numbness of arms and legs, and difficulty in ambulation has now been found in 2007 and confirmed in 2008 to be due to deficiency in copper as a result of overdose in zinc, on patients who did not have any exposure to zinc except thru the use of one of those denture creams.

"Poorly fitting dentures requiring large amounts of denture cream to provide a sufficient seal appear to be the common characteristics of patients," quoted WebMD of Hedera and colleagues in their article in the journal *Neurotoxicology*. The alarming report linking since zinc poisoning to dental creams by ABS News brought all this out in the open.

Experts say that many patients with poorly fitting dentures unwittingly use excessive amount that is unsafe, causing zinc toxicity over time with resultant fall in the copper level to an unsafe level. It is most important to follow strictly the instructions on the label of any product about its proper use.

The recommendation is for those concerned to discuss their particular problem with their dentist without delay.

Miscellaneous Health News

People who regularly consume more vegetables and fruits have a lower risk of developing ischemic heart disease (IHD), the condition that leads to heart attack. This was borne out by a European research, published January 19, 2011, in *European Heart Journal.*

"Those who ate at least eight portions of fruit and vegetables a day had a 22% lower risk of dying from IHD than did those who consumed fewer than three portions a day," reported Dr Francesca Crowe of the Cancer Epidemiology Unit at the University of Oxford, UK, as a part of the European Prospective Investigation into Cancer and Nutrition (EPIC) Heart study.

Breast Implant and Cancer

"Patients with either saline or silicone gel-filled breast implants may have a very small but significant risk for a rare cancer called anaplastic large-cell lymphoma (ALCL) adjacent to the implant," according to the January 26, 2011, announcement of the US Food and Drug Administration (FDA).

As the agency investigates the link between the implant and ALCL, it is suggesting to physicians to be suspicious of any fluid accumulation (seroma) around breast implants as possible clue for cancer.

The US-FDA review, which included data published from January 1997 to May 2010, revealed 34 cases of ALCL among those women with breast implants throughout the world. The FDA is not sure, but it could be as high as 60, among the 5 to 10 million breast implants worldwide.

Although the incidence is rare, it is best for women with breast implants to continue their routine medical care and follow-up with their surgeon.

Smoking and Breast Cancer

Women who smoke are at a much higher risk of getting breast cancer, not to mention lung and other forms of cancer.

The study published in the *Archives of Internal Medicine* and aired on CNN pointed out that regular female smokers have a 6% higher risk compared to those who do not smoke. Those who consume a pack daily have 28% increased risk of cancer. The study, which was conducted among 110,000 female nurses, found 8,772 cases of invasive breast cancer over the past 30 years.

Biomarker for Heart Attack

A helpful predictor of heart attack has recently been discovered. It is a protein fragment named Caspase-3 p17, heretofore unknown, found in the blood of heart attack patients, according to Dr. Bruce Liang, director of Pat and Jim Calhoun Cardiology Center in an article published January 11, 2011, in the *Journal of American College of Cardiology*. The coinvestigators were from the Mayo Clinic and the Mayo Medical School in Rochester, Minnesota.

"We've discovered a new biomarker for heart attack, and showed that apoptosis, or a particular kind of cell death, is a cause of heart muscle damage," reported Dr. Liang. "The ability to see a heart attack coming with a simple blood test and to develop new therapies to block apoptosis would enable us to get a head start on treatment and preserve crucial heart muscle and cardiac function."

Detect heart attack early

Today, we have a very sensitive blood test for a protein called cardiac troponin—T (cTnT)—that can confirm if a patient is having an acute heart attack. A more sensitive version of the cTnT could indicate whether a healthy-looking middle-aged person, without symptoms, "has an unrecognized heart disease and an increase risk of dying." This was reported by researchers at the UT Southwestern Medical Center and published December 2, 2010, in the *Journal of the American Medical Association.*

Subjects "with detectable levels of troponin T were nearly seven times more likely to die within six years from heart disease," according to the study.

"This test is among the most powerful predictors of death in general population we've seen so far," stated lead researcher Dr. James de Lemos, associate professor of internal medicine at UT Southwestern.

With this new more sensitive cardiac troponin T (cTnT), physicians can make early diagnosis and prevent countless deaths.

Statins Reduce Cardiac Death

In majority of cases, sudden death from heart disease in low-risk group is surprisingly common. Of course, among the high risk group (those who are smokers, with high blood pressure, diabetes, high blood cholesterol, irregular heart rhythm), the incidence of sudden cardiac death (SCD) is much more frequent.

Sudden cardiac death is defined as "unexpected death from a cardiac etiology after cardiac arrest within 1 hour of the onset of acute symptoms," like chest pains, severe shortness of breath, or collapse. Every year, there are more than 3 million SCDs around the world, including the one in every 1000 persons in the general population in the United States, which statistic is similarly true in other parts of the globe. Arrhythmias—irregularities of the heart rhythm called ventricular tachycardia (VT) and ventricular fibrillation (VF)—are the most common causes among 80% who had severe coronary heart disease and the rest among those with ischemic (lack of blood supply leading to) cardiomyopathy (heart muscle damage).

Studies have been conducted to find out how to protect all these patients, both high and low-risk groups. This 13-year review of clinical data revealed that "statins have been shown to reduce VT/VF and sudden cardiac death only in subjects with underlying coronary artery disease or ischemic cardiomyopathy."

The findings suggest that taking statins (cholesterol-lowering drugs) lowers the risk for sudden cardiac death among those with stable coronary heart disease, compared to those with the same medical condition not on any statin drug.

However, all the medications to lower cholesterol will not provide the optimum benefit to the body unless a low-fat, high-fiber diet and daily exercises are part of the whole healthy lifestyle regimen.

Veggies Protect the Stomach

Those taking NSAID drugs like ibuprofen and other antiarthritis pain medications regularly can be victims of stomach irritation which could result in ulcers and bleeding complication. To prevent stomach ulceration, ingesting 8 to 10 ounces of vegetables a day can work wonders by protecting the stomach wall lining, according to a researcher at Sweden's Uppsala University.

Healthy Dish

Omega-3 fish oil (omega-3 fatty acids DHA and EPA) is a popular supplement to eating fish for its cardio-protective benefit. It can lower blood pressure, help new brain cells regenerate, and reduce the risk of the development of Alzheimer's, minimize inflammation, and is a great aid in the management of cholesterol and arthritis. It also boosts the immune system. When digested, fish oil breaks down to hormonelike ingredients called prostaglandins, which reduces inflammation, like in arthritis (inflammation of the joints). This leads to lesser need for pain medications as it also lubricates the joints. Fish oil is also good for autoimmune diseases. Indeed, a versatile supplement. Daily exercises, eating fish and vegetables at least 3 times a week, and abstaining from red meat and egg yolk is the healthy way to go for children and adults alike.

Sex Could Be Deadly

Sleeping around indiscriminately, or having multiple sex partners, can be hazardous to health and deadly. A perfectly healthy-looking person could be walking around with HIV, chlamydia, gonorrhea, and other STDs (sexually transmitted diseases), including syphilis. And no matter how normal looking the sexual organs of the women or men are, they could be harboring bacteria, fungi, viruses, and sometimes even parasites not obvious to the naked eye. Only a medical checkup and laboratory tests could confirm their presence or absence. STD infections in general, affecting the sexual organs and of the eyes and mouth are common. Be smart. You do not want a 15-minute session of pleasure to risk your health and life for weeks, if not years, of agony and shame. An Internet message said, "Unlike love, herpes is forever." That may sound funny, but herpes is really for keeps. Sex is a major and serious responsibility, not only to our body and health but to our family and friends, to all our loved ones.

Crackling Brain Food

If you want a healthy snack, one that keeps your brain sharp and reduces your risk for the development of Alzheimer's, nothing beats crunchy celery, cucumber, carrot, broccoli, cauliflower, olives, bell peppers, and other veggies. Eating them uncooked preserve all the phytochemicals in them, like luteolin, which prevents brain inflammation, a common condition linked to aging, chronic brain syndrome, multiple sclerosis, etc. So to stay young with a sharper mind, stay away from the high-carbo snacks, including soft drinks and savor the benefits from these crunchy veggies. Even your looks and your complexion will shine, with your favorite moisturizer and without the use of glutathione or other expensive herbal products, which may even be dangerous after chronic use. Veggies are in, especially among teenagers. We adults should learn from the younger generation.

Laughter: A Healer

Living a healthy lifestyle includes laughter. The more we laugh in life, the healthier we are. Indeed laughter is "the best medicine." Laughing increases our T-cells in the body which boost our immunity.

Laughing also lowers the cortisol (stress hormone) level allowing us to minimize stress and its adverse effects on our system. It also blocks out bad emotions within us, giving us a better outlook and perspective in life. Even if nothing is funny, laugh anyway, because the act of laughing in itself brings out all those benefits. And don't worry if people think you are crazy and laugh at you. You are doing them a favor anyway by helping them get healthier.

Antimicrobial Pesticide

Hospitals and other institutions use antimicrobial pesticides (sanitizers, sterilizers, disinfectants) to suppress or destroy harmful bacteria on inanimate objects and surfaces. In the United States, there are about 5,000 antimicrobial pesticides in the form of sprays, gases, powders, or liquids.

In a 5-year study (2002-2007) in four states across the USA, there were 401 acute illnesses affecting workers handling the pesticides in healthcare facilities. Some of the symptoms included eye irritation, throat pain, cough, shortness of breath, skin rash, acute asthmatic attacks. One person in this series died.

While the use of these chemicals for cleaning in public places and at home is commonplace and taken for granted, the danger they pose are real and could be serious in the long run, especially for children.

Magnets: A Scam

One of the most preposterous health claims in the various marketing media is the effectiveness and healing power of magnets (wristbands, bracelets, anklets, necklace, belts) for a multitude of medical conditions. This is nothing but a scam. It is unfortunate that some people are gullible, falling easy prey to unscrupulous vendors of modern "snake oil." Living a healthy lifestyle is all we need to prevent illnesses and stay healthy.

Overweight and Breast Cancer

The obesity hormone called leftin is linked to an increase risk of breast cancer among women. Regular consumption of saturated fats and greater body fats lead to higher level of leftin. A study at the Texas MD Anderson Cancer Center in Houston shows that women who switch to low-fat, high-fiber diet can reduce their leftin level and their risk of developing breast cancer. Leftin level might be a marker for breast cancer. A diet of red meats is associated with many forms of cancers, besides cardiovascular and metabolic diseases.

Fast-food Salads

Most, if not all the fast-food chains, have joined the bandwagon, offering salad on their menu for the health-conscious customers. Are you safer eating these salads? Maybe not, says the Physicians Committee for Responsible Medicine, which came out with a report rating 34 salads from seven restaurants (from Wendy's to Subway). The study showed these salads are no better than their burger because of their high-fat dressing, toppings of cheese, and fried croutons. The PCRM report stated that the "Crispy Chicken Bacon Ranch Salad at McDonald's packs more fat and calories than a Big Mac."

Green leafy vegetable salad with oil and vinegar dressing, minus all the fatty trimmings, is obviously the healthier way to go.

Low Fat or Low Carb

The new findings from the Center for Obesity Research and Education at Temple University, Philadelphia, "have revealed that after a two-year comparison, a low-carb diet fares about as well as a low-fat diet with regards to weight loss, but low-carb improves cardiovascular risk factors more."

Both the blood pressure and cholesterol levels (both cardiovascular risks) fared better with the low-carbohydrate diet, when coupled with an overall healthier lifestyle regimen.

"Put simply—it appears that both diets are equally good for losing weight, but the low-carb diet protects you from potential coronary heart diseases more effectively," the investigators reported.

For those with high serum cholesterol, low-fat diet for weight reduction and overall cardiovascular health is the preferred option. Combining the two diets is certainly even a better alternative.

Obviously, behavioral changes, living a healthy lifestyle, which requires discipline, is the key.

Lifestyle and Stroke

Individuals who choose to live a healthy lifestyle have an 80% lower risk in developing first-time stroke. This was revealed an article in the medical journal STROKE, which reported a review of 795,000 strokes in the United States.

Third on the list, following heart attack and cancer, stroke is the largest cause of major disability and premature death, in the USA.

A healthy lifestyle includes cessation from smoking, strict moderation in alcohol intake, low-fat and low-carb diet (consuming mainly fish, vegetables, fruits, nuts, and grains), daily physical exercise, adequate sleep, rest and relaxation. For those on prescription medications, compliance is essential, including regular medical checkup.

Blood Test for Alzheimer's

To date, physicians are handicapped in diagnosing Alzheimer's dementia until the disease is full-blown, which by then is irreversible and hopeless.

On the horizon is a potential test, a simple blood test, that could detect Alzheimer's real early, before any obvious signs and symptoms show and before any damages in the brain take place.

This new technology "relies on thousands of synthetic molecules to fish for disease-specific antibodies," reported the journal *CELL*.

When proven to work for Alzheimer's, the same technology could also work for the early diagnosis of other diseases, according to Dr. Thomas Kopdadek of the Scripps Research Institute. He and his team took a different approach, where they utilize "a large library of randomly selected, unnatural molecules known as 'peptoids' to screen for antibodies found in the bloodstream of animals or patients with specific diseases." The preliminary results are most encouraging.

A drug to treat Alzheimer's?

Yes. Recently, Forest Pharmaceuticals, Inc. (USA) introduced what the firm describes as "the first and only NMDA-receptor antagonist for the treatment of moderate to severe Alzheimer's disease." The drug is called Namenda (memantine HCl), which in randomized, multicenter, double-blind, parallel group, and placebo-controlled studies showed a "significant effect on cognition and functional ability . . . and other scale parameters, including attention, language, praxis, visuopatial ability, construction, and memory." Activities evaluated were eating, walking, toileting, bathing, grooming, dressing, attention to conversation, household activities, and traveling beyond home. More extensive use and experience with the drug are needed to provide long term results.

Warning signs for stroke and heart attack

Either of these two conditions may occur without any warning. This is why preventive measures, from early childhood onward, to ward off these illnesses are essential, together with preemptive regular medical checkup after the age 40. Earlier for those with strong personal or family history of hypertension, diabetes, high-cholesterol blood level. But the classical warnings of an impending stroke could include numbness or weakness in the face (facial asymmetry), arm, or leg, or both on the same side; confusion; inability to speak; problem with vision of one or both eyes; headache; dizziness; physical imbalance. For heart attack: pressure discomfort tightness or severe squeezing under the breastbone for several minutes, or actual chest pains, pain, and or numbness of one arm, jaw, neck, or stomach; feeling of shortness of breath or an impending doom; cold clammy sweats; nausea; lightheadedness. Any of these symptoms, not necessarily all of them occurring at the same time, are warning signs. But why wait for them? See your physician and practice a healthy lifestyle of abstinence from tobacco, eating healthy, doing daily exercises, and managing your stress with regular relaxation with family and friends.

Simple A1c Test for Prediabetes

Early detection of any disease, including prediabetes, helps prevent the full onset of the disease, in this case, type 2 diabetes. If detected early, prediabetes can be "delayed" or even prevented entirely from becoming full-blown diabetes. And we have such a blood test, called hemoglobin A1c, which measures average blood sugar level over the previous 8-12 weeks, a test that does not even require fasting and one that gives a more global picture of the condition. A1c will tell us if one is prediabetic (borderline, or potential diabetes victim), and this early opportunity will allow physicians to help halt the progression to actual diabetes. About 60 million, a third of the adult Americans, are prediabetic. One third of these individuals will develop into type 2 diabetes in less than a decade, without even knowing they are at high risk. If in doubt, especially those with family history of diabetes, it is prudent to consult with a physician about hemoglobin A1c test to find out about your level risk.

What's To Come

Instead of the cumbersome, uncomfortable diagnostic procedures now available for detecting lung cancer, the University of Texas researchers are developing a new lung cancer test that allows the use of "a simple mouth tissue sample, which compares the changes that takes place 95% of the time in both mouth and lung cells" among those individuals with lung cancer. This would be a fantastic progress in our fight against lung cancer and cancers in general.

A noninvasive "virtual biopsy" technology (using harmless electrical current to better detect skin and cervical cancer and eliminate need for surgical biopsy) has been developed by an Australian scientist.

A new ultrasound, "which can catch tiny tumors earlier," is being evaluated for clinical use in Norway. Second to prevention, catching any cancer in its early stage can lead to complete cure, among most cancers.

Progress in science, in every sphere of human endeavor, benefits mankind as a whole. We are indeed lucky to be living in this world of today, in spite of all its imperfections and problems, most of which are man-made. For world peace and prosperity, where there is no war, poverty, and hunger, all we really need is love, tolerance, and respect for each other. And the best place to start is at our own home.

Useful Websites

Guide to common simple emergencies

http://www.ncemi.org/cse/contents.htm

To calculate cardiovascular risk

http://hp2010.nhlbihin.net/atpiii/calculator.asp

To calculate body mass index (BMI)

http://www.nhlbisupport.com/bmi

To convert measurements

http://www.convert-me.com/en

To get various statistics

http://www.cdc.gov/nchs/fastats/default.htm

Author's Email Address: scalpelpen@gmail.com

Index

Y

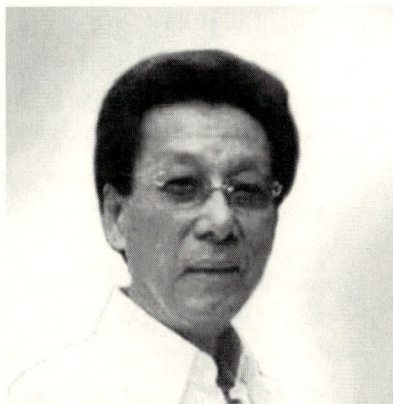

About the Author

Philip S. Chua, MD, FACS, FPCS, is Cardiac Surgeon Emeritus in Northwest Indiana, where he founded in 1972 and later headed the 4-man heart surgery team known as Cardiovascular Surgery Associates. Immediately prior to this, he underwent his Cardiac Surgery Fellowship training under the world-renowned heart transplant surgeon, Denton A. Cooley, MD, FACS, Surgeon-in-Chief and President Emeritus of the Texas Heart Institute in Houston, Texas.

Dr. Chua is a Fellow of the American College of Surgeons, the Philippine College of Surgeons, and the International College of Surgeons. He was Chairman of Cardiac Surgery of the Cebu Cardiovascular Center of the Cebu Doctors' University Hospital in Cebu City, Philippines, from 1997 to 2010, where he shuttled to and from Indiana and Las Vegas almost every two months. He was President and Chief of Staff at St. Mary Medical Center, St. Anthony Medical Center, and The Methodist Hospitals in Northwest Indiana.

Dr. Chua was the founding president of the Denton A. Cooley Cardiovascular Surgical Society, an exclusive professional association of more than 900 cardiac surgeons from more than 52 countries around the world who trained under Dr. Cooley at the prestigious Texas Heart Institute.

In 1989 and again in 1991, he and his associate, Victor K. O'yek, MD, FACS, FRCS, spearheaded a complete heart team from Indiana, and performed 24 coronary bypass surgeries for free before an audience of cardiac surgeons from around China. These surgical demonstrations were done at the First Teaching Hospital of the Beijing Medical University, who formally invited the two surgeons from the United States.

The author is past president of the American Heart Association, Northwest Indiana Chapter. On November 25, 1995, Dr. Chua was honored with the most-coveted Sagamore of the Wabash award, bestowed upon him by then Indiana Governor and now incumbent US Senator, Evan Bayh, for professional excellence, distinguished leadership, and dedicated service to the community.

A noted health columnist, Dr. Chua writes weekly for four newspapers in the United States, three newspapers and one health magazine in the Philippines, and three websites on the internet.

The Chairman of the Filipino United Network-USA, a 501(c)(3) United States advocacy Foundation for good governance and responsible citizenship, Dr. Chua is married to a former classmate, Farida Isip Chua, MD, a retired Pediatrician. They have five children who are all physicians, and four of them married to physicians as well, all residing in the United States, with their ten grandchildren.

On June 14, 2008, this family of eleven physicians was honored in New Jersey with the Peace Award for Excellence, presented by the Honorable Willy Gaa, Philippine Ambassador to the United States, on behalf of the Philippine Economic and Cultural Endowment.

Xlibris Corporation takes pride in publishing this most informative and challenging book, entitled *Let's Stop "Killing" Our Children*, whose poignant message could forever change our role in parenting and society's perspective on health and diseases.

Edwards Brothers, Inc.
Thorofare, NJ USA
January 18, 2012